Advances in Tea Chemistry

Advances in Tea Chemistry

Collection Editors

Yongquan Xu
Ying Gao
Qingqing Cao

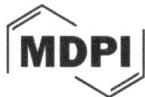

Basel • Beijing • Wuhan • Barcelona • Belgrade • Novi Sad • Cluj • Manchester

Collection Editors

Yongquan Xu
Chinese Academy of
Agricultural Sciences
Hangzhou
China

Ying Gao
Chinese Academy of
Agricultural Sciences
Hangzhou
China

Qingqing Cao
Chinese Academy of
Agricultural Sciences
Hangzhou
China

Editorial Office
MDPI AG
Grosspeteranlage 5
4052 Basel, Switzerland

This is a reprint of the Topical Collection, published open access by the journal *Foods* (ISSN 2304-8158), freely accessible at: https://www.mdpi.com/journal/foods/topical_collections/T707N1G8W4.

For citation purposes, cite each article independently as indicated on the article page online and as indicated below:

Lastname, A.A.; Lastname, B.B. Article Title. *Journal Name* **Year**, *Volume Number*, Page Range.

ISBN 978-3-7258-3035-0 (Hbk)
ISBN 978-3-7258-3036-7 (PDF)
https://doi.org/10.3390/books978-3-7258-3036-7

Cover image courtesy of Yongquan Xu

© 2025 by the authors. Articles in this book are Open Access and distributed under the Creative Commons Attribution (CC BY) license. The book as a whole is distributed by MDPI under the terms and conditions of the Creative Commons Attribution-NonCommercial-NoDerivs (CC BY-NC-ND) license (https://creativecommons.org/licenses/by-nc-nd/4.0/).

Contents

About the Editors vii

Preface ix

Qing-Qing Cao, Ying Gao and Yong-Quan Xu
Advances in Tea Chemistry
Reprinted from: *Foods* 2023, 12, 3944, https://doi.org/10.3390/foods12213944 1

Yuan Chen, Lingling Lai, Youli You, Ruizhen Gao, Jiaxin Xiang, Guojun Wang and Wenquan Yu
Quantitative Analysis of Bioactive Compounds in Commercial Teas: Profiling Catechin Alkaloids, Phenolic Acids, and Flavonols Using Targeted Statistical Approaches
Reprinted from: *Foods* 2023, 12, 3098, https://doi.org/10.3390/foods12163098 3

Wei Wang, Ting Le, Wei-Wei Wang, Jun-Feng Yin and He-Yuan Jiang
The Effects of Structure and Oxidative Polymerization on Antioxidant Activity of Catechins and Polymers
Reprinted from: *Foods* 2023, 12, 4207, https://doi.org/10.3390/foods12234207 16

Yaping Zheng, Kailin Yang, Jie Shen, Xiangdong Chen, Chunnian He and Peigen Xiao
Huangqin Tea Total Flavonoids–Gut Microbiota Interactions: Based on Metabolome and Microbiome Analysis
Reprinted from: *Foods* 2023, 12, 4410, https://doi.org/10.3390/foods12244410 32

Ting Tang, Qing Luo, Liu Yang, Changlun Gao, Caijin Ling and Weibin Wu
Research Review on Quality Detection of Fresh Tea Leaves Based on Spectral Technology
Reprinted from: *Foods* 2024, 13, 25, https://doi.org/10.3390/foods13010025 48

Chun Zou, Xin Zhang, Yongquan Xu and Junfeng Yin
Recent Advances Regarding Polyphenol Oxidase in *Camellia sinensis*: Extraction, Purification, Characterization, and Application
Reprinted from: *Foods* 2024, 13, 545, https://doi.org/10.3390/foods13040545 75

Xing Tian, Haodong Wang, Liang Chen, Hanwen Yuan, Caiyun Peng and Wei Wang
Distinct Changes in Metabolic Profile and Sensory Quality with Different Varieties of *Chrysanthemum* (Juhua) Tea Measured by LC-MS-Based Untargeted Metabolomics and Electronic Tongue
Reprinted from: *Foods* 2024, 13, 1080, https://doi.org/10.3390/foods13071080 89

Jiayu Lu, Zheng Jiang, Jingjie Dang, Dishuai Li, Daixin Yu, Cheng Qu and Qinan Wu
GC–MS Combined with Fast GC E-Nose for the Analysis of Volatile Components of Chamomile (*Matricaria chamomilla* L.)
Reprinted from: *Foods* 2024, 13, 1865, https://doi.org/10.3390/foods13121865 106

Yuan Chen, Changsong Chen, Jiaxing Xiang, Ruizhen Gao, Guojun Wang and Wenquan Yu
Functional Tea Extract Inhibits Cell Growth, Induces Apoptosis, and Causes G0/G1 Arrest in Human Hepatocellular Carcinoma Cell Line Possibly through Reduction in Telomerase Activity
Reprinted from: *Foods* 2024, 13, 1867, https://doi.org/10.3390/foods13121867 122

Yanming Tuo, Xiaofeng Lu, Fang Tao, Marat Tukhvatshin, Fumin Xiang, Xi Wang, et al.
The Potential Mechanisms of Catechins in Tea for Anti-Hypertension: An Integration of Network Pharmacology, Molecular Docking, and Molecular Dynamics Simulation
Reprinted from: *Foods* 2024, 13, 2685, https://doi.org/10.3390/foods13172685 134

Zhiwei Hou, Yugu Jin, Zhe Gu, Ran Zhang, Zhucheng Su and Sitong Liu
^{1}H NMR Spectroscopy Combined with Machine-Learning Algorithm for Origin Recognition of Chinese Famous Green Tea Longjing Tea
Reprinted from: *Foods* **2024**, *13*, 2702, https://doi.org/10.3390/foods13172702 . . . . **149**

Zhihao Ye, Haojie Xu, Yingying Xie, Ziqi Peng, Hongfang Li, Ruyan Hou, et al.
Tea's Characteristic Components Eliminate Acrylamide in the Maillard Model System
Reprinted from: *Foods* **2024**, *13*, 2836, https://doi.org/10.3390/foods13172836 . . . . **162**

Xiaohui Liu, Fabao Dong, Yucai Li, Fu Lu, Botao Wang, Taicen Zhou, et al.
Impact of Mild Field Drought on the Aroma Profile and Metabolic Pathways of Fresh Tea (*Camellia sinensis*) Leaves Using HS-GC-IMS and HS-SPME-GC-MS
Reprinted from: *Foods* **2024**, *13*, 3412, https://doi.org/10.3390/foods13213412 . . . . **173**

About the Editors

Yongquan Xu

Yongquan Xu, professor/doctor in Tea Research Institute, Chinese Academy of Agricultural Sciences, research interests in tea flavor chemistry; tea beverage processing and quality control, has gained over 10 academic grants/ funds, including the grant from the National Natural Science Foundation of China, the Outstanding Youth Fund of Zhejiang Province, and awarded the First Prize of Science and Technology Progress Award of Zhejiang Province as the first contributor.

Ying Gao

Ying Gao, associate professor/doctor in Tea Research Institute, Chinese Academy of Agricultural Sciences, research interests in tea deep processing and diversified utilization, has achieved several grants from the National Natural Science Foundation of China, and awarded the First Prize of Science and Technology Progress Award of Zhejiang Province.

Qingqing Cao

Qingqing Cao, postdoctor in Tea Research Institute, Chinese Academy of Agricultural Sciences, research interests in tea flavor, has obtained two grants from the China Postdoctoral Science Foundation, and awarded the First Prize of Science and Technology Progress Award of Zhejiang Province.

Preface

Tea is well-loved all over the world. Flavor is a leading factor influencing consumer behavior, preferences, and choices of tea. Health-beneficial function is another important reason for its popularity. Nowadays, brewing is not the only way to consume tea. Tea and its extracts are added to foods, beverages, and nutraceuticals.

A great number of secondary metabolites, including flavan-3-ols, phenolic acids, purine alkaloids, tannins, saponins, flavonols and their glycosides, tannins, and saponins, contribute to the flavor and functions of tea. The chemical composition of tea is affected by the origin, variety, postharvest treatment, processing method, storage, and so on. Currently, scientists pay attention to the improvement of tea and tea products with high quality, low cost, and a long shelf life. They also focus on strategies to increase the bioactivity and bioaccessibility of tea because some components in tea are vulnerable and easily degrade after intake.

Thus, we launched the Special Issue "Advances in Tea Chemistry" and invited researchers to contribute original research articles as well review articles. Until now, the Special Issue has collected 13 papers (10 articles, 2 reviews, and 1 editorial) from different universities and research institutes around China and the research fields involved in food science, analytical chemistry, tea processing, flavor chemistry, extraction technology, food functions, risk assessment, and encapsulation technology, etc. Here, we highly appreciate the efforts these contributors have made for the high-quality research on tea chemistry.

Yongquan Xu, Ying Gao, and Qingqing Cao
Collection Editors

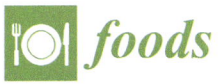

Editorial

Advances in Tea Chemistry

Qing-Qing Cao, Ying Gao * and Yong-Quan Xu *

Tea Research Institute, Chinese Academy of Agricultural Sciences, Key Laboratory of Biology, Genetics and Breeding of Special Economic Animals and Plants, Ministry of Agriculture and Rural Affairs, 9 South Meiling Road, Hangzhou 310008, China; caoqingqing@tricaas.com
* Correspondence: yinggao@tricaas.com (Y.G.); yqx33@126.com (Y.-Q.X.); Tel.: +86-571-86650594 (Y.G.); +86-571-86017633 (Y.-Q.X.)

Citation: Cao, Q.-Q.; Gao, Y.; Xu, Y.-Q. Advances in Tea Chemistry. *Foods* **2023**, *12*, 3944. https://doi.org/10.3390/foods12213944

Received: 17 October 2023
Accepted: 20 October 2023
Published: 28 October 2023

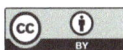

Copyright: © 2023 by the authors. Licensee MDPI, Basel, Switzerland. This article is an open access article distributed under the terms and conditions of the Creative Commons Attribution (CC BY) license (https:// creativecommons.org/licenses/by/ 4.0/).

The origins of tea, a traditional beverage in China, can be traced back to the Shennong period, about 2737 years before the birth of Christ [1]. Nowadays, with more than 2 billion cups consumed daily, tea is recognized as the most popular of the top three non-alcoholic beverages (i.e., tea, coffee, and cocoa), coming second only to water. The tea plant (*Camellia sinensis*) is now grown commercially in more than 60 countries, where it has made great contributions to local economies [2]. According to the statistical data from the UN Food and Agriculture Organization (FAO), the total global production of tea in 2020 was more than 7 million tons, with China, the largest producer, accounting for 42% of that figure [3].

Tea's long history and widespread popularity can be attributed to its unique and gratifying flavor, along with numerous health benefits such as its anti-oxidant, anti-obesity, and anti-microbial properties [4]. An in-depth look reveals that tea contains abundant components with both flavor- and health-enhancing attributes, as well as the already well-known polyphenols, caffeine, and amino acids. These naturally occurring ingredients in tea plants undergo a series of complicated biochemical or physicochemical reactions during tea processing, converting them into new substances that work together to contribute to the final quality of tea-based beverages.

There are six categories of traditional tea in China, popularly known as green tea, yellow tea, white tea, oolong tea, black tea, and dark tea. Due to each one having its own specific manufacturing process, in which the degree of fermentation is a decisive factor, they are very different from one another in terms of their sensory appeal and physicochemical properties. For example, green tea, an unfermented tea variety, usually appears green in color both in terms of its leaves and the final infusion, as well as smelling refreshing and having an umami-dominated flavor. Meanwhile, black tea, with its reddish appearance and caramelized flavor, is made by applying full fermentation. Apart from the traditional teas mentioned above, since 2015 a range of "new tea drinks" have been setting off a burst of enthusiasm among young people around China, even becoming an emerging industry in their own right [5]. New tea drinks are an innovative field of beverage manufacture—with labels invoking fashion, health, and nature—taking traditional tea as their starting point and combining other food ingredients including, but are not limited to, milk, cream, fresh fruits, flowers, and so forth. The new tea industry is burgeoning, yet it has not received the attention it is due from researchers, encompassing topics such as how to successfully blend diverse materials so as to harmoniously shape divergent flavors and functions.

A plethora of studies have been conducted to explore associations between tea's sensory qualities, particularly its flavor, with the chemicals that emerge during tea processing. We have so far detected about 600 volatile components in tea leaves and tea drinks, each of them with different scents, like grassy, woody, floral, etc. [6]. These aromatic compounds gather in different ratios for different teas, then combine to form characteristic aromas. Similarly, the taste of tea or its mouthfeel is induced by non-volatile extracted chemicals in the tea infusion—e.g., the catechins responsible for bitterness and astringency or the theanine that creates an umami taste [4]. The flavor of tea is determined by multiple factors, including aroma and taste or mouthfeel, but we know little about how these things work together. Indeed, the interaction between aroma and taste has been a research challenge even beyond tea.

The healthcare functions of tea come from its rich bioactive ingredients, especially flavonoids. The exploration of tea's functional components has always attracted a great deal of research interest. The therapeutic potentials of quite a few of tea's components have been confirmed repeatedly, and the mechanisms involved, such as EGCG, have also been deeply studied. At the same time, however, the limits of these potentials have also been realized; like the low stability and bioavailability of these components, which limit their utilizability. Moreover, figuring out how to extract, separate, and concentrate those bioactive components in an environmentally friendly, low-cost, and high-performance manner is also worthy of focus.

We launched this Special Issue of Foods, entitled "Advances in Tea Chemistry", with the aim of publishing high-quality research on tea chemistry from a wide range of aspects, including but not limited to the sensory/flavor qualities of tea, tea processing and storage, the extraction, bioactivity, and utilization of functional components from tea, as well as new tea-based beverages or foods. This series will be useful for expanding our understanding of the associations between tea chemistry, flavor, and bioactivity.

Conflicts of Interest: The authors declare no conflict of interest.

References

1. Wambulwa, M.C.; Meegahakumbura, M.K.; Kamunya, S.; Wachira, F.N. From the wild to the cup: Tracking footprints of the tea species in time and space. *Front. Nutr.* **2021**, *8*, 706770. [CrossRef] [PubMed]
2. Drew, L. Making tea. *Nature* **2019**, *566*, S2–S4. [CrossRef] [PubMed]
3. Zhai, X.; Zhang, L.; Granvogl, M.; Ho, C.-T.; Wan, X. Flavor of tea (Camellia sinensis): A review on odorants and analytical techniques. *Compr. Rev. Food Sci. Food Saf.* **2022**, *21*, 3867–3909. [CrossRef]
4. Zhang, L.; Cao, Q.-Q.; Granato, D.; Xu, Y.-Q.; Ho, C.-T. Association between chemistry and taste of tea: A review. *Trends Food Sci. Technol.* **2020**, *101*, 139–149. [CrossRef]
5. Lu, D. Analyze the Marketing Strategies of New-tea Drinks Industry by the SWOT and PEST Tools-Take Nayuki as an Example. In Proceedings of the 2022 7th International Conference on Social Sciences and Economic Development (ICSSED 2022), Wuhan, China, 25–27 March 2022.
6. Zhou, Y.; He, Y.; Zhu, Z. Understanding of formation and change of chiral aroma compounds from tea leaf to tea cup provides essential information for tea quality improvement. *Food Res. Int.* **2023**, *167*, 112703. [CrossRef]

Disclaimer/Publisher's Note: The statements, opinions and data contained in all publications are solely those of the individual author(s) and contributor(s) and not of MDPI and/or the editor(s). MDPI and/or the editor(s) disclaim responsibility for any injury to people or property resulting from any ideas, methods, instructions or products referred to in the content.

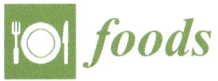

Article

Quantitative Analysis of Bioactive Compounds in Commercial Teas: Profiling Catechin Alkaloids, Phenolic Acids, and Flavonols Using Targeted Statistical Approaches

Yuan Chen [1], Lingling Lai [2], Youli You [3], Ruizhen Gao [1,4], Jiaxin Xiang [1,4], Guojun Wang [5] and Wenquan Yu [1,*]

[1] Fujian Academy of Agricultural Sciences, Fuzhou 350003, China; chenyuan@faas.cn (Y.C.); 18639424217@163.com (R.G.); 19949533447@163.com (J.X.)
[2] Fujian Tea Science Society, Fuzhou 350013, China; lily8011@sina.com
[3] Yongchun County Cultivation Service Center, Quanzhou 362699, China; ycnjz@163.com
[4] College of Horticulture, Fujian Agriculture and Forestry University, Fuzhou 350002, China
[5] Harbor Branch Oceanographic Institute, Florida Atlantic University, Fort Pierce, FL 34946, USA; guojunwang@fau.edu
* Correspondence: wenquan_yu@yeah.net

Abstract: Tea, an extensively consumed and globally popular beverage, has diverse chemical compositions that ascertain its quality and categorization. In this investigation, we formulated an analytical and quantification approach employing reversed-phase ultra-high-performance liquid chromatography (UHPLC) methodology coupled with diode-array detection (DAD) to precisely quantify 20 principal constituents within 121 tea samples spanning 6 distinct variants. The constituents include alkaloids, catechins, flavonols, and phenolic acids. Our findings delineate that the variances in chemical constitution across dissimilar tea types predominantly hinge upon the intricacies of their processing protocols. Notably, green and yellow teas evinced elevated concentrations of total chemical moieties vis à vis other tea classifications. Remarkably divergent levels of alkaloids, catechins, flavonols, and phenolic acids were ascertained among the disparate tea classifications. By leveraging random forest analysis, we ascertained gallocatechin, epigallocatechin gallate, and epicatechin gallate as pivotal biomarkers for effective tea classification within the principal cadre of tea catechins. Our outcomes distinctly underscore substantial dissimilarities in the specific compounds inherent to varying tea categories, as ascertained via the devised and duly validated approach. The implications of this compositional elucidation serve as a pertinent benchmark for the comprehensive assessment and classification of tea specimens.

Keywords: alkaloids; biomarker; catechins; flavonols; tea classification

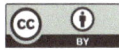

1. Introduction

Tea, obtained from the freshly plucked leaves of *Camellia sinensis*, represents a universally consumed potable [1]. In China, the postharvest processing of *Camellia sinensis* leaves involves a series of six distinct techniques, leading to the production of six types of teas: black tea, green tea, yellow tea, white tea, oolong tea, and dark tea [2,3]. These processing methods have evolved over thousands of years across various regions of China and are generally classified into five categories based on the extent of endogenous enzymatic reactions: (1) non-fermented tea, such as green tea; (2) lightly fermented tea, including yellow tea and white tea; (3) partially fermented tea, represented by oolong tea; (4) fully fermented tea, exemplified by black tea; and (5) post-fermented tea, wherein exogenous microbial fermentation plays a crucial role in the processing. Figure S1 illustrates the distribution of tea types across China. Despite the extensive research conducted on tea and its chemical composition, flavor profiles, and health benefits, there is still much to explore and understand, particularly in relation to the unique chemical profiles of each tea type and their potential implications for human health. The variations in processing techniques and the involvement of different enzymatic reactions and microbial fermentation in tea production contribute to the unique characteristics and properties of each tea variety. Therefore, a comprehensive investigation into the chemical constituents and sensory attributes of these teas is crucial for establishing a deeper understanding of their distinct qualities and potential health implications.

Tea is replete with an array of chemical constituents, prominently inclusive of catechins, phenolic acids, flavonols, and alkaloids, all of which collectively constitute major bioactive constituents [4,5]. These components confer palatability and concurrently confer bioactivities such as antioxidation and antibacterial effects. Fermentation, primarily manifesting as enzymatic oxidation, orchestrates the conversion of tea polyphenols into the corresponding oxidation byproducts, which are eventually activated upon the exposure of tea leaves to ambient humidity and oxygen. The diverse chemical constituents and polyphenol oxidases evident within the six tea types stem from the varying extents of fermentation. Hence, a systematic and exhaustive evaluation of the constituents within the six tea varieties is of paramount significance. Noteworthy endeavors have been directed towards investigating functional constituents, notably catechins, purine alkaloids, and flavonol glycosides, within select Chinese tea variants [6–8]. Notably, tea polyphenols, particularly catechins, undergo oxidative transformations during manufacturing processes, instigated by either moist heat or intrinsic polyphenol oxidases alongside microbial oxidases [9]. Consequently, non-fermented green tea characteristically boasts elevated levels of catechins, with epigallocatechin-3-gallate (EGCG) assuming particular prominence. Modestly fermented white and yellow teas exhibit slightly diminished catechin levels in relation to green tea, thereby facilitating the emergence of theaflavins and thearubigins [10]. Within semi-fermented oolong tea, catechin oxidation transpires solely at the leaf periphery, thereby positioning itself as intermediate to green tea and black tea. Catechin oxidation in dark tea is mediated by microorganisms, ultimately culminating in the generation of theabrownine. Notwithstanding, a comprehensive chemical profiling of Chinese tea remains an outstanding pursuit. A comprehensive and methodical inquiry underpinned by extensive data analysis is pivotal to obviating ambiguities pertaining to the functional constituents of Chinese teas. The standardization of tea quality holds profound ramifications for both tea enterprises and regulatory oversight.

The classification method based on sensory evaluation has a drawback as it lacks quantitative assessment indicators, which leads to difficulties in tea authentication. In contrast, international standards concentrate more on the physical and chemical attributes of tea. The absence of quantitative indicators poses challenges to tea quality control for producers, consumers, and regulatory agencies. In recent years, various analytical techniques, including thin-layer chromatography [11,12], high-performance liquid chromatography [13,14], and ultra-performance liquid chromatography-tandem mass spectrometry [15,16], have been utilized to determine the chemical composition of tea. However, most of these studies have focused on only a few chemical markers from a small number of teas. Thus, a comprehensive analysis of tea using a single analytical method is still missing [17]. To meet international standards, there is an urgent need for analyzing the major chemical constituents of different types of processed teas. In this research, we established an efficient and rapid UHPLC-DAD method for the determination of 20 components, including catechins, alkaloids, phenolic acids, and flavonols, in 121 tea samples from six distinct types of tea. Furthermore, we identified the potential essential chemical components critical for classifying tea types. By performing a principal component analysis on the chemical composition of the six different types of tea leaves, we conducted a classification analysis of the tea sample characteristics.

2. Materials and Methods

2.1. Reagents and Materials

Gallic acid (GA), (−)-gallocatechin (GC), caffeine (CAF), theophylline (THEO), (−)-epigallocatechin (EGC), (+)-catechin (C), chlorogenic acid (CHL), theobromine (TB), caffeic acid (CAA), (−)-epicatechin (EC), (−)-epigallocatechin gallate (EGCG), p-coumaric acid (COU), (−)-gallocatechin gallate (GCG), ferulic acid (FER), sinapic acid (SIN), epicatechin gallate (ECG), rutin (RUT), myricetin (MYR), quercetin (QUE), and kaempferol (KAE) were purchased from Sigma (St. Louis, MO, USA), and the purity of the reagents was above 95%. The acetonitrile (HPLC grade) was purchased from Merck KgaA (Darmstadt, Germany), and all other reagents including methanol and formic acid were purchased from Sinopharm Chemical Reagent Co., Ltd. (Shanghai, China). Ultrapure water was obtained from a Milli-Q water system (Millipore, Bedford, MA, USA). A total of 121 samples covering six different types of teas, including black tea (BT, n = 17), green tea (GT, n = 29), yellow tea (YT, n = 7), white tea (WT, n = 12), oolong tea (OT, n = 42), and dark tea (DT, n = 14), were purchased from local supermarkets in Beijing and Fuzhou, China, and kept in boxes sealed by tin foil at 4 °C.

2.2. Tea Sample Extraction

The sample extraction method was optimized to enhance the efficiency of extracting key constituents in tea. Tea samples underwent initial drying at 35 °C for 2 h, followed by crushing into powders and passage through a 40 mesh screen (304 stainless steel sieve, Yongkang Jielong Industrial and Trade Co., Ltd., Jinhua, China). The selection of this specific mesh screen aimed to optimize the extraction procedure, achieving elevated dissolution rates while minimizing material loss. An aliquot of 0.5 g sample powder was weighed into an Erlenmeyer flask and 10 mL of the methanol-dimethyl sulfoxide mixture (50:50, v/v) was added. The mixture was shaken for 15 min at room temperature and centrifuged at 8000 rpm for 15 min at 4 °C. This extraction process was repeated once. The supernatants from the two extracts were combined, diluted to 50 mL with the methanol-dimethyl sulfoxide mixture (50:50, v/v), and stored at −20 °C until analysis.

2.3. Development of UHPLC-DAD Analytical Method

In this study, a UHPLC-DAD system was employed for the analysis. The instrument used for this analysis was the Ultimate 3000 UHPLC (Thermo Fisher Scientific, Milan, Italy). Prior to UHPLC analysis, the extract was filtered through a 0.22 μm microporous membrane, and 1 μL of the filtered extract was injected into the UHPLC system. Chromatographic separation was performed using a reverse phase column (Merck Lichrospher RP 18, 100 mm × 2.1 mm, 2 μm, Hessian, Germany). Mobile phases A and B were 0.1% formic acid and acetonitrile, respectively [18]. The gradient elution procedure was: 0 min, 93% A; 12 min, 80% A; 16 min, 50% A; 20 min, 93% A. The analysis duration for each specimen was 20 min, inclusive of a 4 min column equilibration period. The column temperature and flow rate were maintained at 30 °C and 0.3 mL min^{-1}, respectively. For detection, two wavelengths, 280 and 340 nm, were compared in this study using the DAD integrated into the UHPLC system. The developed UHPLC method was validated according to ICH guidelines [18] to ensure fulfillment of current regulatory standards.

2.4. Statistical Analysis

Data were presented as mean ± standard deviation and range (min-max). The differences among different groups (>2 groups) were evaluated using ANOVA adjusted by Tukey post hoc test in SPSS software (SPSS for Windows, Release 19.0, SPSS Inc., Chicago, IL, USA). Different lower cases indicate significant differences (p < 0.05). To identify potential chemical biomarkers for the classification of teas, a random forest (RF) algorithm was implemented in the "Random Forest" package [19] under R software (Version 3.5.3, https://www.r-project.org/, accessed on 6 July 2021). RF achieves classification by constructing a series of decision trees. It optimizes the classification by aggregating the inputs across all trees. Although this method cannot be compared to traditional chemometrics, which has a solid statistical foundation, RF possesses several advantages, including excellent predictive capabilities and the ability to balance all variables even in cases of overfitting [20,21]. Principal component analysis (PCA) was used to examine patterns in composition data and to highlight similarities and dissimilarities in the phytochemical contents of the tea products.

3. Results

3.1. Development and Validation of a UHPLC-DAD Analytical Method

The structures of the 20 compounds are displayed in Figure S2. For enhanced precision, we compared the absorption peaks of these compounds at two wavelengths of 280 and 340 nm (Figure 1B). It came to our attention that all components exhibited enhanced sensitivity and reduced interference at 280 nm, signifying their suitability for concurrent determination of the chosen compounds. We then proceeded to verify the reliability of this analysis method. Table 1 illustrated the favorable linearity of all analytes with $R^2 > 0.999$. The relative standard deviations (RSD) were within the range of 0.01–0.31% for intraday assays and 0.42–3.31% for interday assays. Table 1 shows that the limit of detection (LOD) of the analytes was between 0.03 and 2.73 mg/L, alongside the average recovery rate, which ranged from 93.61% to 106.25%. These results indicate that the proposed analysis method was sensitive, precise, and accurate. An analysis of the main chemical components in six different types of teas revealed that green tea contained the highest levels of chemical components (Figure S3).

Table 1. Validation parameters for the UHPLC-DAD method proposed in this study ($n = 6$).

Standard	Calibration Equation	R [a]	LR [b]	intraRSD [c]	interRSD [d]	LOD [e]	REC [f]
GAI	$y = 19681x + 5061.6$	0.9998	0.17–100	0.16	1.57	0.05	99.26
GAL	$y = 17021x - 5572.6$	0.9998	0.10–100	0.26	0.67	0.03	100.80
CAF	$y = 15953x - 948.43$	0.9999	0.63–100	0.21	2.37	0.19	97.44
THE	$y = 1054.4x + 930.46$	0.9991	0.33–100	0.31	0.52	0.10	106.25
EPI	$y = 3799.5x + 759.99$	0.9999	1.17–100	0.15	0.83	0.35	101.73
CAT	$y = 8791.6x - 2528.8$	0.9999	0.60–100	0.13	0.17	0.18	99.20
CHL	$y = 14512x - 426.08$	0.9999	0.50–100	0.13	0.42	0.15	95.92
THO	$y = 20872x + 4110$	0.9999	0.33–100	0.13	1.28	0.10	98.01
CAA	$y = 12547x + 1496$	0.9997	0.43–100	0.13	1.29	0.13	99.71
EPC	$y = 4710.3x + 831.01$	0.9998	1.07–100	0.10	0.86	0.32	101.12
EPG	$y = 7230.3x - 3827.3$	0.9998	0.87–100	0.15	0.47	0.26	100.01
COU	$y = 16970x + 121844$	0.9994	0.63–100	0.17	0.32	0.19	93.61
GAO	$y = 7167.4x - 1372.7$	0.9995	0.43–100	0.15	0.68	0.13	94.48
FER	$y = 17762x + 4688.7$	0.9999	1.00–100	0.08	0.44	0.30	102.63
SIN	$y = 6074.3x + 1169.5$	0.9999	0.37–100	0.06	1.06	0.11	95.24
EPA	$y = 10336x - 2607$	0.9999	1.40–100	0.06	0.68	0.42	105.92
RUT	$y = 2781.4x - 1781.5$	0.9992	0.40–100	0.08	3.31	0.12	100.17
MYR	$y = 4158.4x - 3148.4$	0.9993	0.80–100	0.01	2.53	0.24	96.74
QUE	$y = 4763.1x - 2477.3$	0.9997	9.10–100	0.01	3.71	2.73	96.22
KAE	$y = 7795.4x + 5093.3$	0.9994	2.17–100	0.01	2.87	0.65	100.95

[a] correlation coefficient; [b] linear range (mg/L); [c] relative standard deviation based on intraday assays (%); [d] relative standard deviation based on inter-day assays (%); [e] limit of detection (mg/L); [f] recovery (%). The data presented in mg/L refers to the detection limit of the extraction solution.

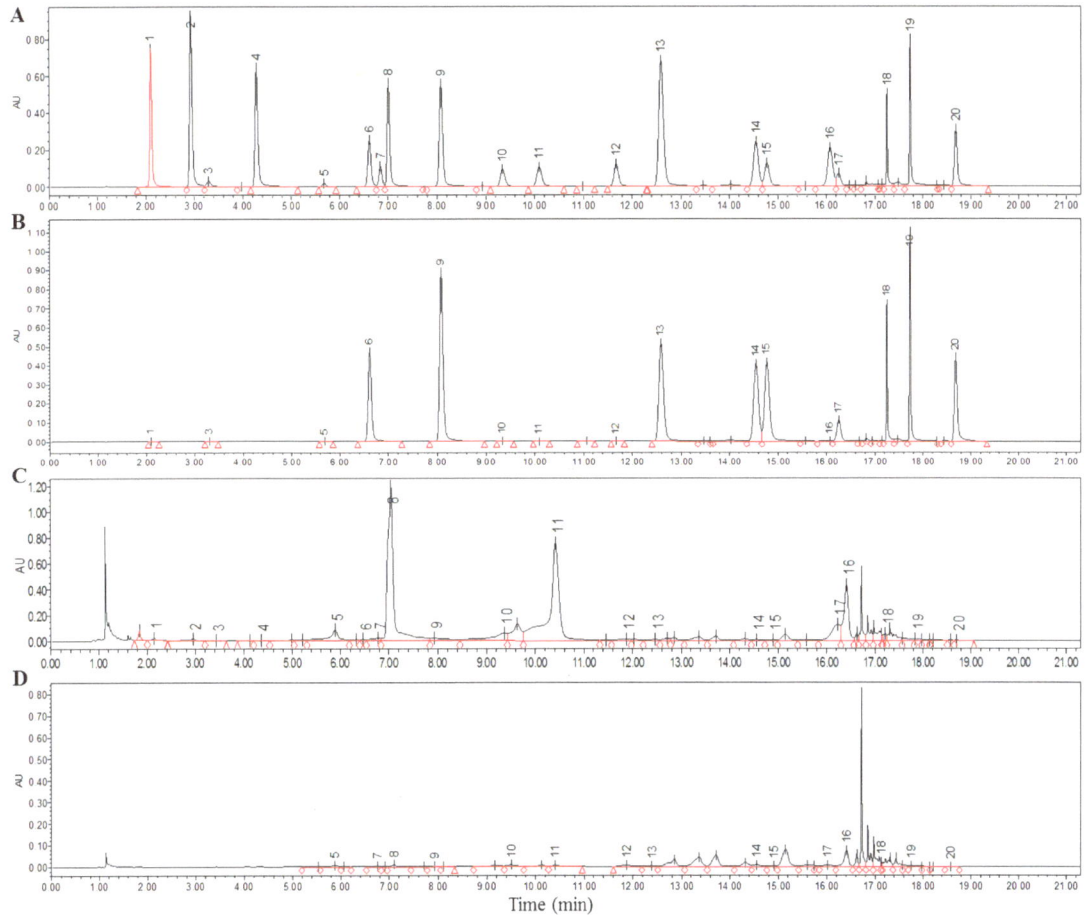

Figure 1. UHPLC-DAD chromatograms of 20 chemical components in tea detected at 280 and 340 nm. (**A**,**B**) A chromatogram of the standard at 280 and 340 nm. (**C**,**D**) A representative chromatogram of the sample at 280 and 340 nm. Component: 1, gallic acid; 2, gallocatechin; 3, caffeine; 4, theophylline; 5, epgallocatechin; 6, catechin; 7, chlorogenic acid; 8, theobromine; 9, caffeic acid; 10, epicatechin; 11, epigallocatechin gallate; 12, coumaric acid; 13, gallocatechin gallate; 14, ferulic acid; 15 sinapic acid; 16, epicatechin gallate; 17, rutin; 18, myricetin; 19, quercetin; 20, kaempferol.

3.2. Comparison of Alkaloids Levels in Six Different Types of Chinese Teas

Our developed method successfully detected three types of alkaloids, namely theophylline (THEO), theobromine (TB), and caffeine (CAF). Remarkably, CAF was the predominant alkaloid in all six types of teas, followed by TB and THEO, indicating that tea processing methods might have had little impact on the alkaloid composition ratio. Nevertheless, our results indicated that different tea types possessed different alkaloid contents. For instance, YT and OT exhibited the highest and lowest TB levels, respectively, while DT showed significantly higher levels of THEO than other tea types ($p < 0.05$, Table 2). Moreover, GT displayed significantly higher levels of CAF compared to OT and WT, and YT exhibited markedly higher TB levels than the other tea types ($p < 0.05$, Table 2). These observations suggested that processing methods may have differentially affected the composition of tea alkaloids, which are known to possess various health-promoting effects.

Table 2. Comparative analysis of alkaloid levels in six different types of teas ($n = 121$), including caffeine (CAF), theophylline (THEO), and theobromine (TB).

Alkaloid	GT ($n = 29$)	YT ($n = 7$)	DT ($n = 14$)	WT ($n = 12$)	OT ($n = 42$)	BT ($n = 17$)	F Value	p Value
Caffine	53.45 ± 22.07 (0–129.8)	39.40 ± 14.49 (13.90–58.66)	35.94 ± 25.26 (0–103.07)	27.85 ± 23.14 (0.01–63.95) [a]	25.98 ± 23.49 (0–147.47) [a]	43.43 ± 29.42 (0–143.89)	3.462	0.006
Percentage of total alkaloids	97.30%	93.84%	95.45%	96.01%	98.03%	97.21%		
Theophylline	0.05 ± 0.05 (0–0.17)	0.07 ± 0.15 (0–0.40)	0.43 ± 0.60 (0–1.63) [a, b]	0.07 ± 0.10 (0–0.34) [c]	0.10 ± 0.22 (0–1.25) [c]	0.06 ± 0.11 (0–0.35) [c]	5.088	0.000
Percentage of total alkaloids	0.10%	0.17%	1.15%	0.23%	0.29%	0.14%		
Theobromine	1.43 ± 0.69 (0.01–2.50)	2.52 ± 1.67 (0.22–4.75) [a]	1.28 ± 0.69 (0.25–2.28) [b]	1.09 ± 0.91 (0.46–3.08) [b]	0.57 ± 0.46 (0.09–2.36) [a, b, c]	1.19 ± 0.80 (0.32–2.79) [b]	10.67	0.000
Percentage of total alkaloids	2.60%	6.00%	3.40%	3.77%	1.68%	2.66%		

Tea type: OT, oolong tea; GT, green tea; WT, white tea; DT, dark tea; YT, yellow tea. Note: Data expressed as mean ± standard deviation and range (min-max). [a, b, c] Values with different letters indicate significant differences ($p < 0.05$) compared to GT, YT, and DT samples using ANOVA and Tukey post hoc test. The results were reported in mg/g to indicate the concentration of compounds in 1 g of tea leaves after conversion.

3.3. Dynamic Changes in Catechins in Six Different Types of Tea

Table 3 illustrates the remarkable effect of tea processing methods on the composition ratio of tea catechins. Our data revealed that GC levels were markedly higher in OT and GT compared to other tea varieties ($p < 0.05$, Table 3). Lower EGC levels were detected in DT and BT, while C levels were relatively higher in WT and GT ($p < 0.05$). Notably, WT exhibited significantly higher EC levels than others ($p < 0.05$). The EGCG content was higher in the GT and YT groups, while it was lower in the DT group ($p < 0.05$). Furthermore, the GCG levels in the GT group were significantly higher compared to the WT, DT, and BT groups, and the ECG levels of the GT tea variety were also the highest ($p < 0.05$). Investigating tea catechin changes can aid in regulating tea quality during thermal processing.

Table 3. Comparative analysis of catechin levels in six different types of teas ($n = 121$), including gallocatechin (GC), epicatechin gallate (EGC), epicatechin (EC), epigallocatechin gallate (EGCG), gallocatechin gallate (GCG), epicatechin gallate (ECG), and catechin (C).

Catechin	GT ($n = 29$)	YT ($n = 7$)	DT ($n = 14$)	WT ($n = 12$)	OT ($n = 42$)	BT ($n = 17$)	F Value	p Value
Gallocatechin	1.55 ± 1.10 (0–4.26)	0.61 ± 0.68 (0–2.00)	0.59 ± 0.29 (0–1.22) [a]	0.42 ± 0.33 (0–0.98) [a]	2.31 ± 1.17 (0–4.95) [a, b, c, d]	0.14 ± 0.21 (0–0.64) [a, e]	20.70	0.000
Percentage of total catechins	1.10%	0.48%	6.62%	0.39%	2.76%	0.47%		
Epicatechin gallate	22.01 ± 18.94 (0.84–79.73)	14.08 ± 10.57 (4.16–30.84)	1.36 ± 1.20 (0–4.26) [a]	26.36 ± 32.27 (0.37–95.89) [c]	20.07 ± 14.00 (0–50.19) [c]	2.50 ± 2.73 (0–8.7) [a, d, e]	6.458	0.000
Percentage of total catechins	15.53%	10.98%	15.20%	24.66%	23.95%	8.18%		
Epicatechin	4.50 ± 2.97 (0.67–14.36)	7.02 ± 3.99 (1.14–13.04)	1.14 ± 0.79 (0–2.37)	26.54 ± 36.68 (0.28–84.48) [a, b, c]	2.62 ± 1.49 (0–6.95) [d]	0.68 ± 0.89 (0.06–3.40) [d]	9.478	0.000
Percentage of total catechins	3.18%	5.47%	12.73%	24.82%	3.13%	2.22%		
Epigallocatechin gallate	83.90 ± 31.65 (46.11–158.61)	82.38 ± 14.08 (65.42–107.9)	3.57 ± 5.04 (0.11–18.87) [a, b]	29.33 ± 30.13 (0.13–78.83) [a]	46.43 ± 19.33 (1.87–86.42) [a, b, c]	23.85 ± 45.66 (0.05–153.58) [a, b]	23.42	0.000
Percentage of total catechins	59.21%	64.21%	39.88%	27.43%	55.41%	78.10%		
Gallocatechin gallate	1.16 ± 0.77 (0.14–2.96)	1.15 ± 0.75 (0.32–2.56)	0.32 ± 0.27 (0.03–1.04) [a]	0.25 ± 0.21 (0–0.55) [a]	0.89 ± 0.94 (0–3.50)	0.10 ± 0.13 (0.01–0.58) [a, b, e]	7.591	0.000
Percentage of total catechins	0.82%	0.90%	3.62%	0.23%	1.06%	0.33%		
Epicatechin gallate	24.94 ± 8.42 (11.89–41.84)	20.66 ± 4.02 (15.25–27.86)	1.40 ± 1.12 (0.04–3.55) [a, b]	18.29 ± 11.45 (3.07–38.27) [c]	10.09 ± 7.44 (0.44–46.60) [a, b, c, d]	2.30 ± 1.54 (0.34–4.84) [a, b, d, e]	34.83	0.000
Percentage of total catechins	17.60%	16.10%	15.64%	17.11%	12.04%	7.53%		
Catechin	3.65 ± 5.83 (0–22.11)	2.39 ± 1.16 (0.78–3.95)	0.57 ± 0.53 (0–1.41)	5.72 ± 15.15 (0.07–53.33)	1.37 ± 2.46 (0–15.31)	0.97 ± 1.19 (0–3.22)	1.809	0.117
Percentage of total catechins	2.57%	1.86%	6.32%	5.35%	1.64%	3.16%		

Tea type: OT, oolong tea; GT, green tea; WT, white tea; DT, dark tea; YT, yellow tea. Note: Data expressed as mean ± standard deviation and range (min-max). [a, b, c, d, e] Values with different letters indicate significant differences ($p < 0.05$) compared to GT, YT, DT, WT, and OT samples using ANOVA and Tukey post hoc test. The results were reported in mg/g to indicate the concentration of compounds in 1 g of tea leaves after conversion.

3.4. Dynamics Changes in Flavonols in Six Different Types of Teas

The tea processing procedures have resulted in a shift in the composition ratio of tea flavonols. As shown in Table 4, OT and WT exhibited a relatively lower proportion of RUT than other tea varieties. WT also contained the lowest level of KAE among all tea types. While BT, GT, and DT demonstrated a higher proportion of QUE, YT had the lowest concentration of QUE. The differences in flavonol levels among the six different tea varieties were not statistically significant (Table 4).

Table 4. Comparative analysis of flavonol levels in six different types of teas (n = 121), including rutin (RUT), myricetin (MYR), quercetin (QUE), and kaempferol (KAE).

Flavonol	GT (n = 29)	YT (n = 7)	DT (n = 14)	WT (n = 12)	OT (n = 42)	BT (n = 17)	F Value	p Value
Rutin	2.82 ± 1.49 (0.12–6.91)	1.31 ± 1 (0.28–3.00)	1.52 ± 1.21 (0.18–3.49)	2.29 ± 1.89 (0.38–5.62)	1.86 ± 2.43 (0.15–15.25)	2.34 ± 1.25 (0.31–4.00)	1.586	0.169
Percentage of total flavonols	75.14%	79.54%	77.98%	59.99%	57.68%	74.91%		
Myricetin	0.67 ± 0.78 (0.01–3.74)	0.29 ± 0.24 (0.01–0.66)	0.24 ± 0.25 (0–0.68)	1.46 ± 1.67 (0.04–4.76)	1.22 ± 3.15 (0–14.95)	0.59 ± 0.64 (0.05–2.22)	0.958	0.446
Percentage of total flavonols	17.99%	17.30%	12.30%	38.24%	37.98%	18.76%		
Quercetrin	0.19 ± 0.86 (0–4.66)	0.02 ± 0.01 (0–0.03)	0.13 ± 0.19 (0.01–0.55)	0.06 ± 0.03 (0–0.10)	0.06 ± 0.10 (0–0.66)	0.11 ± 0.12 (0.01–0.50)	0.372	0.866
Percentage of total flavonols	5.00%	1.12%	6.78%	1.45%	2.00%	3.47%		
Kampferol	0.07 ± 0.08 (0–0.25)	0.03 ± 0.03 (0.01–0.07)	0.06 ± 0.11 (0–0.40)	0.01 ± 0.01 (0–0.03)	0.08 ± 0.08 (0–0.34)	0.09 ± 0.12 (0.01–0.39)	1.631	0.157
Percentage of total flavonols	1.87%	2.04%	2.94%	0.31%	2.34%	2.86%		

Tea type: OT, oolong tea; GT, green tea; WT, white tea; DT, dark tea; YT, yellow tea. Note: Data expressed as mean ± standard deviation and range (min-max). ANOVA and Tukey post hoc tests were used to detect no significant differences in the levels of the four flavonols among the six types of tea. The results were reported in mg/g to indicate the concentration of compounds in 1 g of tea leaves after conversion.

3.5. Dynamics Changes in Phenolic Acids in Six Different Types of Tea

In this study, six phenolic acids, namely gallic acid (GA), coumaric acid (COU), chlorogenic acid (CHL), ferulic acid (FER), sinapic acid (SIN), and caffeic acid (CAA) were identified and analyzed. As presented in Table 5, the composition ratio of these components was significantly influenced by tea processing procedures, which classified teas into distinct chemo-types. It is worth noting that CAA was not detected (as nd). DT, BT, WT, and OT exhibited dormancy with GA, while YT displayed dormancy with CHL. OT and GT contained two major phenolic acids.

Table 5. Comparative analysis of phenolic acids levels in six different types of teas (n = 121), including gallic acid (GA), chlorogenic acid (CHL), ρ-coumaric acid (COU), ferulic acid (FER), sinapic acid (SIN), and caffeic acid (CAA).

Phenolic Acids	GT (n = 29)	YT (n = 7)	DT (n = 14)	WT (n = 12)	OT (n = 42)	BT (n = 17)	F Value	p Value
Gallic acid	0.99 ± 0.52 (0.28–2.51)	1.20 ± 0.66 (0.39–2.03)	4.12 ± 2.89 (1.03–11.57) [a,b]	2.24 ± 0.87 (0.9–3.61) [a,c]	1.12 ± 0.94 (0.07–3.71) [c]	2.54 ± 0.91 (1.23–5.04) [a,c,e]	16.62	0.000
Percentage of total phenolic acids	24.59%	21.95%	92.72%	10.12%	46.18%	38.70%		
Chlorogenic acid	1.50 ± 4.60 (0–22.83)	3.28 ± 2.61 (0.1–7.88)	0.01 ± 0.03 (0–0.09)	19.25 ± 34.50 (0–80.76)	0.15 ± 0.24 (0–1.29) [d]	2.79 ± 11.19 (0–46.2)	5.352	0.000
Percentage of total phenolic acids	37.10%	59.59%	0.29%	86.79%	6.26%	42.42%		
ρ-coumaric acid	0.15 ± 0.13 (0–0.46)	0.09 ± 0.11 (0.01–0.32)	0.08 ± 0.18 (0–0.66)	0.12 ± 0.18 (0–0.63)	0.14 ± 0.32 (0–1.64)	0.80 ± 1.64 (0.03–4.97)	3.179	0.010
Percentage of total flavonols	3.82%	1.55%	1.70%	0.54%	5.63%	12.23%		
Ferulic acid	1.05 ± 2.93 (0–15.05)	0.24 ± 0.35 (0.02–1.02)	0.06 ± 0.05 (0.01–0.18)	0.33 ± 0.34 (0.02–0.96)	0.64 ± 0.52 (0–1.62)	0.13 ± 0.13 (0–0.39)	1.358	0.245
Percentage of total phenolic acids	26.16%	4.45%	1.32%	1.47%	26.41%	1.93%		
Sinapic acid	0.34 ± 0.31 (0.03–1.34)	0.66 ± 0.83 (0.2–2.5)	0.18 ± 0.11 (0.04–0.4)	0.24 ± 0.28 (0–0.88)	0.37 ± 0.36 (0–1.32)	0.31 ± 0.46 (0.02–1.88)	1.741	0.131

Table 5. Cont.

Phenolic Acids	GT (n = 29)	YT (n = 7)	DT (n = 14)	WT (n = 12)	OT (n = 42)	BT (n = 17)	F Value	p Value
Percentage of total phenolic acids	8.34%	12.12%	3.96%	1.08%	15.52%	4.72%		
Caffeic acid	nd	nd	nd	nd	nd	nd		

Tea type: OT, oolong tea; GT, green tea; WT, white tea; DT, dark tea; YT, yellow tea. Note: Data expressed as mean ± standard deviation and range (min-max). [a, b, c, d, e] Values with different letters indicate significant differences ($p < 0.05$) compared to GT, YT, DT, WT, and OT samples using ANOVA and Tukey post hoc test. The results were reported in mg/g to indicate the concentration of compounds in 1 g of tea leaves after conversion.

DT contained a notable quantity of GA, accounting for over 90% of the total phenolic acids, which was significantly higher compared to other tea types ($p < 0.05$, Table 5). A substantial proportion of FER, almost a quarter of the total phenolic acids, was identified in OT and GT (Table 5). Furthermore, the proportion of CHL in GT and YT exceeded that found in other tea types.

3.6. Identification of Potential Biomarkers for Tea Classification Using Random Forests

In this study, the random forests (RF) classifier was employed to distinguish different types of tea and identify possible biomarkers based on 19 detected chemical components (Figure 2A). The results showed that the proposed RF classifier achieved accuracies of 78.57% for BT, 86.21% for GT, 85.71% for OT, 82.35% for BT, 50.00% for WT, and 57.14% for YT (Figure 2B). The overall accuracy of the classifier was 79.34% using 19 identified chemical components. Although the accuracy of the present classifier was still low, especially for WT and YT, the performance could be improved by increasing the number of samples. In addition, GC, EGCG, and ECG, as the main components of tea catechins, were identified as important biomarkers for tea classification (Figure 2C). Moreover, tea catechins had different responses under thermal processing.

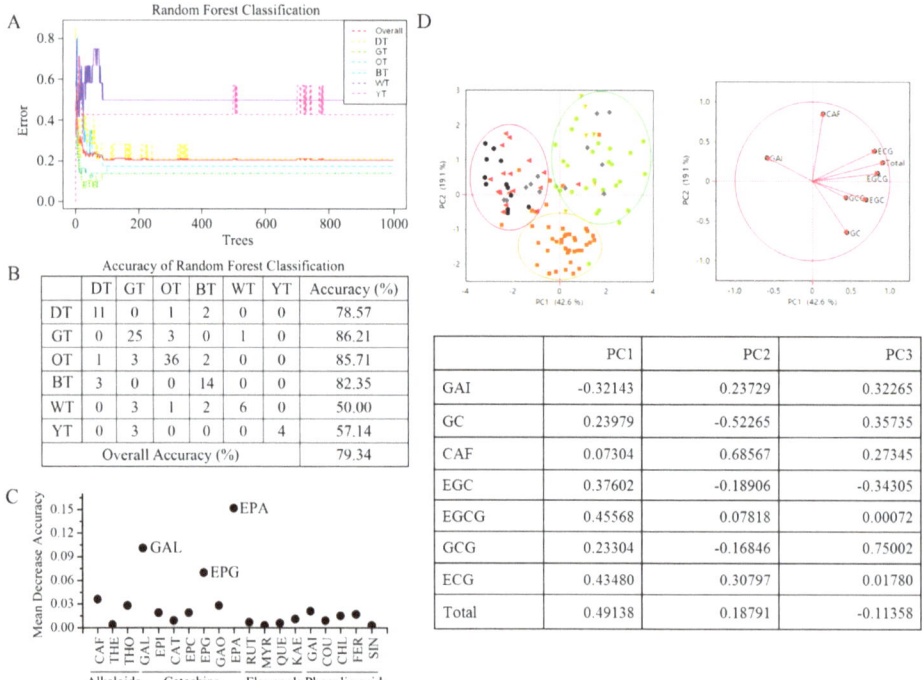

Figure 2. Tea classification based on 19 chemical components using random forests. (**A**) Random forest classification; (**B**) accuracy of random forest classification; (**C**) potential biomarkers identified

by random forests. Component: CAF, caffeine; THEO, theophylline; TB, theobromine; GC, (−)-gallocatechin; EGC, (−)-epigallocatechin; C, (+)-catechin; EC, (−)-epicatechin; EGCG, (−)-epigallocatechin gallate; GCG, (−)-gallocatechin gallate; ECG, epicatechin gallate; RUT, rutin; MYR, myricetin; QUE, quercetin; KAE, kaempferol; GA, gallic acid; COU, coumaric acid; CHL, chlorogenic acid; FER, ferulic acid; SIN, sinapic acid. Tea type: BT, black tea; OT, oolong tea; GT, green tea; WT, white tea; DT, dark tea; YT, yellow tea. (**D**) Principal component analysis (PCA) of 6 types of teas. Black: DT, Red: BT, Green: GT, Yellow: YT, Brown: OT, Gray: WT.

3.7. Principal Component Analysis

Principal component analysis (PCA) was performed on the data obtained from the sample processing of a particular type of tea (Figure 2D). The first principal component (PC1) explained 42.59% of the total variance, while the second principal component (PC2) explained 19.14% of the total variance, and the third principal component (PC3) explained 13.82% of the total variance. Together, PC1, PC2, and PC3 explained a cumulative variance of 75.54%. The results show that the tea samples of six varieties could be classified into three categories based on their fermentation levels. Green tea and yellow tea (non-fermented tea) were categorized together. Oolong tea (semi-fermented tea) was classified separately. Black tea and dark tea (post-fermented tea and fully fermented tea) were grouped together.

4. Discussion

Currently, there is a lack of quantitative methods for classifying tea categories in accordance with tea standards. This study aimed to introduce a quantitative and objective approach to identifying tea categories, thereby establishing a scientific foundation for the development of chemical classification methods for tea. Previous research has demonstrated the efficacy of HPLC-DAD in identifying the distinctive constituents of Laoshan green tea (GT) harvested during both summer and autumn, providing accurate determinations of tea leaves across both seasons [22]. Expanding on this foundation, our objective was to formulate and validate a UHPLC-DAD methodology to concurrently quantify 19 key components, encompassing alkaloids, catechins, flavonols, and phenolic acids, within six differently processed teas. Additionally, we endeavored to pinpoint significant biomarkers for tea classification.

Tea, as a globally consumed beverage, can be classified into six main groups based on the degree of fermentation: green tea (GT), yellow tea (YT), white tea (WT), oolong tea (OT), black tea (BT), and dark tea (DT), in the increasing order of fermentation. The results obtained from our analysis revealed distinct differences in both tea categories and specific compounds as fermentation levels changed. PCA analysis based on these specific compounds also showed good classification results for tea classes with different fermentation levels. These insights contribute to the broader knowledge base surrounding tea, its fermentation process, and its potential implications for health and flavor profiles.

In the present investigation, caffeine was observed to comprise the largest proportion among the six tea types, especially in green tea (GT), which is in accordance with the findings of Boros et al., who extracted caffeine from a variety of teas and reported similar results [23,24]. Interestingly, our results indicated that the processing method for tea leaves had minimal influence on the proportion of alkaloid composition. However, it is worth noting that different alkaloids may react differently to the processing method due to the effects of steeping time, temperature, pH value, and picking time, which all contribute to the chemical composition of tea leaves [25–28].

Catechins are a standard type of flavonoid found in green tea (GT), and it has been observed that green tea contains more catechins than black or oolong teas [29]. The current study also found that green tea has the highest amount of catechins compared to other tea varieties. Previous studies have indicated that unfermented green tea has EGCG as its main component [29,30], while fermented green tea has GC as its main component with less EGCG [2,5]. Our study confirms that green tea has the highest amount of EGCG, with significantly higher levels than other tea types except for yellow tea. Interestingly, our findings show that DT has the lowest amount of EGCG, which may be attributed to the conversion of catechins to theaflavins or theobromine during the fermentation process in black tea, leading to a significant reduction in total catechins (EGCG, ECG, and EGC) [31–33]. Furthermore, different processing methods have been found to affect the ratio of catechin composition in tea leaves, possibly due to the gradual decrease in catechin content and increase in gallic acid content during tea fermentation [5,34]. Another study reported that thermal processing affects the eight catechins in tea differently [35].

Tea flavonols are potent antioxidants that have been shown to protect against cancer and cardiovascular disease [36–38], it is of interest to understand the levels of flavonols in different teas and how processing methods impact flavonol composition. We identified RUT, MYR, QUE, and KAE as the major flavonols in tea leaves, in particular RUT and MYR. Our study found that black tea (BT) had lower total flavonol content compared to other teas, which is consistent with the findings of Selim et al. [39,40]. We also found that the gallic acid (GA) content was the highest in black tea (BT) among the 121 tea samples, previous reports indicated that the increase in gallic acid content coupled with deepening fermentation [41,42].

Previous studies classified black, green, white, yellow, dark, and oolong teas by UV spectroscopy [43]; Ding et al., classified tea quality levels based on CLPSO-SVM using near-infrared spectrum [44]. To further explore the potential biomarkers for tea classification, we identified GC, EGCG, and ECG as important biomarkers for tea classification using UHPLC-DAD quantification combined with RF calculations. Previously, Wang et al., identified the physicochemical components such as catechin and caffeine in yellow tea (YT) using quantitative descriptive analysis (QDA) and partial least squares regression (PLSR). RF, although lacking a comprehensive theoretical foundation comparable to traditional chemometrics, offers advantages such as strong predictive capabilities and balanced handling of all variables even in cases of overfitting [20,21]. Additionally, RF's ability to handle data dimensions without limitations made it a valuable tool for predicting the types of tea accurately. Previous studies have also demonstrated RF's predictive prowess in tea sample analysis. For example, Zheng et al. [45] demonstrated the superior predictive performance of RF compared to other machine learning methods, such as PCA and SVM, in predicting unknown tea samples. Similarly, Xu et al. [46] used RF based on fused signals to achieve the best performance in predicting the concentrations of chemical components in tea. Our study builds upon this knowledge and showcases the potential of RF in further advancing tea classification methodologies.

In conclusion, we have developed a UHPLC-DAD analytical method to simultaneously determine a total of 19 major components in tea, including alkaloids, catechins, flavonols, and phenolic acids. The method has undergone methodological validation, demonstrating sensitivity, stability, and good repeatability in content determination. Significant differences in these components have been observed among the six types of tea studied, with green tea (GT) and yellow tea (YT) exhibiting higher total chemical content compared to the other teas. These observations suggest that the varying degrees of fermentation in the six major tea categories may influence the composition of alkaloids, catechins, flavanols, and phenolic acids in tea leaves. Furthermore, GC, EGCG, and ECG, serving as the principal constituents of catechins in tea, have been identified as important biomarkers for tea classification. The results of PCA analysis reveal the possibility of categorizing these six tea types into three groups based on their fermentation levels. In future work, we plan to establish a tea composition database and develop a standard analytical method for the evaluation and classification of teas.

Supplementary Materials: The following supporting information can be downloaded at: https://www.mdpi.com/article/10.3390/foods12163098/s1, Figure S1: Map of China showing the location of all tea sample collection sites; Figure S2: Chemical structures of phenolic acids, alkaloids, flavonol and flavonol glycosides in oolong tea; Figure S3: Changes of major chemical components in six different types of teas.

Author Contributions: Writing—original draft preparation, Y.C. and L.L.; methodology, Y.C. and L.L.; writing—review and editing, Y.Y., R.G., J.X. and W.Y.; Guide paper writing skills and plan experimental designs, G.W. All authors have read and agreed to the published version of the manuscript.

Funding: This study received financial support from the 5511 Collaborative Innovation Project of germplasm resources nursery (No. XTCXGC 2021019); the free exploration scientific and technological innovation project of Fujian Academy of Agricultural Sciences (No ZYTS 2019019); the Fujian Province Foreign Cooperation Projects, China (No 2021I0034) and the Foreign Cooperation Projects of Fujian Academy of Agricultural Sciences (No. DWHZ-2-22-21).

Data Availability Statement: The datasets used and/or analyzed during the current study are available from the corresponding authors upon reasonable request.

Conflicts of Interest: The authors declare no conflict of interest.

Abbreviations

BT: black tea; OT, oolong tea; GT, green tea; WT, white tea; DT, Red tea; YT, yellow tea; CAF, caffeine; THEO, theophylline; TB, theobromine; GC, gallocatechin; EGC, epigallocatechin; C, catechin; EC, epicatechin; EGCG, epigallocatechin gallate; GCG, gallocatechin gallate; ECG, epicatechin gallate; RUT, rutin; MYR, myricetin; QUE, quercetin; KAE, kaempferol; GA, gallic acid; COU, coumaric acid; CHL, chlorogenic acid; FER, ferluic acid; SIN, sinapic acid.

References

1. Farag, M.A.; Elmetwally, F.; Elghanam, R.; Kamal, N.; Hellal, K.; Hamezah, H.S.; Zhao, C.; Mediani, A. Metabolomics in tea products; a compile of applications for enhancing agricultural traits and quality control analysis of *Camellia sinensis*. *Food Chem.* **2023**, *404 Pt B*, 134628. [CrossRef]
2. Tang, G.Y.; Meng, X.; Gan, R.Y.; Zhao, C.N.; Liu, Q.; Feng, Y.B.; Li, S.; Wei, X.-L.; Atanasov, A.G.; Corke, H.; et al. Health Functions and Related Molecular Mechanisms of Tea Components: An Update Review. *Int. J. Mol. Sci.* **2019**, *20*, 6196. [CrossRef] [PubMed]
3. Wang, Y.; Kan, Z.; Thompson, H.J.; Ling, T.; Ho, C.T.; Li, D.; Wan, X. Impact of Six Typical Processing Methods on the Chemical Composition of Tea Leaves Using a Single Camellia sinensis Cultivar, Longjing 43. *J. Agric. Food Chem.* **2019**, *67*, 5423–5436. [CrossRef]
4. Truong, V.L.; Jeong, W.S. Cellular Defensive Mechanisms of Tea Polyphenols: Structure-Activity Relationship. *Int. J. Mol. Sci.* **2021**, *22*, 9109. [CrossRef] [PubMed]
5. Jiang, H.; Yu, F.; Qin, L.; Zhang, N.; Cao, Q.; Schwab, W.; Li, D.; Song, C. Dynamic change in amino acids, catechins, alkaloids, and gallic acid in six types of tea processed from the same batch of fresh tea (*Camellia sinensis* L.) leaves. *J. Food Compos. Anal.* **2019**, *77*, 28–38. [CrossRef]
6. Chen, S.; Li, M.; Zheng, G.; Wang, T.; Lin, J.; Wang, S.; Wang, X.; Chao, Q.; Cao, S.; Yang, Z.; et al. Metabolite Profiling of 14 Wuyi Rock Tea Cultivars Using UPLC-QTOF MS and UPLC-QqQ MS Combined with Chemometrics. *Molecules* **2018**, *23*, 104. [CrossRef] [PubMed]
7. Rahim, A.A.; Nofrizal, S.; Saad, B. Rapid tea catechins and caffeine determination by HPLC using microwave-assisted extraction and silica monolithic column. *Food Chem.* **2014**, *147*, 262–268. [CrossRef] [PubMed]
8. Stodt, U.; Engelhardt, U.H. Progress in the analysis of selected tea constituents over the past 20 years. *Food Res. Int.* **2013**, *53*, 636–648. [CrossRef]
9. Chen, G.; Yuan, Q.; Saeeduddin, M.; Ou, S.; Zeng, X.; Ye, H. Recent advances in tea polysaccharides: Extraction, purification, physicochemical characterization and bioactivities. *Carbohydr. Polym.* **2016**, *153*, 663–678. [CrossRef]
10. Shitandi, A.A. *Chapter 16—Tea Processing and Its Impact on Catechins, Theaflavin and Thearubigin Formation*; Elsevier Inc.: Amsterdam, The Netherlands, 2013.
11. Tang, C.; Guo, T.; Zhang, Z.; Yang, P.; Song, H. Rapid visualized characterization of phenolic taste compounds in tea extract by high-performance thin-layer chromatography coupled to desorption electrospray ionization mass spectrometry. *Food Chem.* **2021**, *355*, 129555. [CrossRef]
12. Zhao, F.; Qian, J.; Liu, H.; Wang, C.; Wang, X.; Wu, W.; Wang, D.; Cai, C.; Lin, Y. Quantification, identification and comparison of oligopeptides on five tea categories with different fermentation degree by Kjeldahl method and ultra-high performance liquid chromatography coupled with quadrupole-orbitrap ultra-high resolution mass spectrometry. *Food Chem.* **2022**, *378*, 132130. [PubMed]
13. Shirai, N. Organic Acid Analysis in Green Tea Leaves Using High-performance Liquid Chromatography. *J. Oleo Sci.* **2022**, *71*, 1413–1419. [CrossRef] [PubMed]

14. Huang, S.; Zhao, H.; Hu, Y.; Ren, D.; Yi, L. Comprehensive analysis of chemical constituents of tea flowers by ultra-performance liquid chromatography-high resolution mass spectrometry combined with integrated filtering strategy. *Chin. J. Chromatogr.* **2022**, *40*, 242–252. [CrossRef]
15. Keuth, O.; Humpf, H.U.; Furst, P. Determination of pyrrolizidine alkaloids in tea and honey with automated SPE clean-up and ultra-performance liquid chromatography/tandem mass spectrometry. *Food Addit. Contam. Part A Chem. Anal. Control Expo. Risk Assess.* **2022**, *39*, 149–157. [CrossRef]
16. Li, H.; Zhong, Q.; Wang, M.; Luo, F.; Wang, X.; Zhou, L.; Zhang, X. Residue degradation, transfer and risk assessment of pyriproxyfen and its metabolites from tea garden to cup by ultra performance liquid chromatography tandem mass spectrometry. *J. Sci. Food Agric.* **2022**, *102*, 3983–3993. [CrossRef] [PubMed]
17. Zhai, X.; Zhang, L.; Granvogl, M.; Ho, C.T.; Wan, X. Flavor of tea (*Camellia sinensis*): A review on odorants and analytical techniques. *Compr. Rev. Food Sci. Food Saf.* **2022**, *21*, 3867–3909. [CrossRef]
18. Seo, C.S.; Song, K.H. Phytochemical Characterization for Quality Control of Phyllostachys pubescens Leaves Using High-Performance Liquid Chromatography Coupled with Diode Array Detector and Tandem Mass Detector. *Plants* **2021**, *11*, 50. [CrossRef] [PubMed]
19. Liaw, A.; Wiener, M. Classification and regression by randomForest. *R News* **2001**, *2*, 18–22.
20. Breiman, L. Random forests. *Mach. Learn.* **2001**, *45*, 5–32. [CrossRef]
21. Yélamos, I.; Escudero, G.; Graells, M.; Puigjaner, L. Simultaneous fault diagnosis in chemical plants using support Vector Machines. *Comput. Aided Chem. Eng.* **2007**, *24*, 1253–1258.
22. Peng, T.Q.; Yin, X.L.; Gu, H.W.; Sun, W.; Ding, B.; Hu, X.C.; Ma, L.-A.; Wei, S.-D.; Liu, Z.; Ye, S.-Y. HPLC-DAD fingerprints combined with chemometric techniques for the authentication of plucking seasons of Laoshan green tea. *Food Chem.* **2021**, *347*, 128959. [CrossRef] [PubMed]
23. Boros, K.; Jedlinszki, N.; Csupor, D. Theanine and Caffeine Content of Infusions Prepared from Commercial Tea Samples. *Pharmacogn. Mag.* **2016**, *12*, 75–79. [PubMed]
24. Bobkova, A.; Demianova, A.; Belej, L.; Harangozo, L.; Bobko, M.; Jurcaga, L.; Poláková, K.; Božiková, M.; Bilčík, M.; Árvay, J. Detection of Changes in Total Antioxidant Capacity, the Content of Polyphenols, Caffeine, and Heavy Metals of Teas in Relation to Their Origin and Fermentation. *Foods* **2021**, *10*, 1821. [CrossRef] [PubMed]
25. Hajiaghaalipour, F.; Sanusi, J.; Kanthimathi, M.S. Temperature and Time of Steeping Affect the Antioxidant Properties of White, Green, and Black Tea Infusions. *J. Food Sci.* **2016**, *81*, H246–H254. [CrossRef] [PubMed]
26. Wang, M.; Yang, J.; Li, J.; Zhou, X.; Xiao, Y.; Liao, Y.; Tang, J.; Dong, F.; Zeng, L. Effects of temperature and light on quality-related metabolites in tea [*Camellia sinensis* (L.) Kuntze] leaves. *Food Res. Int.* **2022**, *161*, 111882. [CrossRef]
27. Ren, Z.; Chen, Z.; Zhang, Y.; Lin, X.; Weng, W.; Liu, G.; Li, B. Characteristics of Pickering emulsions stabilized by tea water-insoluble protein nanoparticles at different pH values—ScienceDirect. *Food Chem.* **2021**, *375*, 131795. [CrossRef] [PubMed]
28. Wakamatsu, M.; Yamanouchi, H.; Sahara, H.; Iwanaga, T.; Kuroda, R.; Yamamoto, A.; Minami, Y.; Sekijima, M.; Yamada, K.; Kajiya, K. Catechin and caffeine contents in green tea at different harvest periods and their metabolism in miniature swine. *Food Sci. Nutr.* **2019**, *7*, 2769–2778. [CrossRef] [PubMed]
29. Musial, C.; Kuban-Jankowska, A.; Gorska-Ponikowska, M. Beneficial Properties of Green Tea Catechins. *Int. J. Mol. Sci.* **2020**, *21*, 1744. [CrossRef]
30. Farhan, M. Green Tea Catechins: Nature's Way of Preventing and Treating Cancer. *Int. J. Mol. Sci.* **2022**, *23*, 10713. [CrossRef]
31. Tan, J.; Dai, W.; Lu, M.; Lv, H.; Guo, L.; Zhang, Y.; Zhu, Y.; Peng, Q.; Lin, Z. Study of the dynamic changes in the non-volatile chemical constituents of black tea during fermentation processing by a non-targeted metabolomics approach. *Food Res. Int.* **2016**, *79*, 106–113. [CrossRef]
32. Li, L.; Wang, Y.; Cui, Q.; Liu, Y.; Ning, J.; Zhang, Z. Qualitative and quantitative quality evaluation of black tea fermentation through noncontact chemical imaging. *J. Food Compos. Anal.* **2021**, *106*, 104300. [CrossRef]
33. Yang, C.; Zhao, Y.; An, T.; Liu, Z.; Dong, C. Quantitative Prediction and Visualization of Key Physical and Chemical Components in Black Tea Fermentation Using Hyperspectral Imaging. *LWT-Food Sci. Technol.* **2021**, *141*, 110975. [CrossRef]
34. Li, J.; Wu, S.; Yu, Q.; Wang, J.; Deng, Y.; Hua, J.; Zhou, Q.; Yuan, H.; Jiang, Y. Chemical profile of a novel ripened Pu-erh tea and its metabolic conversion during pile fermentation. *Food Chem.* **2022**, *378*, 132126. [CrossRef] [PubMed]
35. Fan, F.Y.; Shi, M.; Nie, Y.; Zhao, Y.; Ye, J.H.; Liang, Y.R. Differential behaviors of tea catechins under thermal processing: Formation of non-enzymatic oligomers. *Food Chem.* **2016**, *196*, 347–354. [CrossRef] [PubMed]
36. Popiolek-Kalisz, J.; Fornal, E. The Impact of Flavonols on Cardiovascular Risk. *Nutrients* **2022**, *14*, 1973. [CrossRef]
37. Kopustinskiene, D.M.; Jakstas, V.; Savickas, A.; Bernatoniene, J. Flavonoids as Anticancer Agents. *Nutrients* **2020**, *12*, 457. [CrossRef]
38. Hazafa, A.; Rehman, K.U.; Jahan, N.; Jabeen, Z. The Role of Polyphenol (Flavonoids) Compounds in the Treatment of Cancer Cells. *Nutr. Cancer* **2020**, *72*, 386–397. [CrossRef]
39. Li, J.; Wang, J.; Yao, Y.; Hua, J.; Zhou, Q.; Jiang, Y.; Deng, Y.; Yang, Y.; Wang, J.; Yuan, H.; et al. Phytochemical comparison of different tea (*Camellia sinensis*) cultivars and its association with sensory quality of finished tea. *LWT-Food Sci. Technol.* **2020**, *117*, 108595. [CrossRef]

40. Selim, D.A.; Shawky, E.; El-Khair, R. Identification of the discriminatory chemical markers of different grades of Sri Lankan white, green and black tea (*Camellia sinenesis* L.) via metabolomics combined to chemometrics. *J. Food Compos. Anal.* **2022**, *109*, 104473. [CrossRef]
41. Kongpichitchoke, T.; Chiu, M.T.; Huang, T.C.; Hsu, J.L. Gallic Acid Content in Taiwanese Teas at Different Degrees of Fermentation and Its Antioxidant Activity by Inhibiting PKCdelta Activation: In Vitro and in Silico Studies. *Molecules* **2016**, *21*, 1346. [CrossRef]
42. Zhang, H.; Liu, Y.Z.; Xu, W.C.; Chen, W.J.; Wu, S.; Huang, Y.Y. Metabolite and Microbiome Profilings of Pickled Tea Elucidate the Role of Anaerobic Fermentation in Promoting High Levels of Gallic Acid Accumulation. *J. Agric. Food Chem.* **2020**, *68*, 13751–13759. [CrossRef] [PubMed]
43. Dankowska, A.; Kowalewski, W. Tea types classification with data fusion of UV-Vis, synchronous fluorescence and NIR spectroscopies and chemometric analysis. *Spectrochim. Acta Part A Mol. Biomol. Spectrosc.* **2019**, *211*, 195–202. [CrossRef] [PubMed]
44. Ding, Y.; Yan, Y.; Li, J.; Chen, X.; Jiang, H. Classification of Tea Quality Levels Using Near-Infrared Spectroscopy Based on CLPSO-SVM. *Foods* **2022**, *11*, 1658. [CrossRef] [PubMed]
45. Zheng, L.; Watson, D.G.; Johnston, B.F.; Clark, R.L.; Edrada-Ebel, R.; Elseheri, W. A chemometric study of chromatograms of tea extracts by correlation optimization warping in conjunction with PCA, support vector machines and random forest data modeling. *Anal. Chim. Acta* **2009**, *642*, 257–265. [CrossRef]
46. Xu, M.; Wang, J.; Zhu, L. The qualitative and quantitative assessment of tea quality based on E-nose, E-tongue and E-eye combined with chemometrics. *Food Chem.* **2019**, *289*, 482–489. [CrossRef]

Disclaimer/Publisher's Note: The statements, opinions and data contained in all publications are solely those of the individual author(s) and contributor(s) and not of MDPI and/or the editor(s). MDPI and/or the editor(s) disclaim responsibility for any injury to people or property resulting from any ideas, methods, instructions or products referred to in the content.

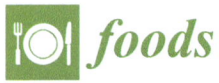

Article

The Effects of Structure and Oxidative Polymerization on Antioxidant Activity of Catechins and Polymers

Wei Wang [1,2,†], Ting Le [1,†], Wei-Wei Wang [1], Jun-Feng Yin [1] and He-Yuan Jiang [1,*]

1 Key Laboratory of Biology, Genetics and Breeding of Special Economic Animals and Plants, Ministry of Agriculture and Rural Affairs, Tea Research Institute, Chinese Academy of Agricultural Sciences, 9 Meiling South Road, Xihu District, Hangzhou 310008, China; ww1040491839@163.com (W.W.); 15968823529@163.com (T.L.)
2 College of Horticulture, Fujian Agriculture and Forestry University, Cangshan District, Fuzhou 350002, China
* Correspondence: jianghy@tricaas.com; Tel.: +86-0571-86650411
† These authors contributed equally to this work.

Abstract: Polyphenols are key free radical scavengers in tea. This study screened the antioxidant active groups of catechins and dimers and analyzed the effects of the degree of oxidative polymerization and oxidative dimerization reaction on their antioxidant activities. ABTS$^{+\cdot}$ free radical scavenging activity, DPPH free radical scavenging activity, and total antioxidant capacity of catechins and polymers were systematically analyzed and compared in this study. Results manifested antioxidant activities of catechins were dominated by B-ring pyrogallol and 3-galloyl, but were not decided by geometrical isomerism. 3-galloyl had a stronger antioxidant activity than B-ring pyrogallol in catechins. The number, not the position, of the galloyl group was positively correlated with the antioxidant activities of theaflavins. Theasinensin A has more active groups than (−)-epigallocatechin gallate and theaflavin-3,3′-digallate, so it had a stronger antioxidant activity. Additionally, the higher the degree of oxidation polymerization, the weaker the antioxidant activities of the samples. The oxidative dimerization reaction hindered the antioxidant activities of the substrate–catechin mixture by reducing the number of active groups of the substrate and increasing the molecular structure size of the product. Overall, pyrogallol and galloyl groups were antioxidant active groups. The degree of oxidative polymerization and the oxidative dimerization reaction weakened the antioxidant activity.

Keywords: antioxidant activity; structure; oxidative dimerization; catechins; polymers

Citation: Wang, W.; Le, T.; Wang, W.-W.; Yin, J.-F.; Jiang, H.-Y. The Effects of Structure and Oxidative Polymerization on Antioxidant Activity of Catechins and Polymers. *Foods* **2023**, *12*, 4207. https://doi.org/10.3390/foods12234207

Academic Editor: Jayani Chandrapala

Received: 30 October 2023
Revised: 16 November 2023
Accepted: 20 November 2023
Published: 22 November 2023

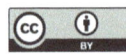

Copyright: © 2023 by the authors. Licensee MDPI, Basel, Switzerland. This article is an open access article distributed under the terms and conditions of the Creative Commons Attribution (CC BY) license (https:// creativecommons.org/licenses/by/ 4.0/).

1. Introduction

Antioxidation refers to resisting the peroxide state of living tissues induced by internal cellular metabolism or external stimuli. In the peroxide state, a balance between generating and eliminating reactive oxygen species (ROS) was broken. ROS content exceeding the scavenging capacity of the defense system will result in oxidative stress damage, such as DNA chain breakage, protein cross-linking, and lipid peroxidation, followed by the imbalance of intracellular metabolism.

One of the mechanisms leading to food spoilage, human diseases, and aging is the imbalance of intracellular metabolism [1,2]. Therefore, there is an urgent need for people to fight against oxidation, which made the search for auxiliary exogenous antioxidants recently become a research hotspot in biochemistry and medicine. As chemical antioxidants, such as butylated hydroxyanisole, may have potential carcinogenic risks in animal experiments [3], the following work is entrusted with a mission to focus on finding green and effective natural substances which have antioxidant properties that can act as substitutes for chemical synthetic antioxidants for safe, sustainable, and healthy development.

Owing to its potential health benefits, tea has long attracted much interest from researchers [4]. Its excellent antioxidant activity has been widely identified [5,6]. Fermentation is the key processing procedure to make black tea, in which the oxidative polymerization of catechins is very active. Oxidative polymerization of catechins is a crucial biochemical reaction to form the characteristics of black tea. When fresh tea leaves are fermented with polyphenol oxidase and peroxidase, catechins will be co-oxidized to form oxidized dimers (such as theaflavins (TFs) and theasinensins (TSs)) and polymers (such as thearubigins (TRs) and theabrownins (TBs)). It is reported that with the increased total phenolic content, the antioxidant activity of black tea is also enhanced [7]. Phenolic compounds were key free radical scavengers [8], such as catechins, TFs, TRs, and TBs [9,10]. In our previous experiments about the antioxidant activity of black tea processing samples, the decreased activity was found to accompany the progression of black tea fermentation. Meanwhile, the catechins content decreased gradually, the dimers' content increased first and decreased later, and the polymer content increased gradually during the fermentation process [11]. Is the reduced antioxidant activity during black tea fermentation due to the lower activity of polymers compared to catechins and dimers or does the oxidative polymerization process reduce it? Additionally, different antioxidant activities of the samples could be found in different antioxidant methods (methods or conditions adopted in each protocol) [12]. It is difficult to generalize conclusions in some cases. Therefore, the antioxidant activities of catechins and their oxidized polymers were systematically studied using the same method in this research to investigate the effects of the degree of oxidation polymerization and the oxidative dimerization reaction on antioxidant activities.

The antioxidant activities of catechins are closely related to their structure, including hydroxyl groups at positions 5 and 7 of the A-ring, an ortho-3'4'-dihydroxyl group (catechol) or 3'4'5'-trihydroxyl group (pyrogall) in the B-ring, and a gallate group located at position 3 of the C-ring (Figure 1) [13]. Structure (quantity and location) could also influence the activity of dimers. Catechins and dimers have regular differences in structure and are natural materials for studying structure–activity relationships. The effective antioxidant active groups in catechins and dimers can be screened through a clever comparison. Catechins are mainly composed of (−)-epigallocatechin gallate (EGCG), (−)-gallocatechin gallate (GCG), (−)-epicatechin gallate (ECG), (−)-catechin gallate (CG), (−)-epigallocatechin (EGC), (−)-gallocatechin (GC), (−)-epicatechin (EC), and (±)-catechin (C) [12]. Catechin was mainly dimerized through benzoquinone and a disproportionation reaction. Among them, the benzoquinone pathway refers to the oxidative polymerization of pyrogallol-type and catechol-type catechins to form TFs [14]. The disproportionation pathway refers to coupling oxidation between pyrogallol-type catechins to form TSs (Figure 2). Four main compounds of TFs are theaflavin (TF), theaflavin-3-gallate (TF-3-G), theaflavin-3'-gallate (TF-3'-G), and Theaflavin-3,3'-digallate (TFDG) [15]. There are many studies about the antioxidant activity of TFs, while that of theasinensin A (TSA) is little, especially in the comparison between TSA and TFs. Due to TSs and TFs being formed competitively during tea processing, it is worth studying which catechin dimer (TSA or TFs) has a stronger antioxidant activity and what their structure–activity relationship is. This is conducive to the targeted regulation of tea processing conditions as it enables us to obtain more dimers with strong antioxidant activities during production.

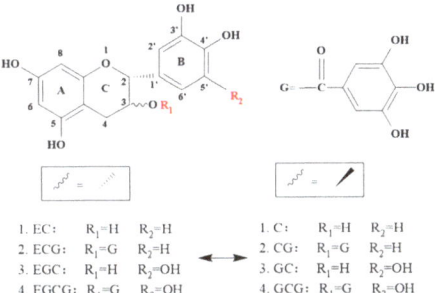

Figure 1. Chemical structure of eight catechins. EC, (−)-epicatechin; ECG, (−)-epicatechin gallate; EGC, (−)-epigallocatechin; EGCG, (−)-epigallocatechin gallate; C, (±)-catechin; CG, (−)-catechin gallate; GC, (−)-gallocatechin; GCG, (−)-gallocatechin gallate.

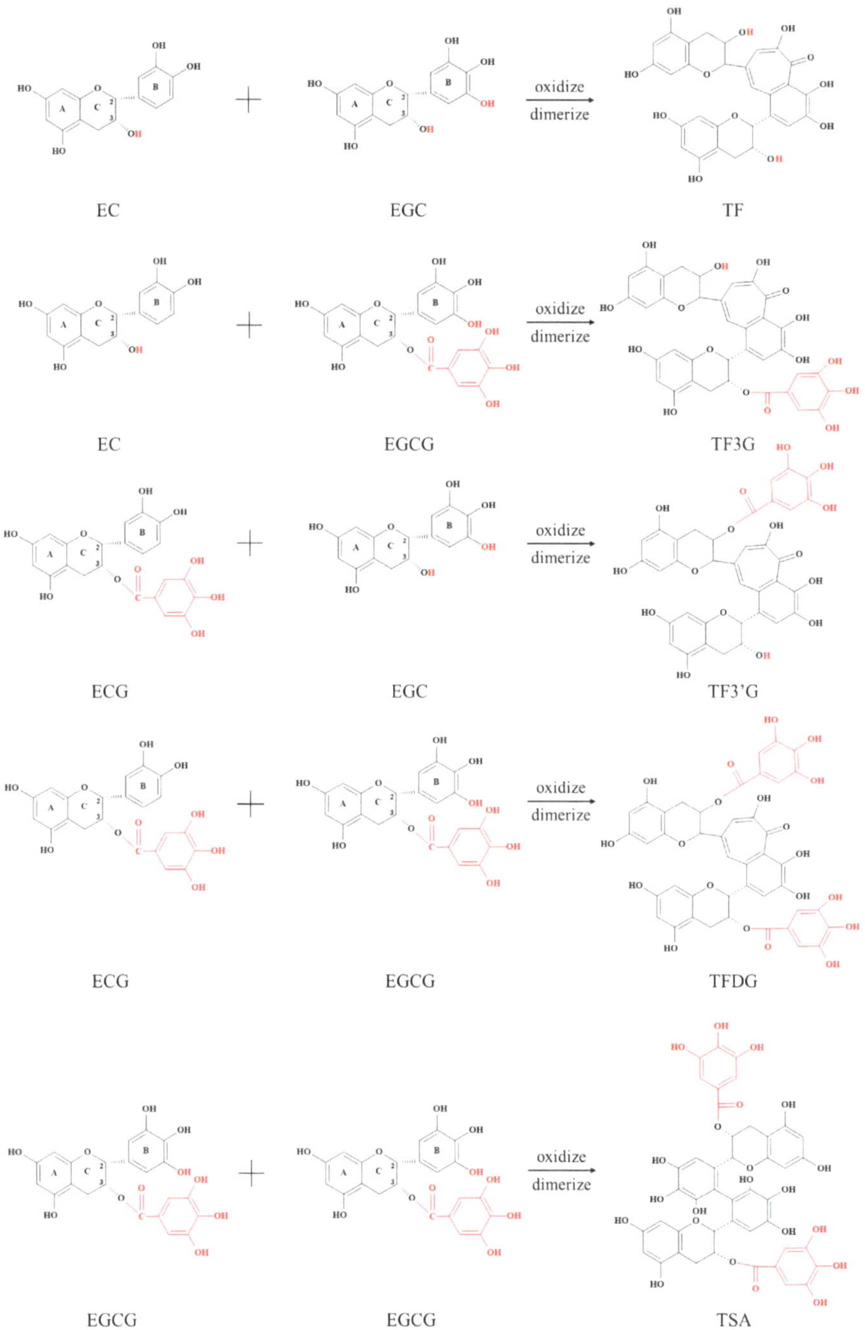

Figure 2. Oxidative dimerization reaction of catechins. TF, theaflavin; TF3G, theaflavin-3-gallate; TF3′G, theaflavin-3′-gallate; TFDG, Theaflavin-3,3′-digallate; TSA, theasinensin A.

Based on these, this study systematically compared and analyzed the antioxidant activities of catechins and their polymers (CTOPs) through three antioxidant methods, exposed the relationship between the degree of oxidative polymerization and antioxidant activity, explored the antioxidant structure–activity relationship by using catechins and dimers with regular differences in structure, and disclosed the effects of the oxidative dimerization reaction on antioxidant activities of a substrate–catechin mixture. Our aim is to find the antioxidant active groups and analyze the effects of the degree of oxidative polymerization and oxidative dimerization reaction on the activity of catechins and polymers to enrich the cognition of the antioxidant activity of tea.

2. Materials and Methods

2.1. Chemicals and Reagents

A total antioxidant capacity assay kit with a ferric-reducing ability of plasma (FRAP) method (S0116) was purchased from Beyotime (Shanghai, China). 2,2′-Azinobis (3-ethylbenzothiazoline-6-sulfonic acid) (ABTS) was purchased from Meryer (Shanghai, China). 1,1-Diphenyl-2-picrylhydrazyl (DPPH) was purchased from Hefei Bomei Biotechnology Co., Ltd. (Hefei, China). Potassium persulfate was purchased from Macklin (Shanghai, China). Methanol was purchased from Merck KGaA (Darmstadt, Germany). 6-Hydroxy-2,5,7,8-tetramethylchroman-2-carboxylic acid (Trolox), C (HPLC $\geq$ 98%), GC (HPLC $\geq$ 98%), CG (HPLC $\geq$ 98%), GCG (HPLC $\geq$ 98%), EC (HPLC $\geq$ 98%), EGC (HPLC $\geq$ 98%), ECG (HPLC $\geq$ 98%), EGCG (HPLC $\geq$ 98%), TF (HPLC $\geq$ 95%), TF-3-G (HPLC $\geq$ 98%), TF-3′-G (HPLC $\geq$ 98%), and TFDG (HPLC $\geq$ 98%) were purchased from Yuanye (Shanghai, China). TSA (HPLC = 91.4%), TRs SII, and TBs were separated and prepared by us.

2.2. Comparison of Antioxidant Activities of CTOPs

A series of mass concentrations were prepared to compare the activities of samples with different degrees of oxidative polymerization. Samples, prepared before use, were dissolved in purified water and diluted to the required concentration.

2.2.1. ABTS$^{+\cdot}$ Free Radical Scavenging Assay

This assay was carried out in line with the procedure as described previously [6], with mild adjustments. ABTS (7 mM) reacted with potassium persulfate (2.45 mM) in equal volumes for 12–16 h in the dark to prepare the ABTS$^{+\cdot}$ stock solution. ABTS$^{+\cdot}$ stock solution was then diluted with methanol to an absorbance of 0.70 ($\pm$0.02) at 734 nm, which was called the ABTS$^{+\cdot}$ reaction solution. The compounds were diluted to five different concentrations in 6.25 µg/mL~200 µg/mL. The ABTS$^{+\cdot}$ reaction solution (4 mL) was added to 100 µL of the compounds, and the blends were left for 10 min at room temperature in the dark. The absorbance was detected at 734 nm using a spectrophotometer (UV 3600, Shimadzu Corporation, Kyoto, Japan). Trolox and water, respectively, were served as the positive and negative controls. Taking ABTS$^{+\cdot}$ free radical scavenging activity (%, Equation (1)) as the ordinate and the mass concentration of the compounds as the abscissa, a linear regression equation was obtained, and the half maximal inhibitory concentration (IC$_{50}$) of each compound was calculated.

$$\text{ABTS}^{+\cdot} \text{ free radical scavenging activity } (\%) = (1 - \text{OD}_{sample}/\text{OD}_{NCK}) \times 100 \quad (1)$$

where OD$_{NCK}$ and OD$_{sample}$ are the absorbance of ultra-pure water and sample, respectively.

2.2.2. DPPH Free Radical Scavenging Assay

This assay was carried out following the procedure reported previously [16], with slight modifications. In brief, 7 mg DPPH was dissolved in 100 mL of methanol to make a DPPH stock solution, and the compounds were diluted to five different concentrations in 50 µg/mL~800 µg/mL. The compound (10 µL) was reacted with 200 µL of a DPPH stock solution for 1 h at room temperature in the dark. The absorbance was detected at 515 nm using a Synergy H1 microplate reader (BioTek Instruments Inc., Winooski, VT, USA). Trolox and water were used as the positive and negative controls, respectively. Taking DPPH free radical scavenging activity (%, Equation (2)) as the ordinate and the mass concentration of the compounds as the abscissa, a linear regression equation was obtained, and the IC_{50} of each compound was calculated.

$$DPPH\ free\ radical\ scavenging\ activity\ (\%) = (1 - OD_{sample}/OD_{NCK}) \times 100 \quad (2)$$

2.2.3. Total Antioxidant Capacity Assay

Referring to the instructions, 180 µL FRAP reagent was reacted with 5 µL compound at 37 °C for 5 min, and the absorbance was detected at 593 nm using a Synergy H1 microplate reader. The mass concentrations of each sample were 1, 0.5, and 0.25 mg/mL. Blank control was water, while positive control was Trolox. The calibration curve was prepared using a $FeSO_4$ standard solution (0.125 mM–4 mM). The ability to reduce iron ions was expressed as mM $FeSO_4$ equivalent antioxidant capacity.

2.3. Structure–Activity Relationship of Catechins and Their Dimers in Antioxidant Activity

Catechins and dimers are natural materials for studying the structure–activity relationship due to their regular differences in structure. Effects of the structure of catechins and dimers on antioxidant activity were studied.

This part mainly explored the effects of geometrical isomerism, B-ring structure, and the number of galloyl groups on the antioxidant activities of catechins. Meanwhile, the number and position of the galloyl group on the antioxidant activities of TFs were also studied. The antioxidant activity of TSA was compared with EGCG and TFDG. The molarities of each compound used in $ABTS^{+\cdot}$ free radical scavenging assay, DPPH free radical scavenging assay, and total antioxidant capacity assay were 100, 400, and 250 µM, respectively. The structural information of compounds is displayed in Table S1. The detection methods of antioxidant activity were similar to those in Section 2.2.

2.4. Influence of Oxidative Dimerization Reaction on the Antioxidant Activity of Catechins and Dimers

This study was carried out following our previous procedure [17]. Catechin dimeric oxidation products (product) are generated with the oxidative dimerization reaction of catechins (substrates). The antioxidant activity between dimers and related substrate monomers or substrate–catechin mixtures was compared next. It could help to learn whether the dimer or substrate–catechin held stronger antioxidant activity and explain the influence of the oxidative dimerization reaction on the antioxidant activity of substrate–catechin mixtures. The substrate–catechins corresponding to each dimer are shown in Figure 2.

The molarities of each compound used in $ABTS^{+\cdot}$ free radical scavenging assay, DPPH free radical scavenging assay, and total antioxidant capacity assay were 100, 100, and 250 µM, respectively. The detection methods of antioxidant activity were similar to those in Section 2.2.

2.5. Statistical Analysis

All results were recorded as means ± standard deviations of at least three replicates. Comparisons between the two groups were performed with Student's *t* test, and one-way analysis of variance with Duncan's post hoc test was performed to measure the significant differences among multiple comparisons between compound effects. $p < 0.05$ and $p < 0.01$ were considered statistically significant.

3. Results

3.1. Comparison of Antioxidant Activities of CTOPs

This section systematically compared the antioxidant activity of CTOPs with three methods. Considering that the molecular weights of TRs, SII, and TBs were difficult to calculate, the activities of CTOPs were compared at a series of mass concentrations rather than molarities.

3.1.1. ABTS$^{+·}$ Free Radical Scavenging Activity

ROS are highly chemically reactive because they contain unpaired electrons. Free radical scavengers or antioxidants can provide electrons and inhibit oxidation. The ABTS$^{+·}$ free radical scavenging assay and DPPH free radical scavenging assay indirectly reflect the antioxidant activity of compounds by detecting the ability of compounds to scavenge free radicals. Among them, the ABTS$^{+·}$ free radical scavenging assay is fit for assessing the ability of compounds as hydrogen/electron donors, and for evaluating the antioxidant activity of compounds [18].

Every sample dose-dependently scavenged the ABTS$^{+·}$ free radical (Figure S1A—Supplementary Materials). IC$_{50}$ of CTOPs were compared in Figure 3A. The ABTS$^{+·}$ free radical scavenging activity of each sample was significantly stronger than Trolox (115 ± 1 µg/mL) except for TBs (186 ± 1 µg/mL), which showed that most of these samples obtained remarkable antioxidant potential. Tested samples could be classified into three categories according to their ABTS$^{+·}$ free radical scavenging activity ($p < 0.05$): catechins, dimers, and polymers. From this view, the ABTS$^{+·}$ free radical scavenging activity was negatively correlated with the degree of oxidative polymerization. At the same time, the ABTS$^{+·}$ free radical scavenging activities of TFs (70 ± 1 µg/mL), TRs SII (90 ± 0 µg/mL) and TBs components isolated from a tea sample also manifested a higher degree of oxidative polymerization, the weaker the ABTS$^{+·}$ free radical scavenging activity of these samples.

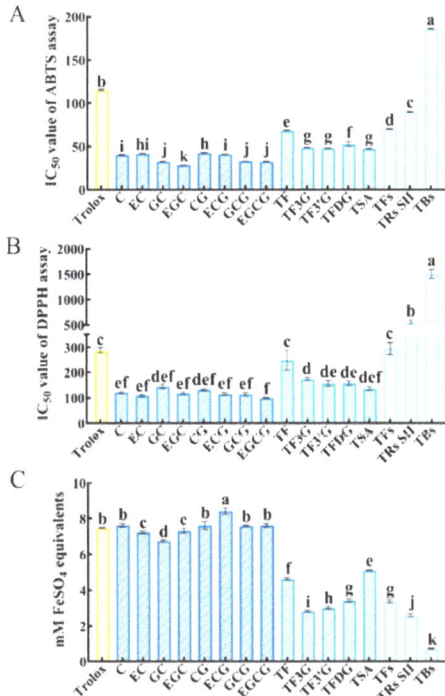

Figure 3. Antioxidant activities of catechins and their polymers (CTOPs) at mass concentrations. (**A**) ABTS$^{+·}$ free radical scavenging activity of CTOPs; (**B**) DPPH free radical scavenging activity of CTOPs; (**C**) total antioxidant capacity of CTOPs. The concentration of samples used in total antioxidant capacity assay was 1 mg/mL. Theaflavins (TFs), thearubigins SII(TRs SII), and theabrownins (TBs) were components isolated from a tea sample using solvent extraction. $^{a-k}$ Different letters above the column indicate significant differences ($p < 0.05$).

3.1.2. DPPH Free Radical Scavenging Activity

DPPH free radical is a neutral free radical with a single electron. When antioxidants are present, the DPPH free radical is eliminated. The scavenging mechanism of DPPH free radicals is mainly hydrogen atom transfer [19].

Similar to the results in the $ABTS^{+\cdot}$ free radical scavenging assay, every sample likewise scavenged the DPPH free radical in a dose-dependent manner (Figure S1B—Supplementary Materials). As shown in Figure 3B, the DPPH free radical scavenging activity of each sample was significantly stronger than Trolox (289 ± 11 µg/mL) except for TF (249 ± 40 µg/mL), TFs (295 ± 24 µg/mL), TRs SII (556 ± 41 µg/mL), and TBs (1505 ± 88 µg/mL). The DPPH free radical scavenging activities of catechins were stronger than those of dimers, followed by polymers. While that of TFs were significantly stronger than TRs SII, followed by TBs. These results signaled the capacity of CTOPs to clear away DPPH free radicals that were negatively related to the degree of oxidative polymerization.

3.1.3. Total Antioxidant Capacity

In the total antioxidant capacity assay with the FRAP method, ferric lessening ability was used to represent the total antioxidant capacity. Every sample reduced Fe^{3+}-TPTZ in a dose-dependent manner (Figure S1C—Supplementary Materials). At the same concentration, the total antioxidant capacity of different samples was compared (Figure 3C).

At the concentration of 1 mg/mL, the total antioxidant capacity of ECG (8.41 ± 0.17 mM $FeSO_4$ equivalents) was significantly stronger than Trolox (7.48 ± 0.03 mM $FeSO_4$ equivalents). No significant difference was discovered among GCG (7.59 ± 0.03 mM $FeSO_4$ equivalents), EGCG (7.61 ± 0.1 mM $FeSO_4$ equivalents), CG (7.61 ± 0.21 mM $FeSO_4$ equivalents), C (7.62 ± 0.1 mM $FeSO_4$ equivalents), and Trolox, while the total antioxidant capacities of other samples were significantly weaker than Trolox. Compared with the above two antioxidant indexes, the total antioxidant capacities of CTOPs were relatively lower (number of samples that obtained a stronger antioxidant activity than Trolox). The total antioxidant capacities of catechins were significantly stronger than those of dimers, followed by polymers. The total antioxidant capacities of TFs (3.37 ± 0.07 mM $FeSO_4$ equivalents) were also significantly stronger than TRs SII (2.6 ± 0.09 mM $FeSO_4$ equivalents), followed by TBs (0.72 ± 0.02 mM $FeSO_4$ equivalents). These results implied the higher the degree of oxidative polymerization, the weaker the total antioxidant capacity of the samples. At a concentration of 0.5 mg/mL and 0.25 mg/mL (Figure S2—Supplymentary Materials), the total antioxidant capacities of dimers and polymers were also significantly weaker than Trolox, while most of the catechins did not obtain values significantly lower than Trolox. The total antioxidant capacities of catechins were significantly stronger than dimers, followed by polymers. The total antioxidant capacities of TFs were significantly stronger than TRs SII, followed by TBs. All these results were consistent with that at 1 mg/mL.

In conclusion, compared with Trolox, a commonly used positive control in the antioxidant assay, CTOPs showed stronger $ABTS^{+\cdot}$ free radical scavenging activities except for TBs as well as DPPH free radical scavenging activities except for TF, TFs, TRs SII, and TBs at mass concentration. The total antioxidant capacities of dimers and polymers were significantly weaker than Trolox, but most of the catechins were did not obtain values significantly lower than Trolox. Therefore, CTOPs possessed outstanding antioxidant activities to some extent. Studies have demonstrated that polyphenols are the main constituents of antioxidant activities in tea. The higher content of polyphenolic compounds existing in green teas made green tea extract show a more effective antioxidant activity [20]. Catechins have outstanding antioxidant activities [5] and the contents of catechins positively correlates with antioxidant activities [21]. Additionally, Chen et al. [8] found that catechin-oxidized polymers also have strong free radical scavenging activities, which was not much different from substrate–catechins.

The results of different antioxidant methods were contradictory, mainly involving the comparison of different catechins or TFs. For example, the $ABTS^{+\cdot}$ free radical scavenging activity of TFDG was significantly weaker than TF-3′-G, while the total antioxidant capacity of TFDG was significantly stronger than TF-3′-G. There was no significant difference in the DPPH· free radical scavenging activity between TFDG and TF-3′-G. ABTS$^{+·}$ is a free radical with a positive charge. The ABTS$^{+·}$ free radical scavenging assay detects the power of the ABTS$^{+·}$ to abstract an electron or a hydrogen atom from the compound [5]. DPPH is a neutral free radical that could take in an electron of hydrogen radical to turn into a diamagnetic molecule [19]. Total antioxidant capacity assay with the FRAP method reflects the ferric-reducing ability of the sample, which mainly reflects the ability of electron transfer, one of the mechanisms of free radical scavenging. Therefore, the differences in the above results are derived from the diverse principles of these antioxidant methods. DPPH and ABTS$^{+·}$ free radicals are chemical free radicals that are not naturally present in food or the human body and are far from the biological environment. Therefore, in addition to testing the ABTS$^{+·}$ free radical scavenging ability, DPPH free radical scavenging ability, and iron chelating ability of active ingredients, in future studies, we will also detect the antioxidant enzyme activity, ROS content, and oxidation product content in the body to verify the main conclusions obtained in this experiment.

Notably, although some small diversities in the results of three antioxidant methods were presented, a general trend in antioxidant activities could be concluded, i.e., when comparing the antioxidant activities of CTOPs at mass concentrations, the higher the degree of oxidative polymerization, the weaker the ABTS$^{+·}$ free radical scavenging activity, DPPH free radical scavenging activity, and total antioxidant capacity of the samples. This was consistent with the results of Wang et al. [11] detected with the FRAP method. This study compared the antioxidant activity of catechins, dimers, and polymers at mass concentrations, which could help explain the antioxidant activities among different teas, such as green tea and black tea. The comparison among tea extracts (a mixture of many components) are usually carried out at the mass concentrations. Carloni et al. [5] tested the antioxidant activities of green, white, and black teas made of the same tea cultivar, and they found that the antioxidant activity of green tea was significantly stronger than black tea in the ABTS, ORAC, and LDL assays. As is widely known, green tea has more catechins than black tea because fermentation lessens catechin levels in the latter tea as catechins are converted to TFs and TRs. Therefore, the conclusion of Carloni et al. [5] was further demonstrated from the compound aspect in our results. Another study marked that at the same mass concentration, TFs isolated from black tea exhibited more antioxidant activities compared to TRs [22], which was also consistent with our results. Based on the above results and discussion, the decline of the antioxidant activity during black tea fermentation was at least partly due to the antioxidant activity of polymers being weaker than dimers, while that of dimers was weaker than catechins at mass concentrations (Figure S4).

In addition, the antioxidant activity seemed not to be simply influenced by the molarity of the sample. The molecular weight of EGCG is 458 g/mol, which is larger than EC (290 g/mol). At the same mass concentration, the molarity of EGCG is less than EC, but the antioxidant activity of EGCG was stronger than EC in every assay. Therefore, the higher antioxidant activity of EGCG could be caused by other reasons, such as the number and position of active groups. The same phenomenon was found in dimers. The antioxidant activity of TSA (914 g/mol), a compound with the highest molecular weight within the tested dimers, was significantly stronger than TF (565 g/mol) except for the total antioxidant capacity at 0.5 mg/mL. The influence of structure on the antioxidation activity of catechins and dimers will be studied in the following experiments.

3.2. Structure–Activity Relationship of Catechins in Antioxidant Activity

Catechins with a 2-phenyl benzo-pyran structure, belonging to flavanols, consist of three basic rings: A, B, and C [14]. The structural diversities of the 8 common catechins mainly exist in the B ring and C ring as shown in Figure 1. A pairwise comparison of catechins facilitated the discovery of the effects of structure on antioxidant activity.

3.2.1. Screening of Antioxidant Active Group

The antioxidant activities between C and GCG or EC and EGCG were compared (Figure 4A); this was the comparison between catechins comprising a B-ring catechol but no 3-galloy and catechins simultaneously having a B-ring pyrogallol and 3-galloyl (Table S1). Results of the three antioxidant methods showed that the activity of GCG was significantly stronger than C, while that of EGCG was significantly stronger than EC, which proved that pyrogallol in the B-ring and 3-galloyl were possible antioxidant active groups of catechins.

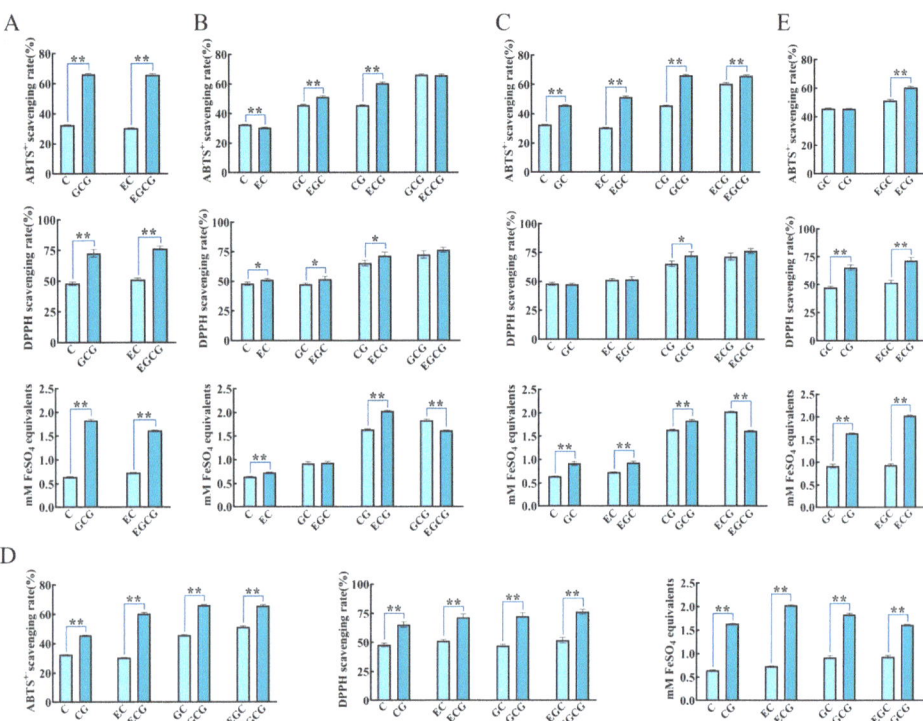

Figure 4. Structure–activity relationship of catechins with regard to antioxidant activities. (**A**) Screening of antioxidant active group. Effect of geometrical isomerism (**B**), B ring structure (**C**), and 3-galloyl groups (**D**) on antioxidant activities of catechins. (**E**) The dominant active group of catechins in antioxidant activity. ** $p < 0.01$. * $p < 0.05$.

3.2.2. Influence of Geometrical Isomerism on Catechins' Antioxidant Activity

Cis-catechins were compared with their corresponding trans-catechins to probe into the influence of geometrical isomerism on the activity of catechins (Figure 4B). In terms of the scavenging ABTS$^{+\cdot}$ free radical, C, EGC, and ECG were significantly stronger than EC, GC, and CG, respectively. There was no significant difference between GCG and EGCG. With regard to the scavenging DPPH free radicals, EC, EGC, and ECG were significantly stronger than C, GC, and CG, respectively. No significant differences was discovered between GCG and EGCG. The total antioxidant capacity of EC, ECG, and GCG was significantly stronger than C, CG, and EGCG, respectively. Moreover, GC and EGC had no significant differences between each other. To sum up, the comparison of antioxidant activities between cis-catechin and its corresponding trans-catechin had no accordant rule in different indexes. Therefore, geometrical isomerism was regarded as not an independent and critical factor affecting the antioxidant activities of catechins. Our results were confirmed by a previous report to a certain extent. Xu et al. [23] compared the antioxidant activity of tea epicatechins with their epimers through LDL oxidation, DPPH free radical assays, and a FRAP assay. They found that the majority of the noted diversities between epi-catechins and their corresponding epimers were tiny, even though they were occasionally statistically significant. Nevertheless, some studies offered different conclusions. Cis-catechins were more efficient in clearing away free radicals at high concentrations, while trans-catechins displayed stronger scavenging activities for macromolecular free radicals than cis-catechins at low concentrations [24–26]. Whether the above variant results are caused by discrepant sample concentrations and antioxidant models needs to be further verified.

3.2.3. Influence of B Ring Structure on Catechins' Antioxidant Activity

The phenolic hydroxyl group has a strong hydrogen-donating property, which can capture free radicals in the reaction system to achieve an antioxidant effect [27]. Both catechol and pyrogallol were disclosed as crucial substructures in heightening the antioxidant capacities of phenolic compounds [8]. Catechol and pyrogallol, which were stronger antioxidant substructures, will be studied in this experiment (Figure 4C).

In three indicators, the activity of GCG was significantly stronger than CG. The ABTS$^{+\cdot}$ free radical scavenging activity and total antioxidant capacity of GC and EGC were significantly stronger than C and EC, respectively. The ABTS$^{+\cdot}$ free radical scavenging activity of EGCG was significantly stronger than ECG, but the total antioxidant capacity of ECG was significantly stronger than EGCG. There were no significant differences between GC and C or EGC and EC or EGCG and ECG on the DPPH free radical scavenging activity. The above results hinted that pyrogallol was the stronger antioxidant substructure in the B-ring of catechins compared with catechol (except for the total antioxidant capacity of ECG and EGCG). This corresponded with the report of No et al. [28], which clearly showed that the pyrogallol in the catechin B-ring is the key structure for cleaning free radicals.

3.2.4. Influence of 3-Galloyl Group on Catechins' Antioxidant Activity

Catechins with a 3-galloyl group were compared with catechins without this group to confirm the antioxidant effect of 3-galloyl in catechins (Figure 4D).

In three indicators, the antioxidant activities of CG, ECG, GCG, and EGCG were significantly stronger than C, EC, GC, and EGC, respectively. These clear and coincident results adequately displayed that the 3-galloyl group heightened the antioxidant activity of catechins. This was consistent with a previous report, which indicated that the 3-galloyl group of ECG and GCG is the most vital structure for scavenging free radicals [28].

Based on the results of Sections 3.2.2–3.2.4, compared with other catechins, EGCG and GCG containing B-ring pyrogallol and 3-galloyl at the same time possessed stronger antioxidant activities at molarity, which corresponds in with the results in the literature [13,29].

3.2.5. The Dominant Active Group of Catechins in Antioxidant Activity

As exposed in Sections 3.2.3 and 3.2.4, B-ring pyrogallol and 3-galloyl were key antioxidant groups in catechins. An interesting question was whether B-ring pyrogallol or 3-galloyl had stronger antioxidant activities. To answer this question, ECG was compared with EGC, and CG was compared with GC (Figure 4E).

Results of the three antioxidant methods displayed that ECG had a significantly stronger activity than EGC. Additionally, the DPPH free radical scavenging activity and total antioxidant capacity of CG were significantly stronger than GC. No significant differences in ABTS$^{+\cdot}$ free radical scavenging activities were presented between CG and GC. The conclusion based on the above results was that 3-galloyl was a stronger antioxidant group in catechins than B-ring pyrogallol. Almajano et al. [29] reported that in the ABTS$^{+\cdot}$ radical scavenging assay, ORAC assay, and FRAP assay, the antioxidant activity of catechins was in the following order: ECG ≈ EGCG > EGC > EC (0.5 mM). The stronger antioxidant activity of ECG compared with EGC was consistent with our results.

3.3. Structure–Activity Relationship of Dimers in Antioxidant Activity

The structure–activity relationship obtained from catechin results was further verified by studying the influence of chemical structure on the activity of dimers. As dimers of catechins, TFs have a benzotropolone skeleton structure, while TSs possess a double flavanol skeleton structure. TFs and TSs contain different amounts of phenolic hydroxyl groups. In TFs, in addition to the original two phenolic hydroxyl groups on the A ring of each substrate–catechin, the structure formed by the B rings of two substrate–catechins through the benzoquinone pathway contains three hydroxyl groups. In TSs, in addition to the original two phenolic hydroxyl groups on the A ring of each substrate–catechin, the structure formed by the B rings of two substrate–catechins through the disproportionation pathway contains six phenolic hydroxyl groups [30]. The chemical structures of TFs and TSA are shown in Figure 2.

3.3.1. Influence of Number and Position of Galloyl Group on Antioxidant Activities of TFs

The influence of the number and position of the galloyl group on the antioxidant activities of TFs was studied (Figure 5A). In terms of scavenging $ABTS^{+\cdot}$ and DPPH free radicals, TFDG showed a significantly stronger activity than TF-3′-G and TF-3-G, followed by TF. In terms of the ferric-reducing ability, TFDG had a significantly stronger activity than TF-3′-G and TF, while there were no significant differences between TFDG and TF-3-G or TF-3′-G and TF-3-G or TF-3′-G and TF. These results agreed with the results of the catechins in Section 3.2.4: the galloyl group was the vital antioxidant group and its number was positively correlated to this activity. Similar results have been reported in relation to the antioxidant activities of TFs (TF, TF-3-G, TF-3′-G, TFDG) strengthening when increasing the amount of gallate groups [19,31,32].

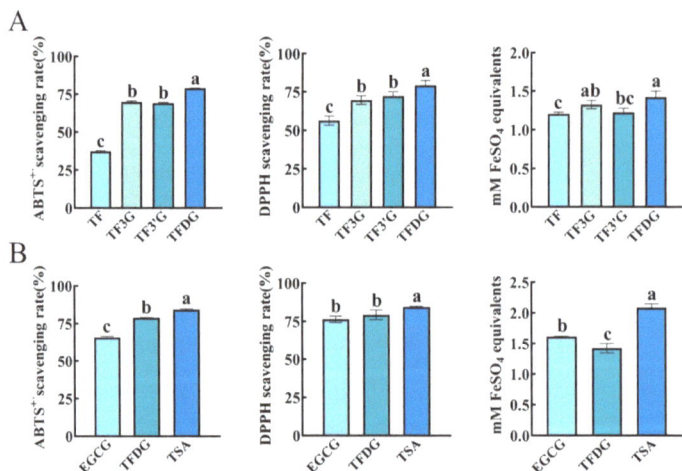

Figure 5. Structure–activity relationship of TFs and TSA with regard to antioxidant activities. (**A**) Antioxidant activities of TFs being influenced by the number but not the position of galloyl group; (**B**) antioxidant activity of TSA. ^{a,b,c} Different letters above the column indicate significant differences ($p < 0.05$).

Leung et al. [31] reported that there is no difference in the inhibitory activity of Cu^{2+}-mediated LDL oxidation between TF-3-G and TF-3′-G. Also, the position of the galloyl group did not affect the $ABTS^{+\cdot}$ free radical scavenging activity, DPPH free radical scavenging activity, and total antioxidant capacity in our results. Wu et al. [32] found that a superoxide radical, singlet oxygen ($^1O_2$), and H_2O_2 scavenging activity of TF-3′-G was stronger than that of TF-3-G, suggesting that the 3′-position gallate group in TFs may play a vital role in heightening their antioxidant activities. The reason for these differences in the above reports is unclear at present. One thing is for sure, TFDG, which simultaneously possesses 3- and 3′-galloyl groups, exhibited the strongest antioxidant activity in TFs.

3.3.2. Antioxidant Activity of TSA Compared with EGCG and TFDG

TSA is the star compound of catechin dimers and has received widespread attention from researchers since its discovery.

When compared at molarity, EGCG and TFDG were the representatives with the strongest antioxidant activity in catechins and TFs, respectively. It was shown that in three antioxidant methods, the activity of TSA was significantly stronger than TFDG and EGCG (Figure 5B). When considering the theory of structure, TSA possesses two galloyl groups and two pyrogallol groups (EGCG has one galloyl group and one pyrogallol group, while TFDG has two galloyl groups and no pyrogallol group), and the number of phenolic hydroxyl groups (16/molecule) is bigger than that of EGCG (8/molecule) and TFDG (13/molecule), which may result in a more prominent activity of TSA than EGCG and TFDG. Yoshino et al. [33] confirmed that TSs could chelate Fe^{2+} much stronger than EGCG, while O_2^--scavenging activities of TSs were also better or nearly similar to that of EGCG. The results of the lipid peroxidation evaluation system showed that TSs had an excellent ability to inhibit lipid peroxidation compared with other polyphenols, and the effect was not much different from that of EGCG [34]. It is worth noting that the antioxidant activity of TSA was firstly compared with eight catechins and four TFs in this study, and TSA had the strongest antioxidant activity in all compounds (Figure S3—Supplementary Materials).

3.4. Influence of Oxidative Dimerization on the Antioxidant Activity of the Substrate Mixture

Firstly, the antioxidant activity between the product and related substrate monomer was compared (Figure 6). The $ABTS^{+\cdot}$ free radical scavenging activity of TF between EC and EGC was significantly different. There was no significant difference among TF, EC, and EGC in the DPPH free radical scavenging activity. The total antioxidant capacity of TF was significantly stronger than EC and EGC. The $ABTS^{+\cdot}$ free radical scavenging activity of TF-3-G was significantly stronger than EC and EGCG. The DPPH free radical scavenging activity of TF-3-G was significantly stronger than EC and was not significant difference in relation to EGCG. The total antioxidant capacity of TF-3-G between EC and EGCG was significantly different. The $ABTS^{+\cdot}$ and DPPH free radical scavenging activity of TF-3′-G was significantly stronger than EGC and ECG. The total antioxidant capacity of TF-3′-G between EGC and ECG was significantly different. The $ABTS^{+\cdot}$ and DPPH free radical scavenging activity of TFDG was significantly stronger than ECG and EGCG. However, the total antioxidant capacity of TFDG was significantly weaker than ECG and EGCG. The antioxidant activities of TSA in the three methods were significantly stronger than EGCG. The comparison of the antioxidant activity between product and substrate monomers varied in different indexes, but, mostly, the activity of dimers was not less than that of catechins. Jovanovic et al. [35] found that TF scavenged superoxide radicals at a higher rate than EGCG. Leung et al. [31] used Cu^{2+}-mediated oxidation of human LDL as a model and confirmed that TFs have at least the same antioxidant capacities as catechins. Electroanalytical data revealed that TF had a stronger antioxidant potential and was a better copper chelator than EGCG after an interaction with copper [36]. There are also studies showing that EGCG has a stronger antioxidant capacity than TFs [37,38]. Hydrogen peroxide, hydroxyl radicals, peroxide anions, and superoxide anions are well-known reactive oxygen species (ROS). Lin et al. [37] reported that the superoxide scavenging abilities of theaflavins and EGCG are as follows: EGCG > TF-3-G > TF > TF-3,3′-G. However, in the present study, the restraint ability of xanthine oxidase activity was as follows: TF-3,3′-G > TF-3-G > EGCG > TF. Moreover, the order of H_2O_2 scavenging ability was TF-3-G > TF-3,3′-G > TF > EGCG, i.e., the antioxidant activity of dimers was not less than that of their individual substrate–catechin mixture. Leung et al. [31] also reported that in protecting human LDL from oxidation on the molar basis they gained the following ability: TF = EC

> EGC, TF-3-G = EGCG > EC, ECG > TF-3′-G > EGC, TFDG > ECG, and TFDG > EGCG. Therefore, although the antioxidant activity of dimers was not more than any catechin, a stronger activity was found in dimers compared with their individual substrate–catechin mixture in the vast majority of experiments, which was consistent with our conclusion.

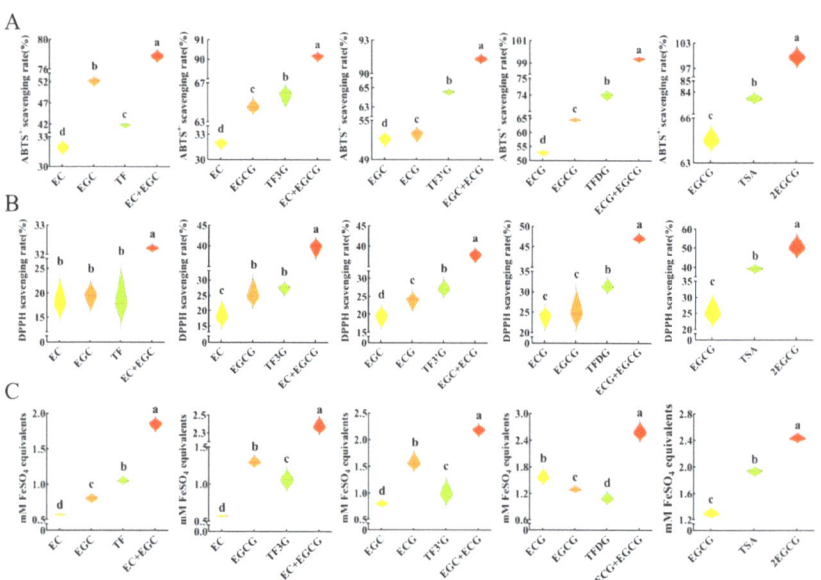

Figure 6. Effects of the oxidative dimerization reaction on the antioxidant activity of substrate–catechin mixture. The molarities of each compound used in ABTS$^{+\cdot}$ free radical scavenging assay (**A**), DPPH free radical scavenging assay (**B**), and total antioxidant capacity assay (**C**) were 100, 100, and 250 µM, respectively. [a,b,c,d] Different letters above the violin indicate significant differences ($p < 0.05$).

The antioxidant activity between the product and substrate mixture was then compared (Figure 6). It is interesting to note that the substrate mixture had a significantly stronger antioxidant activity than the product in all results. For example, the antioxidant activities of ECG + EGCG were significantly stronger than those of TFDG in three methods. Under the premise that the activity of dimer was not weaker than that of the related substrate monomer (in most cases), this result disclosed that the oxidative dimerization reaction hindered the antioxidant activity of the substrate–catechin mixture, which was another reason why the antioxidant activity during black tea fermentation declined (Figure S4).

Due to the presence of multiple hydroxyl groups in the structure of the galloyl group and pyrogallol, the number of galloyl groups, pyrogallols, and hydroxyl groups could be used to explain the differences between the activity of dimers and their substrates as well as the effects of the oxidative dimerization reaction on the antioxidant activity of catechins. TSA has twice as many galloyl groups, pyrogallols, and hydroxyl groups as its substrate EGCG; thus, TSA was significantly more active than EGCG at the same molarity. However, the activity of the one-molecule TSA was significantly weaker than that of the two-molecule EGCG. Hence, the antioxidant activity of the compound was not only affected by the number of its antioxidant active groups but could also be affected by the size of its molecular structure and the spatial location of its active groups. In addition, by analyzing the structure of TFs and their substrates, it was discovered that the number of galloyl groups in TFs is the sum of the two substrates, pyrogallol does not exist in TFs but lies in pyrogallol-type catechins which are the substrate of TFs, and the number of hydroxyl groups in TFs is greater than that of the substrate monomers but less than the sum of the two substrates. In short, the oxidative dimerization reaction weakens the antioxidant activity of the substrate–catechin mixture by reducing the number of active groups of the substrate and increasing the molecular structure size of the product.

4. Conclusions

The effects of structures on the antioxidant activities of catechins and dimers was revealed, and the antioxidant active groups were screened in this study. Antioxidant activities of catechins were dominated by B-ring pyrogallol and 3-galloyl, but were not decided by geometrical isomerism. 3-galloyl was a stronger antioxidant group than B-ring pyrogallol in catechins. The number, not the position, of the galloyl group was positively correlated with the antioxidant activities of TFs. TSA has more antioxidant active groups (galloyl groups, pyrogallol groups, and phenolic hydroxyl groups) than EGCG and TFDG; thus, TSA had a stronger antioxidant activity. Additionally, this study found that the higher the degree of oxidation polymerization, the weaker the $ABTS^{+\cdot}$ free radical scavenging activity, DPPH free radical scavenging activity, and total antioxidant capacity of the samples. Under the premise that the antioxidant activities of dimers were greater than or equal to that of their substrate–catechin monomers (most of the time), the oxidative dimerization process significantly impaired the antioxidant activities of the substrate–catechin mixture (Table 1). Therefore, the degree of oxidative polymerization and oxidative dimerization reaction are not conducive to the antioxidant activity, which could reveal the mechanism of the descending antioxidant activity during the fermentation of black tea (Figure S4). Furthermore, the oxidative dimerization reaction weakened the antioxidant activity of the substrate–catechin mixture by reducing the number of active groups of the substrate and increasing the molecular structure size of the product. To sum up, the antioxidant active groups of catechins and dimers were screened and the effects of the degree of oxidative polymerization and oxidative dimerization reaction on their antioxidant activities was analyzed in this study, which could enrich the knowledge of the antioxidant activities of catechins and polymers.

Table 1. Effects of structure and oxidative polymerization on antioxidant activities of catechins, dimers, and polymers.

	Indexes	Antioxidant Activity (DPPH, $ABTS^{+\cdot}$ and Total Antioxidant Capacity Assay in Non-Cellular System)
Structure–activity relationship of catechins	Geometrical isomerism Catechol or pyrogallol in B-ring 3-galloyl group Dominant active group	Not an independent interfering factor Pyrogallol stronger than catechol 3-Galloyl group stronger than the no-galloyl group 3-Galloyl group
Structure–activity relationship of dimers	Number of galloyl groups in TFs Position of galloyl groups in TFs Structure of TSA	Positively correlated with activities No influence Possessing strong activity at molarity due to having rich active groups
Oxidative polymerization	Dimers vs. substrate monomer Dimers vs. substrate mixture Degree of oxidation polymerization (mass concentration)	Dimers greater than or equal to the substrate monomer (in most cases) Dimers weaker than the substrate mixture ($p < 0.05$) Not positively correlated with the activity

Supplementary Materials: The following supporting information can be downloaded at: https://www.mdpi.com/article/10.3390/foods12234207/s1, Table S1: Catechins and TFs used in structure–activity relationship assay. Figure S1: Dose–effect relationship of antioxidant activities of catechins and their oxidized polymers (CTOPs); Figure S2: Total antioxidant capacity assay with FRAP method at 0.5 mg/mL and 0.25 mg/mL; Figure S3: Comparison of antioxidant activities of catechins and their dimers at molarity; Figure S4: Declining mechanism of antioxidant activity during black tea fermentation.

Author Contributions: W.W.: conceptualization, validation, formal analysis, investigation, writing—original draft, and visualization; T.L.: investigation, methodology, validation, data curation, formal analysis, writing—original draft, and visualization; W.-W.W.: validation, formal analysis, and resources; J.-F.Y.: resources; H.-Y.J.: conceptualization, supervision, funding acquisition, and writing—review and editing. All authors have read and agreed to the published version of the manuscript.

Funding: This research was funded by the National Natural Science Foundation of China (32372766), the Key Research and Development Program of Zhejiang Province (projects no. 2022C02033-3 and no. 2023C02040) and the Science and Technology Innovation Project of Chinese Academy of Agricultural Sciences (CAAS-ASTIP-2023-TRICAAS).

Data Availability Statement: The data are contained within this article and the Supplementary Materials.

Acknowledgments: We would like to thank Chenyang Shao for providing assistance in writing this paper.

Conflicts of Interest: The authors declare no conflict of interest.

References

1. Dröge, W. Free Radicals in the Physiological Control of Cell Function. *Physiol. Rev.* **2002**, *82*, 47–95. [CrossRef]
2. Kaufmann, J.A.; Bickford, P.C.; Taglialatela, G. Free radical-dependent changes in constitutive Nuclear factor kappa B in the aged hippocampus. *NeuroReport* **2002**, *13*, 1917–1920. [CrossRef]
3. Williams, G.M.; Iatropoulos, M.J.; Whysner, J. Safety assessment of butylated hydroxyanisole and butylated hydroxytoluene as antioxidant food additives. *Food Chem. Toxicol.* **1999**, *37*, 1027–1038. [CrossRef]
4. Zhang, H.; Qi, R.; Mine, Y. The impact of oolong and black tea polyphenols on human health. *Food Biosci.* **2019**, *29*, 55–61. [CrossRef]
5. Carloni, P.; Tiano, L.; Padella, L.; Bacchetti, T.; Customu, C.; Kay, A.; Damiani, E. Antioxidant activity of white, green and black tea obtained from the same tea cultivar. *Food Res. Int.* **2013**, *53*, 900–908. [CrossRef]
6. Xu, Y.-Q.; Zou, C.; Gao, Y.; Chen, J.-X.; Wang, F.; Chen, G.-S.; Yin, J.-F. Effect of the type of brewing water on the chemical composition, sensory quality and antioxidant capacity of Chinese teas. *Food Chem.* **2017**, *236*, 142–151. [CrossRef]
7. Koch, W.; Kukula-Koch, W.; Komsta, Ł. Black Tea Samples Origin Discrimination Using Analytical Investigations of Secondary Metabolites, Antiradical Scavenging Activity and Chemometric Approach. *Molecules* **2018**, *23*, 2093. [CrossRef]
8. Chen, N.; Han, B.; Fan, X.; Cai, F.; Ren, F.; Xu, M.; Zhong, J.; Zhang, Y.; Ren, D.; Yi, L. Uncovering the antioxidant characteristics of black tea by coupling in vitro free radical scavenging assay with UHPLC–HRMS analysis. *J. Chromatogr. B* **2020**, *1145*, 122092. [CrossRef]
9. Qu, F.; Zeng, W.; Tong, X.; Feng, W.; Chen, Y.; Ni, D. The new insight into the influence of fermentation temperature on quality and bioactivities of black tea. *LWT* **2020**, *117*, 108646. [CrossRef]
10. Liu, S.; Huang, H. Assessments of antioxidant effect of black tea extract and its rationals by erythrocyte haemolysis assay, plasma oxidation assay and cellular antioxidant activity (CAA) assay. *J. Funct. Foods* **2015**, *18*, 1095–1105. [CrossRef]
11. Wang, W.; Le, T.; Wang, W.; Yu, L.; Yang, L.; Jiang, H. Effects of key components on the antioxidant activity of black tea. *Foods* **2023**, *12*, 3134. [CrossRef]
12. Xu, Y.-Q.; Gao, Y.; Granato, D. Effects of epigallocatechin gallate, epigallocatechin and epicatechin gallate on the chemical and cell-based antioxidant activity, sensory properties, and cytotoxicity of a catechin-free model beverage. *Food Chem.* **2021**, *339*, 128060. [CrossRef]
13. He, J.; Xu, L.; Yang, L.; Wang, X. Epigallocatechin Gallate Is the Most Effective Catechin Against Antioxidant Stress via Hydrogen Peroxide and Radical Scavenging Activity. *Med. Sci. Monit.* **2018**, *24*, 8198–8206. [CrossRef]
14. Fu, J.; Jiang, H.; Zhang, J.; Shi, L.; Wang, W. Recent progress in synthesis of oxidized dimeric catechin catalyzed by exogenous polyphenol oxidase. *Food Sci.* **2019**, *40*, 274–280. [CrossRef]
15. Lun Su, Y.; Leung, L.K.; Huang, Y.; Chen, Z.-Y. Stability of tea theaflavins and catechins. *Food Chem.* **2003**, *83*, 189–195. [CrossRef]
16. Sui, X.; Dong, X.; Zhou, W. Combined effect of pH and high temperature on the stability and antioxidant capacity of two anthocyanins in aqueous solution. *Food Chem.* **2014**, *163*, 163–170. [CrossRef]
17. Wang, W.; Chen, L.; Wang, W.; Zhang, J.; Engelhardt, U.H.; Jiang, H. Effect of active groups and oxidative dimerization on the antimelanogenic activity of catechins and their dimeric oxidation products. *J. Agric. Food Chem.* **2022**, *70*, 1304–1315. [CrossRef]
18. Re, R.; Pellegrini, N.; Proteggente, A.; Pannala, A.; Yang, M.; Rice-Evans, C. Antioxidant activity applying an improved ABTS radical cation decolorization assay. *Free Radic. Biol. Med.* **1999**, *26*, 1231–1237. [CrossRef]
19. Yang, Z.; Jie, G.; Dong, F.; Xu, Y.; Watanabe, N.; Tu, Y. Radical-scavenging abilities and antioxidant properties of theaflavins and their gallate esters in H2O2-mediated oxidative damage system in the HPF-1 cells. *Toxicology in Vitro* **2008**, *22*, 1250–1256. [CrossRef]
20. Shah, S.; Gani, A.; Ahmad, M.; Shah, A.; Gani, A.; Masoodi, F.A. In Vitro antioxidant and antiproliferative activity of microwave-extracted green tea and black tea (*Camellia sinensis*): A comparative study. *Nutrafoods* **2015**, *14*, 207–215. [CrossRef]
21. Gramza-Michalowska, A.; Korczak, J. Polyphenols-Potential Food Improvement Factor. *Am. J. Food Technol.* **2007**, *2*, 662–670. [CrossRef]
22. Imran, A.; Arshad, M.U.; Arshad, M.S.; Imran, M.; Saeed, F.; Sohaib, M. Lipid peroxidation diminishing perspective of isolated theaflavins and thearubigins from black tea in arginine induced renal malfunctional rats. *Lipids Health Dis.* **2018**, *17*, 157. [CrossRef]

23. Xu, J.-Z.; Yeung, S.Y.V.; Chang, Q.; Huang, Y.; Chen, Z.-Y. Comparison of antioxidant activity and bioavailability of tea epicatechins with their epimers. *Br. J. Nutr.* **2004**, *91*, 873–881. [CrossRef]
24. Guo, Q.; Zhao, B.; Shen, S.; Hou, J.; Hu, J.; Xin, W. ESR study on the structure–antioxidant activity relationship of tea catechins and their epimers. *Biochim. Et Biophys. Acta (BBA) Gen. Subj.* **1999**, *1427*, 13–23. [CrossRef]
25. Kobayashi, M.; Unno, T.; Suzuki, Y.; Nozawa, A.; Sagesaka, Y.; Kakuda, T.; Ikeda, I. Heat-Epimerized Tea Catechins Have the Same Cholesterol-Lowering Activity as Green Tea Catechins in Cholesterol-Fed Rats. *Biosci. Biotechnol. Biochem.* **2005**, *69*, 2455–2458. [CrossRef]
26. Yang, X.Q. *Tea Polyphenol Chemistry*; Shanghai Science and Technology Press: Shanghai, China, 2003.
27. Wu, S.S. Development of Novel Catechin Esters and Evaluation of their Antioxidant Activity. Master's Thesis, Zhejiang University, Hangzhou, China, 2018.
28. No, J.K.; Soung, D.Y.; Kim, Y.J.; Shim, K.H.; Jun, Y.S.; Rhee, S.H.; Yokozawa, T.; Chung, H.Y. Inhibition of tyrosinase by green tea components. *Life Sci.* **1999**, *65*, PL241–PL246. [CrossRef]
29. Almajano, M.P.; Delgado, M.E.; Gordon, M.H. Albumin causes a synergistic increase in the antioxidant activity of green tea catechins in oil-in-water emulsions. *Food Chem.* **2007**, *102*, 1375–1382. [CrossRef]
30. Shi, L.T.; Jiang, H.Y.; Zhang, J.Y.; Wang, W.W.; Cui, H.C. Review on enzymatic synthesis mechanism and functional activity of theasinensins. *J. Food Saf. Qual.* **2018**, *9*, 223–228. (In Chinese) [CrossRef]
31. Leung, L.K.; Su, Y.; Zhang, Z.; Chen, Z.-Y.; Huang, Y.; Chen, R. Theaflavins in Black Tea and Catechins in Green Tea Are Equally Effective Antioxidants. *J. Nutr.* **2001**, *131*, 2248–2251. [CrossRef]
32. Wu, Y.-y.; Li, W.; Xu, Y.; Jin, E.-h.; Tu, Y.-y. Evaluation of the antioxidant effects of four main theaflavin derivatives through chemiluminescence and DNA damage analyses. *J. Zhejiang Univ. SCIENCE B* **2011**, *12*, 744–751. [CrossRef]
33. Yoshino, K.; Suzuki, M.; Sasaki, K.; Miyase, T.; Sano, M. Formation of antioxidants from (−)-epigallocatechin gallate in mild alkaline fluids, such as authentic intestinal juice and mouse plasma. *J. Nutr. Biochem.* **1999**, *10*, 223–229. [CrossRef]
34. Hashimoto, F.; Ono, M.; Masuoka, C.; Ito, Y.; Sakata, Y.; Shimizu, K.; Nonaka, G.-i.; Nishioka, I.; Nohara, T. Evaluation of the Anti-oxidative Effect (in vitro) of Tea Polyphenols. *Biosci. Biotechnol. Biochem.* **2003**, *67*, 396–401. [CrossRef]
35. Jovanovic, S.V.; Hara, Y.; Steenken, S.; Simic, M.G. Antioxidant Potential of Theaflavins. A Pulse Radiolysis Study. *J. Am. Chem. Soc.* **1997**, *119*, 5337–5343. [CrossRef]
36. Sharma, N.; Phan, H.T.; Chikae, M.; Takamura, Y.; Azo-Oussou, A.F.; Vestergaard, M.d.C. Black tea polyphenol theaflavin as promising antioxidant and potential copper chelator. *J. Sci. Food Agric.* **2020**, *100*, 3126–3135. [CrossRef]
37. Lin, J.-K.; Chen, P.-C.; Ho, C.-T.; Lin-Shiau, S.-Y. Inhibition of Xanthine Oxidase and Suppression of Intracellular Reactive Oxygen Species in HL-60 Cells by Theaflavin-3,3′-digallate, (−)-Epigallocatechin-3-gallate, and Propyl Gallate. *J. Agric. Food Chem.* **2000**, *48*, 2736–2743. [CrossRef]
38. Zhang, J.; Huang, J.A.; Cai, S.X.; Yi, X.Q.; Liu, J.J.; Wang, Y.Z.; Tian, L.L.; Liu, Z.H. Theaflavins and EGCG protect SH-SY5Y cells from oxidative damage induced by amyloid-β 1-42 and inhibit the level of Aβ42 in vivo and in vitro. *J. Tea Sci.* **2016**, *36*, 655–662. (In Chinese) [CrossRef]

Disclaimer/Publisher's Note: The statements, opinions and data contained in all publications are solely those of the individual author(s) and contributor(s) and not of MDPI and/or the editor(s). MDPI and/or the editor(s) disclaim responsibility for any injury to people or property resulting from any ideas, methods, instructions or products referred to in the content.

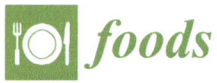

Article

Huangqin Tea Total Flavonoids–Gut Microbiota Interactions: Based on Metabolome and Microbiome Analysis

Yaping Zheng [1,2,†], Kailin Yang [1,2,†], Jie Shen [3], Xiangdong Chen [1,2], Chunnian He [1,2,*] and Peigen Xiao [1,2]

[1] Institute of Medicinal Plant Development, Chinese Academy of Medical Sciences, Peking Union Medical College, Beijing 100193, China; zyp0316@163.com (Y.Z.); yangkailin199908@163.com (K.Y.); xdchen@implad.ac.cn (X.C.); pgxiao@implad.ac.cn (P.X.)
[2] Key Laboratory of Bioactive Substances and Resources Utilisation of Chinese Herbal Medicine, Ministry of Education, Beijing 100193, China
[3] School of Medical Laboratory, Weifang Medical University, Weifang 261053, China; jieshen0817@163.com
* Correspondence: cnhe@implad.ac.cn; Tel./Fax: +86-10-57833165
[†] These authors contributed equally to this work.

Abstract: Huangqin tea (HQT), a Non-*Camellia* Tea derived from the aerial parts of *Scutellaria baicalensis*, is widely used in the north of China. The intervention effects of HQT on intestinal inflammation and tumors have been found recently, but the active ingredient and mechanism of action remain unclear. This study aimed to investigate the interactions between the potential flavonoid active components and gut microbiota through culture experiments in vitro combined with HPLC-UV, UPLC-QTOF-MS, and 16S rDNA sequencing technology. The results showed that the HQT total flavonoids were mainly composed of isocarthamidin-7-O-β-D-glucuronide, carthamidin-7-O-β-D-glucuronide, scutellarin, and others, which interact closely with gut microbiota. After 48 h, the primary flavonoid glycosides transformed into corresponding aglycones with varying degrees of deglycosylation. The composition of the intestinal microbiota was changed significantly. The beneficial bacteria, such as *Enterococcus* and *Parabacteroides*, were promoted, while the harmful bacteria, such as *Shigella*, were inhibited. The functional prediction results have indicated notable regulatory effects exerted by total flavonoids and scutellarin on various pathways, including purine metabolism and aminoacyl-tRNA biosynthesis, among others, to play a role in the intervention of inflammation and tumor-related diseases. These findings provided valuable insights for further in-depth research and investigation of the active ingredients, metabolic processes, and mechanisms of HQT.

Keywords: Huangqin tea; gut microbiota; metabolic transformation; the total flavonoids; interaction

Citation: Zheng, Y.; Yang, K.; Shen, J.; Chen, X.; He, C.; Xiao, P. Huangqin Tea Total Flavonoids–Gut Microbiota Interactions: Based on Metabolome and Microbiome Analysis. *Foods* **2023**, *12*, 4410. https://doi.org/10.3390/foods12244410

Academic Editor: Xiaonan Lu

Received: 7 November 2023
Revised: 27 November 2023
Accepted: 1 December 2023
Published: 7 December 2023

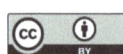

Copyright: © 2023 by the authors. Licensee MDPI, Basel, Switzerland. This article is an open access article distributed under the terms and conditions of the Creative Commons Attribution (CC BY) license (https://creativecommons.org/licenses/by/4.0/).

1. Introduction

The gut microbiota is a complex ecosystem consisting of various microflora that reside in the human gut, which plays a crucial role in digesting food, synthesizing essential vitamins, and regulating the function of the immune system [1]. The composition of the intestinal flora can be influenced by various factors, and diet is widely recognized as the most significant driver in shaping the gut microbiota. In the long term, dietary adjustments were the most effective and healthy approach to modulating and intervening in the intestinal flora [2]. Most Chinese herbal medicines are commonly administered orally, particularly those that can be consumed as tea. The interaction between drugs and the gut microbiota is of significant importance in the processes of digestion, absorption, and metabolism [3,4]. Recently, there has been attention given to the interaction between medicinal substances in traditional Chinese medicine (TCM) and the gut microbiota. However, the specific mechanism by which different types of TCM teas interact with intestinal microorganisms has yet to be revealed [5].

Huangqin tea (HQT) is primarily derived from the stem and leaves of *Scutellaria baicalensis*. As a common Non-*Camellia* Tea, it has been traditionally used in northern and southwest China and possesses distinct properties. The aboveground parts of *S. baicalensis* have heat-clearing, dampness-reducing, fire-reducing, and detoxifying effects. Research indicates that the aerial parts of *S. baicalensis* mainly contain flavonoids and volatile components [6]. Modern studies demonstrated it had various bioactive properties, such as anti-inflammatory, anti-tumor, analgesic, and antipyretic, as well as anti-resistant pathogenic microorganisms [7–11]. Previous studies have reported that baicalin, a compound found in *S. baicalensis*, can be metabolized to baicalein through the intestinal microflora to exert the chemical prevention of colorectal cancer in vivo [12]. Our group's previous study found that HQT had an obvious intervention effect in the colorectal precancerous lesions induced by azoxymethane (AMO) in rats. It can modulate the intestinal microflora structure in diseased rats and improve the host's metabolic disturbance. Therefore, it can be seen that the efficacy of HQT is closely related to the gut microbes, and the primary active constituents of HQT are likely to be flavonoids [13]. However, the specific interaction and underlying mechanism of HQT with intestinal microbes have yet to be fully elucidated. Further research is required to investigate and understand the intricate relationship between HQT and the intestinal microbiota. Clarifying this interaction and mechanism would provide valuable insights into the therapeutic effects of HQT and its potential applications in promoting gut health.

In this study, high-performance liquid chromatography (HPLC), ultra-performance liquid chromatography–quadrupole time-of-flight–mass spectrometry (UPLC-Q-TOF-MS), and 16S rDNA sequencing technology were used to investigate the pharmacodynamic ingredients of HQT and the interaction between normal mouse gut microbes and the total flavonoids. From the perspective of prevention, this study aims to elucidate the material basis of HQT and its significant potential value to prevent colorectal cancer and provide a scientific foundation for the development of functional food based on total flavonoids of HQT.

2. Materials and Methods

2.1. Plant Materials, Chemicals, and Reagents

The *S. baicalensis* stem and leaf were collected from the Institute of Medicinal Plants, Chinese Academy of Medical Sciences in September 2021. The voucher specimens were identified and verified by Professor Chunnian He from the Institute of Medicinal Plant Development (IMPLAD) and then deposited in Pharmacophylogeny Centre of IMPALD in Beijing, China. Scutellarin, apigetrin, baicalin, and isoscutellarein 8-O-β-D-glucuronide were purchased from National Institutes for Food and Drug Control. Isocarthamidin-7-O-β-D-glucuronide and carthamidin-7-O-β-D-glucuronide were isolated from *S. baicalensis* in our laboratory and achieved a purity >95% after UV, IR, and NMR detection [6]. For UPLC-Q-TOF-MS and HPLC-UV analysis, chromatographic-grade methanol, acetonitrile, and formic acid were purchased from Thermo Fisher Scientific (Waltham, MA, USA). All solutions were prepared with ultrapure water (Milli-Q, Millipore Company, Billerica, MA, USA). AB—8 macroporous resin was purchased from Shanghai Macklin Biochemical Co., Ltd. (Shanghai, China). GAM anaerobic culture medium, anaerobic culture bag, anaerobic gas production package, and anaerobic indicator were purchased from Qingdao Hi-tech Industrial Park Hope Bio-technology Co., Ltd. (Qingdao, China). A total of 10 male Kunming mice (8 weeks) were purchased from Sibeifu Biotechnology Co., Ltd. (Beijing, China). The experimental animals were provided free access to food and water at a constant temperature ($25 \pm 2\ °C$) and humidity ($55 \pm 10\%$) on a 12 h light/dark cycle for 3 weeks.

2.2. The HQT Total Flavonoids Preparation

The stems and leaves of *S. baicalensis* were cut into 1–2 cm and dried. Plant samples (1 kg) were soaked in 1200 mL of deionized water for 30 min, heated and refluxed for 60 min, and filtered. Then, they were extracted twice with 1000 mL and 800 mL of deionized water, combined with filtrate, vacuum-concentrated to $0.42\ g \cdot mL^{-1}$ (SP Genevac Rocket Synergy, Genevac, UK), and concentrated hydrochloric acid was added to adjust the pH to 2–3. The AB-8 macroporous resin was used to purify the solution after loading the liquid.

After adding, the liquid absorbed for 2 h. Sugars and other impurities were removed using deionized water (9 L), followed by elution with 70% ethanol (15 L). The eluent was collected, and the ethanol was recovered under reduced pressure. The samples were frozen in −20 °C refrigerator overnight for 24 h, then freeze-drying (Lyovapor L-300, BUCHI, Flawil, Switzerland) to obtain the HQT total flavonoids (125.0 g, yield 12.50%).

2.3. Determination Content of HQT Total Flavonoids

The major chemical components of HQT total flavonoids were analyzed using HPLC (Thermo U3000, Waltham, MA, USA) [6], as well as the content of six major flavonoids—isocarthamidin-7-O-β-D-glucuronide, carthamidin-7-O-β-D-glucuronide, scutellarin, apigetrin, baicalin, and isoscutellarein 8-O-β-D-glucuronide—in the HQT total flavonoids.

2.4. The Metabolic Transformation of Gut Microbiota In Vitro

The total flavonoids solution, 2.5 mg/mL, was prepared using sterile water. Scutellarin was prepared using DMSO and subsequently diluted to 0.25 mg/mL with sterile water. To ensure sterility, the GAM anaerobic culture medium and other experimental materials underwent sterilization in autoclave sterilizer (MLS 375, Panasonic, Osaka, Japan) at 121 °C and 0.120 MPa for 15 min. The fresh feces from healthy mice were collected and mixed with sterile saline at 1:4 (w/v) and centrifuged at 4000 r/min (TG 16 G, Tianjin, China) for 10 min (4 °C). After centrifugation, the supernatant was removed, mixed with culture medium (1:9, v/v), and incubated in an incubator (SPX-50B, Shanghai Lichen Technology Co., Ltd., Shanghai, China) for 48 h (37 °C) to obtain the blank incubation solution. Additionally, the blank culture solution was prepared using normal saline according to the same method described above. The HQT total flavonoids solution was mixed with the incubation solution (1:8, v/v), then further cultured as the total flavonoids conversion group (Group 1). Other groups were prepared in the same proportion. The scutellarin control group (Group 2) combined the scutellarin control solution with the gut microbiota incubation solution. The blank control group (Group 3) consisted of sterile water mixed with the intestinal incubation solution. The sterile total flavonoids control group (Group 4) was created by combining the total flavonoids solution with the blank medium. The blank sterile group (Group 5) was formed by mixing sterile water with the blank medium. Lastly, the drug group (Group 6) was prepared by combining the total flavonoids solution with sterile water. For each group, three samples were prepared in parallel. The groups were placed in anaerobic bags and incubated at 37 °C. Samples were collected at various time points: 0 h, 4 h, 24 h, 36 h, 48 h, and 72 h. For each time point, 750 µL gut microbiota samples were taken and mixed with an equal volume of ice methanol. The mixture was centrifuged at 13,000 r/min for 10 min (4 °C), and the resulting supernatant was collected for analysis using HPLC under the same chromatographic conditions described in Section 2.3. Additionally, groups 1, 2, and 3 were also analyzed using UPLC-Q-TOF-MS [14]. After sampling, the samples were separated and stored at −80 °C.

2.5. 16S rDNA Sequencing Technology

16S rRNA amplicon sequencing was performed for three parallel 0 h and 48 h samples of the total flavonoids conversion group (Group 1), the scutellarin control group (Group 2), and the blank control group (Group 3) under item "2.4". Total DNA was extracted from the samples, and the full length of 16S rDNA was amplified using specific primers. After purifying and quantifying the amplified products, the full-length sequences were selected for sequencing using the universal primer 27F(AG RGTTTGA TYNTGGCTCAG and 1492R (TASGGHTACCTTGTTASGACTT) [15]. The PCR amplification was performed using the New England Biolabs Phusion® High-Fidelity PCR Master Mix with GC Buffer and the efficient fidelity enzyme. After amplification, library construction was carried out. The library was then subjected to quality detection using Qubit, and the insert size was assessed using the Agilent 2100 system, followed by sequencing using the PacBio platform. After sequencing the data using the PacBio platform, the DADA2 method was employed for data processing. This involved removing, correcting, reducing noise, and eliminating chimeras to obtain the ASV (amplicon sequence variant) sequences and their corresponding abundance information. To ensure the accuracy and reliability of the information analysis results, the original data underwent assembly and filtering to obtain valid data.

2.6. Statistical Analysis

The data were presented as the mean ± standard deviation (SD). Statistical analysis was conducted using IBM SPSS 23 software (IBM Software, New York, NY, USA), and the graphs were generated using GraphPad Prism 9 software (GraphPad Software, San Diego, CA, USA). The statistical significance of the data was assessed using one-way ANOVA followed by Duncan's test. A value of $p < 0.05$ was considered statistically significant.

3. Results

3.1. The Content Determination of the Total Flavonoids Sites of HQT

The contents of six major flavonoids in the total flavonoids sites of HQT were determined by HPLC. Table 1 and Figure 1 showed the content determination results of isocarthamidin-7-O-β-D-glucuronide, carthamidin-7-O-β-D-glucuronide, scutellarin, apigetrin, baicalin, and isoscutellarein 8-O-β-D-glucuronide. As can be seen in Table 1, the content of total flavonoids in HQT exceeded 54.51%.

Table 1. The contents of six major flavonoids in the total flavonoid sites of HQT.

NO.	Compound	Content (mg/g)
1	Isocarthamidin-7-O-β-D-glucuronide	242.99 ± 9.16
2	Carthamidin-7-O-β-D-glucuronide	161.23 ± 15.75
3	Scutellarin	91.50 ± 3.30
4	Apigetrin	9.79 ± 1.57
5	Baicalin	7.48 ± 0.65
6	Isoscutellarein 8-O-β-D-glucuronide	32.08 ± 3.71

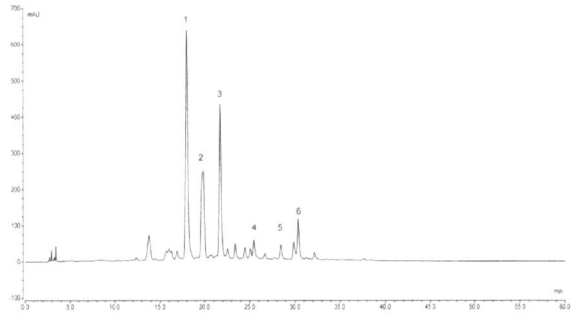

Figure 1. The HPLC chromatogram of of six major flavonoids in the total flavonoid sites of HQT. (1: isocarthamidin-7-O-β-D-glucuronide, 2: carthamidin-7-O-β-D-glucuronide, 3: scutellarin, 4: apigetrin, 5: baicalin, 6: isoscutellarein 8-O-β-D-glucuronide).

3.2. The Metabolic Transformation of the Mouse Gut Microbiota In Vitro

In this study, the anaerobic temperature incubation system of mouse gut microbiota was established successfully in vitro. The results presented in Table 2 demonstrate a decrease in the concentration of total flavonoids and scutellarin in the incubation solution after 72 h in the total flavonoids conversion group (Group 1) and the scutellarin control group (Group 2). However, the concentration of total flavonoids in the blank culture medium remained relatively stable during the same period. Additionally, it can be seen that the peaks of isocarthamidin-7-O-β-D-glucuronide, carthamidin-7-O-β-D-glucuronide, and scutellarin were significantly decreased with time in Figure 2a. This decrease was accompanied by the gradual emergence of peaks D, E, and F, which exhibited a substantial increase in content. Furthermore, Figure 2b shows that the content of scutellarin in Group 2 gradually decreased, and the new peak gradually increased.

Table 2. The transformation concentration of total flavonoids and scutellarin in the mouse intestinal microflora incubation solution for 72 h. (Group 1: the total flavonoids conversion group, Group 2: the scutellarin control group, and Group 4: the sterile total flavonoids control group).

Time (h)	Concentrations (µg/mL)		
	Group 1	Group 2	Group 4
0	140.67	14.07	140.67
4	124.08	11.81	139.22
24	91.60	4.71	139.57
36	67.54	1.61	139.88
48	51.69	0	139.95
72	23.47	0	139.51

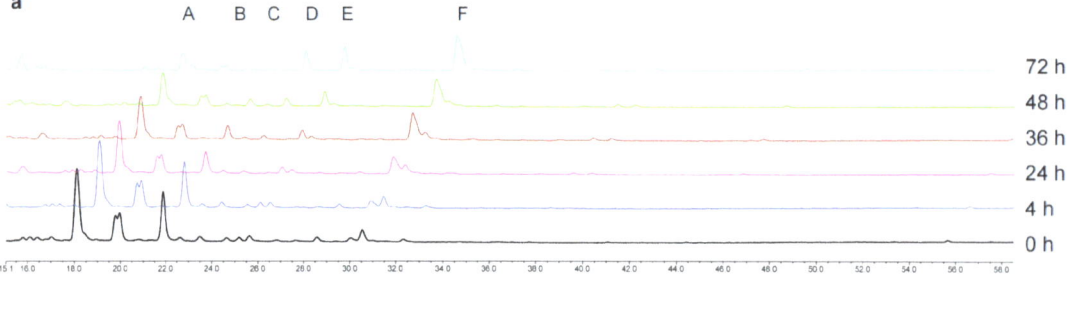

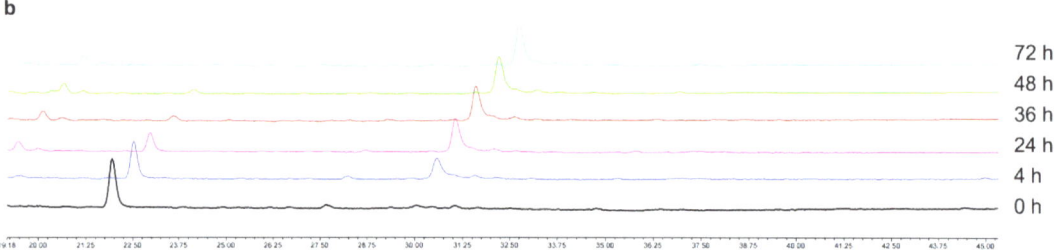

Figure 2. The HPLC plot of the total flavonoids conversion group and the scutellarin control group at different time points. (**a**) The HPLC plot of the total flavonoids conversion group; (**b**) The HPLC plot of the scutellarin control group. (Peak A: isocarthamidin-7-O-β-D-glucuronide. Peak B: carthamidin-7-O-β-D-glucuronide. Peak C: scutellarin. Peak D, E and F: These were the newly generated peaks during the transformation process).

According to the determination results presented in Section 3.1, isocarthamidin-7-O-β-D-glucuronide, carthamidin-7-O-β-D-glucuronide, and scutellarin accounted for 91.1% of the total flavonoids of HQT. Therefore, to better monitor the changes in the total flavonoids content, these three compounds were selected as the key components to calculate the conversion rate of total flavonoids in the gut microbiota incubation solution and draw the time–conversion rate curve in the study. Figure 3a illustrates that the conversion rate curve of these three flavonoid components exhibited an increasing trend. Notably, the conversion rate of scutellarin was higher than that of the other two components in the total flavonoids, reaching over 80% after 48 h of incubation, while the conversion rate of isocarthamidin-7-O-β-D-glucuronide was the lowest. In Figure 3b, the initial content of scutellarin at 0 h was set as 100%; almost all of the scutellarin had been converted into its microbiota metabolites after 48 h.

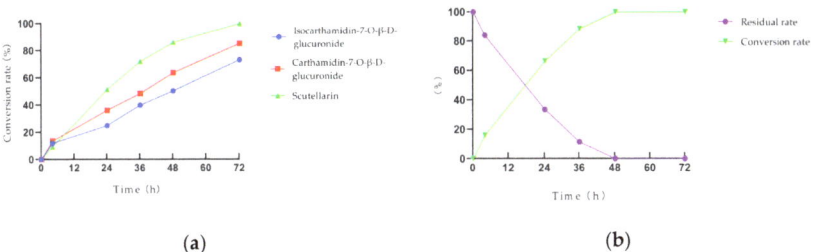

Figure 3. The conversion rate curve of drugs in the gut microbiota incubation solution. (**a**) The conversion rate curve of the three major flavonoid components of the total flavonoids conversion group; (**b**) The conversion rate curve of scutellarin in the scutellarin control group.

3.3. Metabolite Identification of Intestinal Microbiota Based on UPLC-Q-TOF-MS

To investigate the metabolites of total flavonoids in the gut microbiota, we conducted UPLC-Q-TOF-MS analysis and generated a base peak ion (BPI) plot of the sample, which is presented in Figure 4. Figure S1 shows the BPI plots of the blank control group. Table 3 provides detailed information on the formula, retention time, molecular weight, and secondary fragmentation of the compounds. Upon identification and analysis, the main flavonoids were transformed into their respective components. Figure 4a demonstrates that during the initial stage, four components were detectable: isocarthamidin-7-O-β-D-glucuronide, carthamidin-7-O-β-D-glucuronide scutellarin, and isoscutellarein 8-O-β-D-glucuronide. Their numbers were given as I, II, III, and IV, respectively. Most flavonoid components are commonly found in the form of glycosides. Previous studies have demonstrated that deglycosylation of glucoside flavonoids mainly occurs in the gut [16]. Figure 4b and Table 3 shows that four flavonoid components lose one part of glucuronide, transformed into its corresponding glycoside, isocarthamidin, carthamidin, scutellarein, and isoscutellarein.

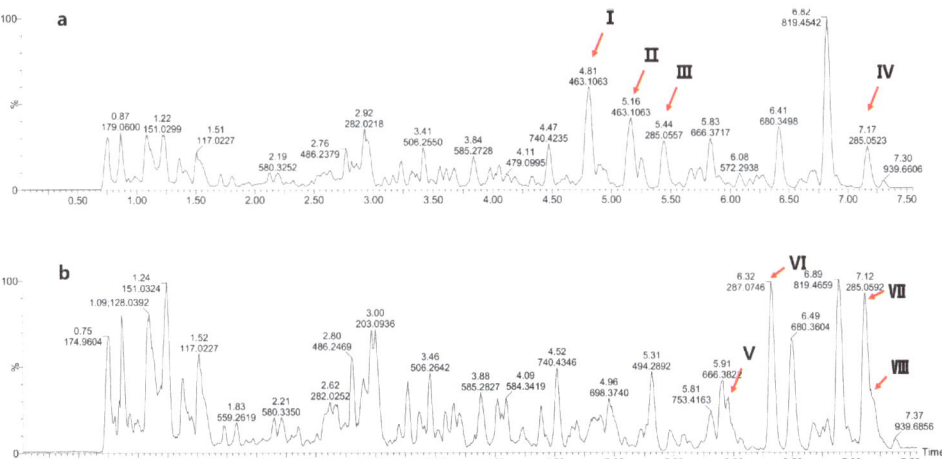

Figure 4. The BPI plots of the total flavonoids conversion group (Group 1) at 0 h and 72 h. (**a**) The BPI plot of Group 1 at 0 h; (**b**) The BPI plot of Group 1 at 72 h. (The numbers of peaks in figure is the same as in Table 3).

Table 3. The fragmentation of the compounds of the total flavonoids conversion group at 0 h and 72 h.

No.	Compound	Formula	Retention Time (min)	m/z	[M-H]-	Fragmentation Ions	Intensity 0 h/72 h
I	Isocarthamidin-7-O-β-D-glucuronide	$C_{21}H_{20}O_{12}$	4.810	464.1070	463.1063	287.0677	523,873/2604
II	Carthamidin-7-O-β-D-glucuronide	$C_{21}H_{20}O_{12}$	5.160	464.1070	463.1063	287.0711, 202.1172	513,752/2442
III	Scutellarin	$C_{21}H_{18}O_{12}$	5.438	462.0935	461.0949	285.0557	182,889/1087
IV	Isoscutellarein-8-β-glucuronide	$C_{21}H_{18}O_{12}$	7.166	462.0935	461.0905	285.0552	266,004/721
V	Isocarthamidin	$C_{15}H_{12}O_6$	5.945	288.0745	287.0746	-	3060/238,199
VI	Carthamidin	$C_{15}H_{12}O_6$	6.324	288.0745	287.0746	-	3964/449,457
VII	Scutellarein	$C_{15}H_{12}O_6$	7.116	286.0625	285.0591	-	6206/367,239
VIII	Isoscutellarein	$C_{15}H_{12}O_6$	7.187	286.0591	285.0591	253.064	18,127/15,2855

3.4. The Analysis of Gut Microbiotaoperational Taxonomic Units (OTUs)

To analyze the effect of the total flavonoids and scutellarin on the intestinal microbiota of mice, the characteristics and common taxa of the different treatment groups are represented in Venn diagrams, as shown in Figure 5. After 48 h, the OTUs decreased from 330 to 322 in the blank control group. This suggested that a few intestinal microbiota may be inhibited upon separation from the intestinal environment. The OTUs in both the total flavonoids conversion group and the scutellarin control group decreased further after incubation, with an 18% decrease in the former and a 17% decrease in the latter. This observation suggested that total flavonoids and scutellarin may exert antibacterial effects on certain intestinal microbiota in vitro.

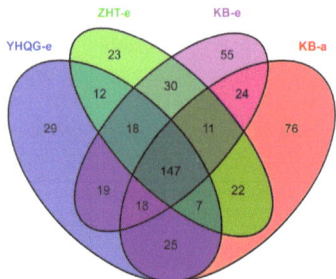

Figure 5. The OTUs Venn diagram for each group. (KB-a: the blank control group at 0 h, KB-e: the blank control group at 48 h, ZHT-e: the total flavonoids conversion group at 48 h, YHQG-e: the scutellarin control group at 48 h).

3.5. The Intestinal Microbiota α Diversity and β Diversity Analysis

Alpha diversity analysis was conducted to assess the sequencing volume's adequacy in capturing all taxa and indirectly measuring species richness in the sample. In Figure 6a, the dilution curve's slope approached 0, indicating that the sequencing depth effectively accounted for all species in the sample. Subsequently, the α diversity index was analyzed by using the Tukey test and the Kruskal–Wallis rank-sum test. The results are shown in Figure 6b,c as well as Table S1.

The pielou and Shannon indexes of the three groups were increased after 48 h of culture. Specifically, the indexes in ZHT-e presented significance ($p < 0.05$). These findings suggested that the total flavonoids in HQT may have the potential to enhance the uniformity of species distribution and the overall community diversity of the intestinal microbiota in normal mice.

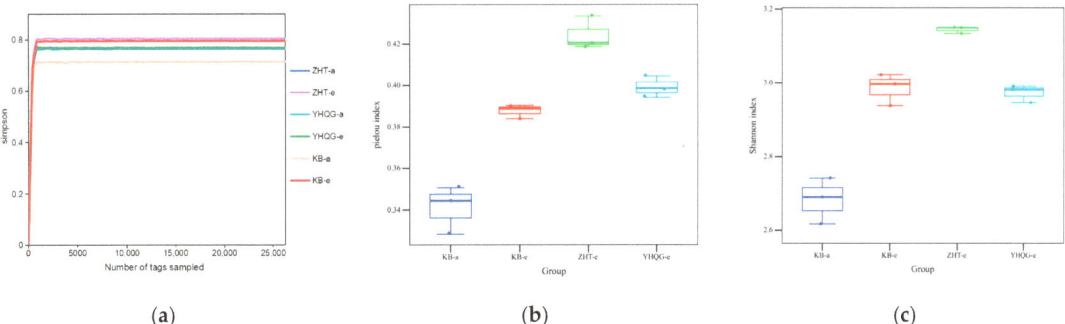

Figure 6. The gut microbial α diversity analysis. (**a**) The dilution curve of Simpson index; (**b**) The box plots of Pielou index in different groups; (**c**) The box plots of Shannon index in different groups. (KB-a: the blank control group at 0 h, KB-e: the blank control group at 48 h, ZHT-a: the total flavonoids conversion group at 0 h, ZHT-e: the total flavonoids conversion group at 48 h, YHQG-a: the scutellarin control group at 0 h, and YHQG-e: the scutellarin control group at 48 h).

Beta diversity analysis can assess the variation in microbial composition among different samples. In this study, we analyzed the composition of mouse intestinal microbiota using principal coordinate analysis (PCoA). As shown in Figure 7, each group formed clusters at 0 h, suggesting that the initial structural composition of each group was relatively similar during the early stage of transformation. After 48 h of anaerobic culture, the blank control group, the total flavonoids conversion group, and the scutellarin control group exhibited distinct clusters in comparison to the three groups at 0 h. This suggested that the bacterial composition of each group underwent changes during the culture period, and there were significant differences between the groups. This finding further supported that the composition of gut microbes underwent significant changes following treatment with total flavonoids and scutellarin compared to the blank control group.

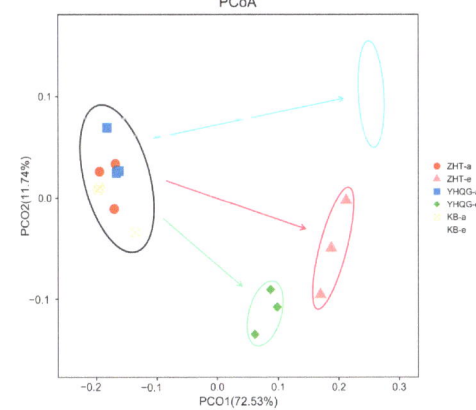

Figure 7. The PCoA analysis of the gut microbiota based on the species abundance ($n = 3$). (KB-a: the blank control group at 0 h, KB-e: the blank control group at 48 h, ZHT-a: the total flavonoids conversion group at 0 h, ZHT-e: the total flavonoids conversion group at 48 h, YHQG-e: the scutellarin control group at 0 h, and YHQG-e: the scutellarin control group at 48 h).

3.6. Analysis of the Microbiota Community Composition

The analysis of the species distribution of mouse gut microbiota showed that the distribution of the top 10 species in relative abundance at the phylum level and genus level varied after 48 h of incubation. Hence, the discrepancies in the gut microbiota among the various groups were visualized.

In Figure 8a, at the taxonomic phylum level, *Firmicutes* and *Proteobacteria* in the total flavonoids conversion group and scutellarin control group changed significantly compared to the blank control group. In addition, at the taxonomic genus level, *Enterococcus* was the most abundant genus in each group in Figure 8b. *Enterococcus* in the blank control group and the total flavonoids conversion group significantly reduced after 48 h ($p < 0.01$) compared with the blank control group at 0 h in Figure 8d. Interestingly, in the scutellarin control group, the abundance of *Enterococcus* remained relatively stable throughout the period. In Figure 8d, after the culture, the levels of *Enterococcus* were found to be highest in the YHQG-e group, followed by the ZHT-e group, and finally, the KB-e group. These findings suggested that scutellarin can help to keep the abundance of *Enterococcus* within the gut microbiota. Apart from its probiotic potential, studies have shown that *Enterococcus* can synthesize exopolysaccharides with various bioactive properties, which possess antioxidant, antibacterial, anti-biofilm, antitumor, immunological, and anti-diabetic activities [17]. This indicated that *Enterococcus* has a wide range of potential health benefits and therapeutic applications. Notably, the levels of *Shigella* were significantly reduced in the total flavonoids conversion group and scutellarin control group. The finding suggested that total flavonoids and scutellarin have inhibitory effects on *Shigella*. According to Figure 8d, it is also found that the abundance of *Parabacteroides*, *Butyricimonas*, and *Phocaeicola* increased following intervention with total flavonoids compared to the other groups. Additionally, the intervention of scutellarin led to an increase in the abundance of *Bacteroides*, *Ligilactobacillus*, *Enterococcus*, and *Muribaculum*.

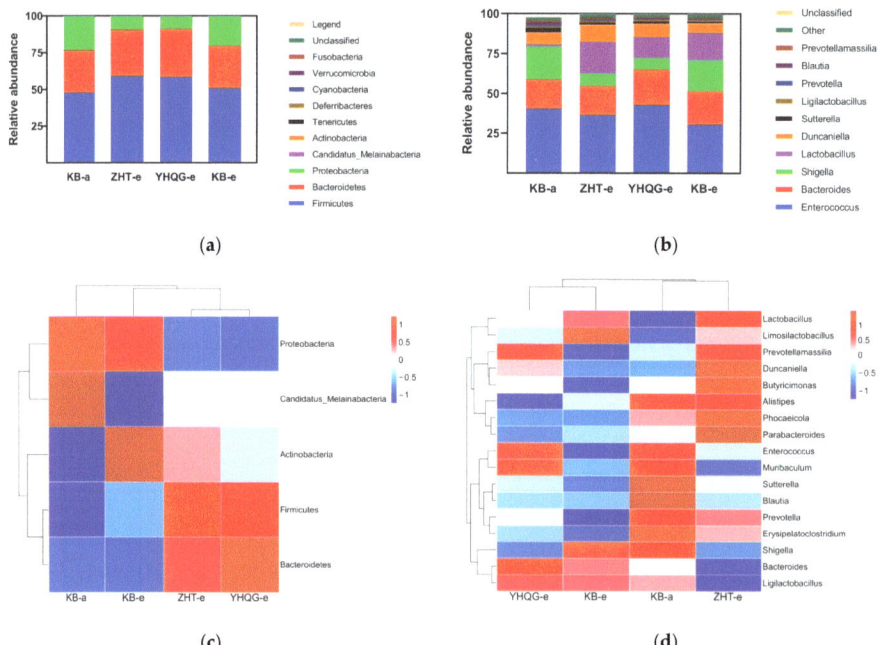

Figure 8. The analysis of relative abundance of gut microbiota species in three groups at phylum and genus levels. (**a**) The species stacking map of the relative abundance at the phylum level. (**b**) The species stacking map of the relative abundance at the genus level. (**c**) The heatmap of differential gut bacterial taxa at phylum level. (**d**) The heatmap of differential gut bacterial taxa at genus level. (KB-a: the blank control group at 0 h, KB-e: the blank control group at 48 h, ZHT-e: the total flavonoids conversion group at 48 h, and YHQG-e: the scutellarin control group at 48 h).

3.7. The Differential Bacterial Screening Results

The linear discriminant analysis (LEfSe, linear discriminant analysis effect size) combining the rank sum test and discriminant analysis was used to identify significantly changing microbial taxa. The cladogram illustrated the taxonomic distribution of labeled species in each group, with larger circles indicating a higher degree of enrichment. The threshold for linear discriminant analysis (LDA) was set at a value greater than 4, with $p < 0.05$.

In this study, 59 distinct bacterial taxa were selected, which encompassed 3 phyla, 7 classes, 7 orders, 12 families, 12 genera, and 18 species (refer to Figure 9). The length of each bar in the chart indicates the effect size of the corresponding taxa. Prior to the transformation, *Enterococcaceae*, *Sutterellaceae*, *Lachnospiraceae*, and *Morganellaceae* were predominantly enriched. After 48 h, the blank control group exhibited the highest abundance of *Lactobacillaceae* and *Bifidobacteriaceae*. Meanwhile, the total flavonoids conversion group was predominantly enriched with *Muribaculaceae*, *Bacteroidaceae*, *Rikenellaceae*, *Prevotellaceae*, and *Erysipelotrichaceae*. The scutellarin control group primarily influenced *Prevotellamassilia*.

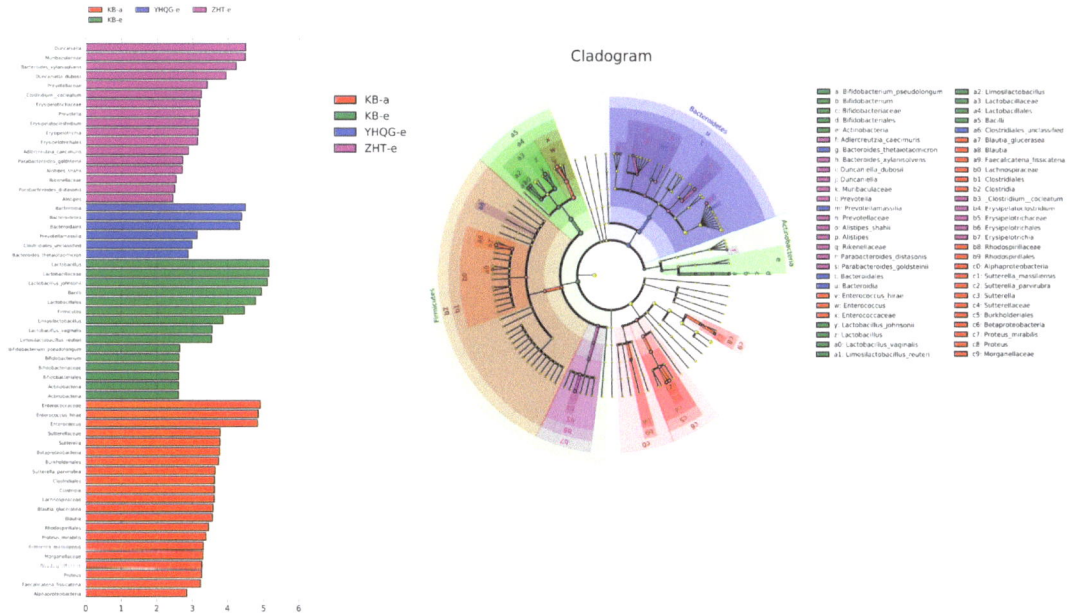

Figure 9. The LEfSe analysis bar chart (**left**) and evolutionary clade chart (**right**) (LDA > 2 and $p < 0.05$). In the evolutionary clade gram, circles radiating from inside to outside represent the taxonomic level from phylum to genus (or species). Each small circle at different taxonomic level represents a classification at the level; the small circle diameter is proportional to the relative abundance size. Red nodes represent differential species biomarkers that played an important role in the red group (KB-a: the blank control group at 0 h), green nodes represent differential species biomarkers that played an important role in the green group (KB-e: the blank control group at 48 h), blue nodes represent differential species biomarkers that played an important role in the blue group (YHQG-e: the scutellarin control group at 48 h), and purple nodes represent differential species biomarkers that played an important role in the purple group (ZHT-e: the total flavonoids conversion group at 48 h).

3.8. The Prediction Results of Gut Microbial Function

Tax4Fun [18] was a functional prediction tool based on the SILVA [19] database. It primarily focuses on the functional annotation of sequenced and annotated prokaryotic genomes in the KEGG database for functional prediction for the OTUs information. The SILVA database, which is rapidly updated, offers a significant advantage in terms of the accuracy of functional prediction results. Consequently, it enables us to gain more comprehensive insights into the gut microbiota community.

In KEGG pathway analysis, the functions of lever 1 mainly included metabolism, cellular processes, and human diseases. Level 2 involved membrane transport, carbohydrate metabolism, and amino acid metabolism. Level 3 were transporters, ABC transporters, and ribosomes. In Figure S2, we identified six primary differential pathways according to the KEGG database. Additionally, we found 36 secondary differential pathways and 259 tertiary differential pathways within the same database. According to Figure S2, compared with the blank control group, the scutellarin control group exhibited significant up-regulation in several metabolic pathways, including Purine metabolism, Aminoacyl-tRNA biosynthesis, Pyrimidine metabolism, two-component system, starch and sucrose metabolism, and ribosome. In the total flavonoids conversion group, several metabolic pathways, including Aminoacyl-tRNA biosynthesis, Nicotinate and nicotinamide metabolism, homologous recombination, Histidine metabolism, and DNA replication, exhibited significant differences compared with the blank control group.

4. Discussion

HQT derived from the aerial parts part of *Scutellaria baicalensis*, which had significant application potential. It has a longstanding tradition of being consumed as a tea in the northern and southwestern regions of China. Our previous experiments found that HQT had an obvious intervention effect in the colorectal precancerous lesions induced by AMO in rats. Additionally, the inhibitory effect on aberrant crypt foci (ACF) formation was primarily attributed to the influence of HQT on the intestinal microflora [13]. Therefore, we explored the interaction of total flavonoids and normal mouse intestinal microflora based on the in vitro transformation system in this study.

The predominant components of the total flavonoids in HQT were isocarthamidin-7-O-β-D-glucuronide, carthamidin-7-O-β-D-glucuronide, and scutellarin. We investigated the transformation of total flavonoids by the intestinal microflora of normal mice through anaerobic culture in vitro. According to the conversion curve, the conversion rate of scutellarin consistently exceeded that of isocarthamidin-7-O-β-D-glucuronide and carthamidin-7-O-β-D-glucuronide in the total flavonoids conversion group. Furthermore, after 72 h, scutellarin in the total flavonoids was nearly completely transformed into its metabolites. Further, the UPLC-Q-TOF-MS analysis of the total flavonoids conversion group revealed a conversion of the primary flavonoid glycosides in the total flavonoids into their respective glycosides within the bacterial culture system. Current findings indicated that the metabolic processes conducted by intestinal microflora typically involve deglycosylation, demethylation, reduction, and cyclic fission reactions [20,21]. The biotransformation of flavonoids in vivo was a highly complex process that encompassed the involvement of multiple organs and diverse enzymes. According to recent investigations, upon entering and being transported into the liver, the drug underwent further coupling reactions, such as sulfation and methylation, resulting in the formation of many conjugates [16]. Most O-glycosides of flavonoids underwent O-deglycosylation when acted upon by intestinal bacteria [22]. In this study, isocarthamidin-7-O-β-D-glucuronide, carthamidin-7-O-β-D-glucuronide, scutellarin, and isoscutellarein 8-O-β-D-glucuronide detected in 0 h group by UPLC-Q-TOF-MS were O-glycosides. Through fragment ion identification, it was found that in the intestinal bacteria culture system in this study, the O-glycoside compounds in HQT were converted into corresponding glycoelements by deglycosylation, and this result was consistent with the previous report. Most natural flavonoids predominantly existed as glycosides, rendering them poorly absorbed in the small intestine. Consequently, they transited to the colon in their glycoside form and hydrolyzed into aglycones by the intestinal microflora. Subsequently, these compounds underwent further metabolism, leading to the formation of various metabolites and phenolic acids, which could be more efficiently absorbed by the human body [23]. Hence, the total flavonoids of HQT facilitated their absorption by the gut microbiota, obtaining better effects. This observation underscored the pivotal role played by the intestinal flora in this process.

Based on the sequencing results, the total flavonoids and scutellarin led to slightly lower OUTs compared to the blank control group. This observation suggested that total flavonoids and scutellarin may exert a certain inhibitory effect on individual bacteria [24]. In the warm incubation system outside the body, the absence of regulatory mechanisms for intestinal environment homeostasis led to slight inhibitory effects at the OUTs level. The Pielou and Simpson indices of the total flavonoids conversion group revealed higher values compared to those of the blank control group in Figure 6b,c after 48 h, suggesting that the distribution of the mouse intestinal microbiota may be more uniform in that group. According to the PCoA, the intestinal microbiota structure exhibited significant changes following the intervention of total flavonoids and scutellarin. These findings suggested that the intervention of total flavonoids can facilitate a more uniform distribution of microflora and regulate the microflora structure. To gain deeper insights into the structure of the microflora, we conducted an analysis of the microbial community composition.

At the phylum level, *Firmicutes* and *Proteobacteria* exhibited similar variation tendencies in the total flavonoids conversion group and scutellarin control group. This observation suggested that the effect of total flavonoids and scutellarin on the normal gut microbiota was moderate. This finding further reflected that consuming HQT did not excessively disrupt the balance of normal intestinal microbiota in the human body. At the genus level, total flavonoids and scutellarin increased the abundance of *Enterococcus* while inhibiting the growth of *Shigella*. *Enterococcus* is a naturally occurring component of the human microbiota and is abundant in the intestine, where it plays a crucial role in the digestive system [25]. In addition, *Enterococcus* species were commonly utilized as probiotic food additives or recommended as supplements for the management of intestinal dysbiosis and other ailments [26]. Conversely, extensive research indicated that *Shigella* was a prevalent pathogen responsible for bacterial dysentery in humans. It had the ability to evade immune defenses quickly and induce hemorrhagic diarrhea and severe intestinal inflammation [27]. The total flavonoids and scutellarin might promote the growth of beneficial bacteria, maintain the stability of the intestinal environment, have a certain inhibitory effect on pathogenic bacteria, and reduce the occurrence of digestive system diseases.

In Figure 8d, the abundance of *Parabacteroides*, *Butyricimonas*, and *Phocaeicola* was upregulated under the intervention of total flavonoids. *Parabacteroides* are key members of the human gut microbiota, which have the physiological characteristics of carbohydrate metabolism and secretion of short-chain fatty acids (SCFAs). As a potential probiotic bacterium, its species has potential therapeutic effects in metabolic, inflammatory, and neoplastic diseases [28–31]. The upregulation of *Butyricimonas* abundance can enhance the function of fatty acid biosynthesis, increase the production of SCFAs, and promote the synthesis of butyrate [32]. Recent studies have found that *Phocaeicola* strains can help maintain the epithelial barrier by regulating cytokine levels and the secretion of SCFAs, thereby improving dextran sodium sulfate-induced colitis in mice [33]. And studies have found that increasing the production of SCFAs contributes to the protective effects of probiotics against intestinal and brain health [34]. The results of this study showed that the total flavonoids may effectively increase the abundance of dominant bacteria, enable the intestine to better secrete SCFAs, enhance the protective effect on the intestine, maintain the integrity of the intestinal epithelial barrier, and promote the synthesis of butyrate and provide energy for the intestine. In the previous experiments of our lab, we found that the abundance of related bacteria producing both butyrate and SCFAs increased under the intervention of HQT, which was similar to the results in this study [14]. After transformation, the abundance of *Bacteroides*, *Ligilactobacillus*, *Enterococcus*, and *Muribaculum* was upregulated in the scutellarin control group. Studies reported that *Bacteroides* played a key role in regulating the human immune system, mainly in maintaining the stability of the immune system, anti-inflammatory and anti-tumor systems, and other aspects [35]. As beneficial bacteria, many *Ligilactobacillus* strains exhibited functional properties with health benefits, such as antimicrobial activity, immune effects, and the ability to modulate the gut microbiota [36]. Scutellarin may exert an anti-inflammatory function by promoting the abundance of beneficial bacteria and regulating the immune system function, as well as playing a certain preventive or therapeutic role in the premalignant stage.

The LEfSe analysis showed that *Muribaculaceae*, *Bacteroidaceae*, *Rikenellaceae*, and *Prevotellaceae* were the dominant bacteria in the total flavonoids conversion group, most of which were beneficial bacteria. It has been reported that *Muribaculaceae* can exert beneficial effects on intestinal ecology by regulating immunity and intestinal homeostasis, increasing the output of intestinal beneficial metabolites, prolonging the life span of mice, and inhibiting CD8 + T cell activation to tolerate immune stimulation, and is negatively correlated with inflammatory response [37,38]. In addition, experiments have proved that *Rikenellaceae* and *Bacteroidaceae*, as probiotics, had good anti-inflammatory effects, and *Rikenellaceae* can also protect cells from oxidative stress by neutralizing cytotoxic reactive oxygen species and enhancing the barrier function of intestinal epithelial cells [39–41]. *Erysipelotrichaceae* was important in the immune response, which was highly immunogenic. The bacteria can also produce SCFAs, such as butyric acid, through dietary fiber fermentation [42]. SCFAs induced protective immune responses by producing anti-inflammatory cytokines TGF-β and IL-10 and enhancing epithelial barrier function [43,44]. The scutellarin control group mainly included the dominant gut microbiota, such as *Prevotellaceae* and *Clostridiales*. Animal experiments have demonstrated that *Prevotellaceae* can inhibit the development of inflammatory arthritis in mice and regulate the host immune response [45]. *Clostridiales*, on the other hand, are beneficial for overall health and exhibit an effective anti-tumor response independent of anti-PD-1 immunotherapy by activating CD8 + T cells [46,47]. Therefore, scutellarin may potentially enhance its anti-inflammatory function by promoting the growth of these dominant bacteria, thereby aiding in the regulation and activation of the immune system.

The gut microbial function prediction results showed that the YHQG group was significantly up-regulated in several metabolic pathways, including Purine metabolism, Aminoacyl-tRNA biosynthesis, Pyrimidine metabolism, and starch and sucrose metabolism. It has been demonstrated that Lactobacillus plays a key role in the Purine metabolism pathway [48]. Based on the analysis of gut microbiota structure, it was observed that the total flavonoids conversion group and scutellarin control group increased *Lactobacillus* abundance after transformation. Hence, we speculated that the main component regulating the Purine metabolism pathway in the total flavonoids group was scutellarin. Relative to the KB group, the total flavonoids conversion group showed significant upregulation in several pathways, including Aminoacyl-tRNA biosynthesis, Nicotinate and nicotinamide metabolism, homologous recombination, Histidine metabolism, and DNA replication. Multiple studies have provided evidence that Aminoacyl-tRNA biosynthesis was a biosynthetic pathway enriched with metabolites associated with CRC [49]. The involvement of relevant synthetases in Aminoacyl-tRNA biosynthesis implies that HQT total flavonoids might disrupt CRC development by influencing these synthetases within the Aminoacyl-tRNA biosynthesis pathway.

5. Conclusions

In this study, the total flavonoids were obtained through a process involving water frying and macroporous resin purification. The quantification of the main flavonoids was performed using HPLC (yield 12.50%, content 54.51%). The present study investigated the interaction between the HQT total flavonoids and the gut microbiota. Moreover, the transformation analysis demonstrated that the cultured intestinal bacteria were capable of metabolizing the total flavonoids and converting them into the corresponding aglucons. According to the results of intestinal group sequencing, it was observed that the total flavonoids have the ability to enhance the growth of dominant intestinal microflora. Additionally, they significantly increased the abundance of beneficial bacteria such as *Enterococcus* and *Lactobacillus*. This finding suggested that total flavonoids can potentially contribute to regulating the human immune response, exhibiting antimicrobial and antioxidant properties, as well as demonstrating anti-tumor effects [50].

The functional prediction results revealed significant regulatory effects of total flavonoids and scutellarin on various pathways, including Purine metabolism, Aminoacyl-tRNA biosynthesis, Pyrimidine metabolism, Nicotinate and nicotinamide metabolism, homologous recombination, and Histidine metabolism. These findings provided valuable insights for further in-depth research and investigation. According to this study, it was found that the total flavonoids of HQT could potentially serve as the primary active component responsible for its intervention effect on the intestinal microbiota. This finding not only provides a new perspective to reveal the mechanism behind the prevention of inflammatory and tumor-related diseases, particularly colorectal cancer (CRC), through interventions in the gut microbiota but also offers a fresh perspective on this topic.

Supplementary Materials: The following supporting information can be downloaded at: https://www.mdpi.com/article/10.3390/foods12244410/s1, Supplementary Figure S1. The BPI plots of the blank control group (Group 3) at 0 h and 72 h. (a) The BPI plot of Group 3 at 0 h; (b) The BPI plot of Group 3 at 72 h; Supplementary Figure S2. Analysis of TaxFun4 function prediction differences in KEGG pathway (A: After 48 h, variation analysis between KB-e (the blank control group at 48 h) and YHQG-e (the scutellarin control group at 48 h), B: After 48 h, variation analysis between KB-e (the blank control group at 48 h) and ZHT-e (the total flavonoids conversion group at 48 h); Supplementary Table S1. The α diversity index for each group. (KB-a: the blank control group at 0 h, KB-e: the blank control group at 48 h, ZHT-e: the total flavonoids conversion group at 48 h, and YHQG-e: the scutellarin control group at 48 h).

Author Contributions: Conceptualization, C.H. and P.X.; methodology, Y.Z. and K.Y.; software, J.S.; validation, Y.Z. and K.Y.; formal analysis, Y.Z. and K.Y.; investigation, Y.Z. and K.Y.; resources, C.H. and X.C.; writing—original draft preparation, Y.Z. and K.Y.; writing—review and editing, J.S. and C.H.; visualization, Y.Z. and K.Y.; funding acquisition, C.H. and P.X. All authors have read and agreed to the published version of the manuscript.

Funding: This research was funded by the Innovation Team and Talents Cultivation Program of the National Administration of Traditional Chinese Medicine (No. ZYYCXTD-D-202005), the Science & Technology Fundamental Resources Investigation Program (No.2022FY101000) and the CAMS Innovation Fund for Medical Sciences (CIFMS) ID: 2021-I2M-1-071 and 2022-I2M-2-001.

Institutional Review Board Statement: This research was approved by the Committee on Care and Use of Laboratory Animals of the IMPLAD (the approval code of the animal experiments was SLXD-20211101013).

Data Availability Statement: The data used to support the findings of this study can be made available by the corresponding author upon request.

Conflicts of Interest: The authors declare no conflict of interest.

References

1. De Vos, W.M.; Tilg, H.; Van Hul, M.; Cani, P.D. Gut microbiome and health: Mechanistic insights. *Gut* **2022**, *71*, 1020–1032. [CrossRef] [PubMed]
2. Power, S.E.; O'Toole, P.W.; Stanton, C.; Ross, R.P.; Fitzgerald, G.F. Intestinal microbiota, diet and health. *Br. J. Nutr.* **2014**, *111*, 387–402. [CrossRef] [PubMed]
3. Gong, X.; Li, X.; Bo, A.; Shi, R.; Li, Q.; Lei, L.; Zhang, L.; Li, M. The interactions between gut microbiota and bioactive ingredients of traditional Chinese medicines: A review. *Pharmacol. Res.* **2020**, *157*, 104824. [CrossRef] [PubMed]
4. Yin, L.; Xia, W.; Huang, G.; Xiao, W. Research progress on correlation between traditional Chinese medicine-gut microbiota and host's own metabolic immune homeostasis. *Chin. Herb. Med.* **2022**, *53*, 2526–2538.
5. Men, W.; Chen, Y.; Li, Y.; Yang, Q.; Weng, X.; Gong, Z.; Zhang, R.; Zhu, X. Research Progress of Biotransformation on Effective Ingredients of Chinese Medicine via Intestinal Bacteria. *Chin. J. Exp. Tradit. Med. Formulae* **2015**, *21*, 229–234.
6. Shen, J. Study on Quality Assessment of the Aerial Parts of Scutellaria baicalensis Georgi and a Primary Pharmacophylogenetic Investigation in the Genus Scutellaria. Master's Thesis, Peking Union Medical College, Beijing China, 2018.
7. Wang, X.; Xie, L.; Long, J.; Liu, K.; Lu, J.; Liang, Y.; Gao, L.; Dai, X. Therapeutic effect of baicalin on inflammatory bowel disease: A review. *J. Ethnopharmacol.* **2022**, *283*, 114749. [CrossRef]
8. Xiang, L.; Gao, Y.; Chen, S.; Sun, J.; Wu, J.; Meng, X. Therapeutic potential of *Scutellaria baicalensis* Georgi in lung cancer therapy. *Phytomed. Int. J. Phytother. Phytopharm.* **2022**, *95*, 153727. [CrossRef] [PubMed]

9. Shin, H.S.; Bae, M.J.; Choi, D.W.; Shon, D.H. Skullcap (*Scutellaria baicalensis*) extract and its active compound, wogonin, inhibit ovalbumin-induced Th2-mediated response. *Molecules* **2014**, *19*, 2536–2545. [CrossRef]
10. Cheng, C.S.; Chen, J.; Tan, H.Y.; Wang, N.; Chen, Z.; Feng, Y. *Scutellaria baicalensis* and Cancer Treatment: Recent Progress and Perspectives in Biomedical and Clinical Studies. *Am. J. Chin. Med.* **2018**, *46*, 25–54. [CrossRef] [PubMed]
11. Zhao, T.; Tang, H.; Xie, L.; Zheng, Y.; Ma, Z.; Sun, Q.; Li, X. *Scutellaria baicalensis* Georgi. (Lamiaceae): A review of its traditional uses, botany, phytochemistry, pharmacology and toxicology. *J. Pharm. Pharmacol.* **2019**, *71*, 1353–1369. [CrossRef] [PubMed]
12. Wang, C.Z.; Zhang, C.F.; Chen, L.; Anderson, S.; Lu, F.; Yuan, C. Colon cancer chemopreventive effects of baicalein, an active enteric microbiome metabolite from baicalin. *Int. J. Oncol.* **2015**, *47*, 1749–1758. [CrossRef]
13. Shen, J.; Li, P.; Liu, S.; Liu, Q.; Li, Y.; Zhang, Z.; Yang, C.; Hu, M.; Sun, Y.; He, C.; et al. The chemopreventive effects of Huangqin-tea against AOM-induced preneoplastic colonic aberrant crypt foci in rats and omics analysis. *Food Funct.* **2020**, *11*, 9634–9650. [CrossRef]
14. Shen, J. The Pharmcophylogenetic Investigation of the Genus *Scutellaria* L. in China. Ph.D. Thesis, Peking Union Medical College, Beijing, China, 2021.
15. An, G. Characterization of a Murine Model for Encephalitozoon hellem Infection after Dexamethasone Immunosuppression. *Microorganisms* **2020**, *8*, 1891. [CrossRef]
16. Murota, K.; Nakamura, Y.; Uehara, M. Flavonoid metabolism: The interaction of metabolites and gut microbiota. *Biosci. Biotechnol. Biochem.* **2018**, *82*, 600–610. [CrossRef] [PubMed]
17. Kavitake, D.; Devi, P.B.; Delattre, C.; Reddy, G.B.; Shetty, P.H. Exopolysaccharides produced by Enterococcus genus—An overview. *Int. J. Biol. Macromol.* **2023**, *226*, 111–120. [CrossRef]
18. Aßhauer, K.P.; Wemheuer, B.; Daniel, R.; Meinicke, P. Tax4Fun: Predicting functional profiles from metagenomic 16S rRNA data. *Bioinformatics* **2015**, *31*, 2882–2884. [CrossRef]
19. Pruesse, E. SILVA: A comprehensive online resource for quality checked and aligned ribosomal RNA sequence data compatible with ARB. *Nucleic Acids Res.* **2007**, *35*, 7188–7196. [CrossRef] [PubMed]
20. Braune, A.; Blaut, M. Bacterial species involved in the conversion of dietary flavonoids in the human gut. *Gut Microbes* **2016**, *7*, 216–234. [CrossRef] [PubMed]
21. Riva, A.; Kolimár, D.; Spittler, A.; Wisgrill, L.; Herbold, C.W.; Abrankó, L.; BerrY, D. Conversion of Rutin, a Prevalent Dietary Flavonol, by the Human Gut Microbiota. *Front. Microbiol.* **2020**, *11*, 585428. [CrossRef] [PubMed]
22. Yu, H.; Zheng, R.; Su, W.; Xing, J.; Wang, Y. Metabolism characteristics and pharmacological insights of flavonoids based on the intestinal bacteria. *J. Pharm.* **2021**, *56*, 1748 + 1757–1768.
23. Chen, L.; Cao, H.; Huang, Q.; Xiao, J.; Teng, H. Absorption, metabolism and bioavailability of flavonoids: A review. *Crit. Rev. Food Sci. Nutr.* **2022**, *62*, 7730–7742. [CrossRef]
24. Zhang, L. Reaserch on the Stems and Leaves of *Scutellaria baicalensis* with Anti-Bacterial and Anti-Inflammation Properties and its Effects on Mice Mastitis. Master's thesis, Nanjing University of Traditional Chinese Medicine, Nanjing China, 2019.
25. Qin, J.; Li, R.; Raes, J.; Arumugam, M.; Burgdorf, K.S.; Manichanh, C.; Nielsen, T.; Pons, N.; Levenez, F.; Yamada, T.; et al. A human gut microbial gene catalogue established by metagenomic sequencing. *Nature* **2010**, *464*, 59–65. [CrossRef]
26. Krawczyk, B.; Wityk, P.; Gałęcka, M.; Michalik, M. The Many Faces of *Enterococcus* spp.—Commensal, Probiotic and Opportunistic Pathogen. *Microorganisms* **2021**, *9*, 1900. [CrossRef] [PubMed]
27. Liu, G.; Pilla, G.; Tang, C.M. *Shigella* host: Pathogen interactions: Keeping bacteria in the loop. *Cell. Microbiol.* **2019**, *21*, e13062. [CrossRef]
28. Wu, W.K.K. *Parabacteroides distasonis*: An emerging probiotic? *Gut* **2023**, *72*, 1635–1636. [CrossRef]
29. Zhao, Q.; Dai, M.; Huang, R.; Duan, J.; Zhang, T.; Bao, W.; Zhang, J.; Gui, S.; Xia, S.; Dai, C.; et al. *Parabacteroides distasonis* ameliorates hepatic fibrosis potentially via modulating intestinal bile acid metabolism and hepatocyte pyroptosis in male mice. *Nat. Commun.* **2023**, *14*, 1829. [CrossRef]
30. Wang, K.; Liao, M.; Zhou, N.; Bao, L.; Ma, K.; Zheng, Z.; Wang, Y.; Liu, C.; Wang, W.; Wang, J.; et al. *Parabacteroides distasonis* Alleviates Obesity and Metabolic Dysfunctions via Production of Succinate and Secondary Bile Acids. *Cell Rep.* **2019**, *26*, 222–235.e5. [CrossRef]
31. Lei, Y.; Tang, L.; Liu, S.; Hu, S.; Wu, L.; Liu, Y.; Yang, M.; Huang, S.; Tang, X.; Tang, T.; et al. *Parabacteroides* produces acetate to alleviate heparanase-exacerbated acute pancreatitis through reducing neutrophil infiltration. *Microbiome* **2021**, *9*, 115. [CrossRef] [PubMed]
32. Hu, Q.; Yu, L.; Zhai, Q.; Zhao, J.; Tian, F. Anti-Inflammatory, Barrier Maintenance, and Gut Microbiome Modulation Effects of Saccharomyces cerevisiae QHNLD8L1 on DSS-Induced Ulcerative Colitis in Mice. *Int. J. Mol. Sci.* **2023**, *24*, 6721. [CrossRef]
33. Sun, Z.; Jiang, X.; Wang, B.; Tian, F.; Zhang, H.; Yu, L. Novel Phocaeicola Strain Ameliorates Dextran Sulfate Sodium-induced Colitis in Mice. *Curr. Microbiol.* **2022**, *79*, 393. [CrossRef] [PubMed]
34. Bloemendaal, M.; Szopinska-Tokov, J.; Belzer, C.; Boverhoff, D.; Papalini, S.; Michels, F.; Hemert, S.; Vasquez, A.A.; Aarts, E. Probiotics-induced changes in gut microbial composition and its effects on cognitive performance after stress: Exploratory analyses. *Transl. Psychiatry* **2021**, *11*, 300. [CrossRef] [PubMed]
35. Zafar, H.; Saier, M.H., Jr. Gut Bacteroides species in health and disease. *Gut Microbes* **2021**, *13*, 1848158. [CrossRef] [PubMed]
36. Guerrero Sanchez, M.; Passot, S.; Campoy, S.; Olivares, M.; Fonseca, F. *Ligilactobacillus salivarius* functionalities, applications, and manufacturing challenges. *Appl. Microbiol. Biotechnol.* **2022**, *106*, 57–80. [CrossRef] [PubMed]

37. Liang, H.; Song, H.; Zhang, X.; Song, G.; Wang, Y.; Wang, Y.; Ding, X.; Duan, X.; Li, L.; Sun, T.; et al. Metformin attenuated sepsis-related liver injury by modulating gut microbiota. *Emerg. Microbes Infect.* **2022**, *11*, 815–828. [CrossRef] [PubMed]
38. Hao, H.; Zhang, X.; Tong, L.; Liu, Q.; Liang, X.; Bu, Y.; Gong, P.; Liu, T.; Zhang, L.; Xia, Y.; et al. Effect of Extracellular Vesicles Derived From Lactobacillus plantarum Q7 on Gut Microbiota and Ulcerative Colitis in Mice. *Front. Immunol.* **2021**, *12*, 777147. [CrossRef] [PubMed]
39. Dong, L.; Du, H.; Zhang, M.; Xu, H.; Pu, X.; Chen, Q.; Luo, R.; Hu, Y.; Wang, Y.; Tu, H.; et al. Anti-inflammatory effect of Rhein on ulcerative colitis via inhibiting PI3K/Akt/mTOR signaling pathway and regulating gut microbiota. *Phytother. Res. PTR* **2022**, *36*, 2081–2094. [CrossRef] [PubMed]
40. Shabbir, U.; Rubab, M.; Daliri, E.B.; Chelliah, R.; Javed, A.; Oh, D.H. Curcumin, Quercetin, Catechins and Metabolic Diseases: The Role of Gut Microbiota. *Nutrients* **2021**, *13*, 206. [CrossRef]
41. Wang, T.; Han, J.; Dai, H.; Sun, J.; Ren, J.; Wang, W.; Qiao, S.; Liu, C.; Sun, L.; Liu, S.; et al. Polysaccharides from *Lyophyllum decastes* reduce obesity by altering gut microbiota and increasing energy expenditure. *Carbohydr. Polym.* **2022**, *295*, 119862. [CrossRef] [PubMed]
42. Mao, J.; Wang, D.; Long, J.; Yang, X.; Lin, J.; Song, Y.; Xie, F.; Xun, Z.; Wang, Y.; Wang, Y.; et al. Gut microbiome is associated with the clinical response to anti-PD-1 based immunotherapy in hepatobiliary cancers. *J. Immunother. Cancer* **2021**, *9*, e003334. [CrossRef]
43. Rooks, M.G.; Garrett, W.S. Gut microbiota, metabolites and host immunity. *Nat. Rev. Immunol.* **2016**, *16*, 341–352. [CrossRef]
44. Furusawa, Y.; Obata, Y.; Fukuda, S.; Endo, T.A.; Nakata, G.; Takahashi, D.; Nakanishi, Y.; Uetake, C.; Kato, K.; Kato, T.; et al. Commensal microbe-derived butyrate induces the differentiation of colonic regulatory T cells. *Nature* **2013**, *504*, 446–450. [CrossRef] [PubMed]
45. Bertelsen, A.; Elborn, J.S.; Schock, B.C. Microbial interaction: *Prevotella* spp. reduce P. aeruginosa induced inflammation in cystic fibrosis bronchial epithelial cells. *J. Cyst. Fibros. Off. J. Eur. Cyst. Fibros. Soc.* **2021**, *20*, 682–691. [CrossRef] [PubMed]
46. Lan, Y.; Sun, Q.; Ma, Z.; Chang, L.; Peng, J.; Zhang, M.; Sun, Q.; Qiao, R.; Hou, X.; Ding, X.; et al. Seabuckthorn polysaccharide ameliorates high-fat diet-induced obesity by gut microbiota-SCFAs-liver axis. *Food Funct.* **2022**, *13*, 2925–2937. [CrossRef]
47. Montalban-Arques, A.; Katkeviciute, E.; Busenhart, P.; Bircher, A.; Wirbel, J.; Zeller, G.; Morsy, Y.; Borsig, L.; Garzon, J.F.; Muller, A.; et al. Commensal Clostridiales strains mediate effective anti-cancer immune response against solid tumors. *Cell Host Microbe* **2021**, *29*, 1573–1588.e7. [CrossRef]
48. Wu, J.; Wei, Z.; Cheng, P.; Cheng, Q.; Xu, F.; Yang, Y.; Wang, A.; Chen, W.; Sun, Z.; Lu, Y. Rhein modulates host purine metabolism in intestine through gut microbiota and ameliorates experimental colitis. *Theranostics* **2020**, *10*, 10665–10679. [CrossRef] [PubMed]
49. Coker, O.O.; Liu, C.; Wu, W.K.K.; Wong, S.H.; Jia, W.; Sung, J.; Yu, J. Altered gut metabolites and microbiota interactions are implicated in colorectal carcinogenesis and can be non-invasive diagnostic biomarkers. *Microbiome* **2022**, *10*, 35. [CrossRef] [PubMed]
50. Wang, X.; Zhang, P.; Zhang, X. Probiotics Regulate Gut Microbiota: An Effective Method to Improve Immunity. *Molecules* **2021**, *26*, 6076. [CrossRef] [PubMed]

Disclaimer/Publisher's Note: The statements, opinions and data contained in all publications are solely those of the individual author(s) and contributor(s) and not of MDPI and/or the editor(s). MDPI and/or the editor(s) disclaim responsibility for any injury to people or property resulting from any ideas, methods, instructions or products referred to in the content.

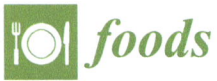

Review

Research Review on Quality Detection of Fresh Tea Leaves Based on Spectral Technology

Ting Tang [1], Qing Luo [1], Liu Yang [1], Changlun Gao [1], Caijin Ling [2,*] and Weibin Wu [1,*]

[1] College of Engineering, South China Agricultural University, Guangzhou 510642, China; 20203163056@stu.scau.edu.cn (T.T.); luoyq@scau.edu.cn (Q.L.); yl1009496755@163.com (L.Y.); gao666@stu.scau.edu.cn (C.G.)

[2] Tea Research Institute, Guangdong Academy of Agricultural Sciences, Guangzhou 510640, China

* Correspondence: lingcaijin@163.com (C.L.); wuweibin@scau.edu.cn (W.W.)

Abstract: As the raw material for tea making, the quality of tea leaves directly affects the quality of finished tea. The quality of fresh tea leaves is mainly assessed by manual judgment or physical and chemical testing of the content of internal components. Physical and chemical methods are more mature, and the test results are more accurate and objective, but traditional chemical methods for measuring the biochemical indexes of tea leaves are time-consuming, labor-costly, complicated, and destructive. With the rapid development of imaging and spectroscopic technology, spectroscopic technology as an emerging technology has been widely used in rapid non-destructive testing of the quality and safety of agricultural products. Due to the existence of spectral information with a low signal-to-noise ratio, high information redundancy, and strong autocorrelation, scholars have conducted a series of studies on spectral data preprocessing. The correlation between spectral data and target data is improved by smoothing noise reduction, correction, extraction of feature bands, and so on, to construct a stable, highly accurate estimation or discrimination model with strong generalization ability. There have been more research papers published on spectroscopic techniques to detect the quality of tea fresh leaves. This study summarizes the principles, analytical methods, and applications of Hyperspectral imaging (HSI) in the nondestructive testing of the quality and safety of fresh tea leaves for the purpose of tracking the latest research advances at home and abroad. At the same time, the principles and applications of other spectroscopic techniques including Near-infrared spectroscopy (NIRS), Mid-infrared spectroscopy (MIRS), Raman spectroscopy (RS), and other spectroscopic techniques for non-destructive testing of quality and safety of fresh tea leaves are also briefly introduced. Finally, in terms of technical obstacles and practical applications, the challenges and development trends of spectral analysis technology in the nondestructive assessment of tea leaf quality are examined.

Keywords: fresh tea leaves; hyperspectral imaging technology; spectroscopy; analytic method

Citation: Tang, T.; Luo, Q.; Yang, L.; Gao, C.; Ling, C.; Wu, W. Research Review on Quality Detection of Fresh Tea Leaves Based on Spectral Technology. Foods 2024, 13, 25. https://doi.org/10.3390/foods13010025

Academic Editor: Corrado Costa

Received: 22 November 2023
Revised: 13 December 2023
Accepted: 18 December 2023
Published: 20 December 2023

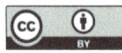

Copyright: © 2023 by the authors. Licensee MDPI, Basel, Switzerland. This article is an open access article distributed under the terms and conditions of the Creative Commons Attribution (CC BY) license (https:// creativecommons.org/licenses/by/ 4.0/).

1. Introduction

The tea tree belongs to the tea group of plants in the genus Camellias of the family Camelliaceae. Tea tree is an important economic crop. Especially for the current stage of China, the tea industry is an important treasure to promote China's agricultural economic development and rural revitalization. China has a long history of tea culture and is a large country in terms of plantation production and consumption. According to the statistics of the China Tea Circulation Association, from 2011 to 2022, the area of tea plantation, the total annual output of dry gross tea, and the total annual output value of dry gross tea have increased by 157.6%, 196.0%, and 404.2%, respectively [1]. There are more than 700 known chemical components in tea. These include primary metabolites of proteins, sugars, fats, and secondary metabolites in the tea tree—polyphenols, pigments, theanines, alkaloids, aromatic substances, and saponins. They not only affect the formation of tea color, aroma, and flavor but also play an important role in the nutritional and health effects of tea [2]. Tea's main uses include waking up, sleeping, relieving fever, aiding in digestion, decreasing gas, expectoration, treating fistulas, facilitating urination, facilitating the large intestine, decreasing miasma, clearing the head and eyes, helping with dysentery, facilitating the small intestine, decreasing headaches, sores, stroke, and sunstroke, aiding in sobriety, and so on [3]. Often used as an herbal remedy throughout history, tea has evolved into a popular beverage that has tremendous economic, health, and cultural value in the marketplace. With the spread and development of tea culture, consumers are demanding more and more regarding the quality of tea. Nowadays, the quality of tea is mainly assessed by sensory review, physical and chemical testing, and emerging technological testing [4].

The sensory quality of tea refers to the comprehensive effect of the many compounds in tea, especially the substances that can be dissolved in tea broth, on the sensory stimulation of the human body. It is mainly composed of appearance, color, aroma, taste, and other factors. Shape and color are the external factors of tea quality, while aroma and taste are the internal core quality factors of tea. The evaluation of tea quality through the sensory review method requires the reviewer to undergo a long period of training and a lot of experience. In addition, the review results are subject to a review of the environment, individual sensory sensitivity differences, and other factors of interference and influence, resulting in the review of the results possessing strong subjectivity. Physical testing techniques mainly include the use of an electronic balance and oven to determine the quality and moisture content of tea leaves. The observation and analysis of the phenotype and structure of tea leaves have been carried out using a microscope [5,6]. Conventional chemical detection techniques mainly include High-Performance Liquid Chromatography (HPLC), Gas Chromatography (GC), Mass Spectrometry (MS), Gas Chromatography-Mass Spectrometry (GC-MS), and the titrimetric method [7]. They are diagnostic analytical methods to detect the content of compounds in tea at the molecular level. These are usually used in combination with emerging techniques such as HSI, MIRS, RS, NIRS, and other scientific techniques. Physicochemical testing techniques are more mature, with more accurate and objective results, which are necessary for the quantitative evaluation of tea quality. However, traditional chemical methods need to be coupled with chemical reagents to titrate the reaction or need to be observed and analyzed with the aid of chromatographic instruments to analyze tea broth preparation after extraction and separation [8]. This method of measuring plant biochemical indicators is time-consuming, labor-costly, and complicated to operate [9]. As a result, the realization and development of tea quality monitoring has been severely constrained. In recent years, researchers have been exploring fast and accurate techniques to monitor tea quality. RGB imaging, multispectral imaging, HSI, nuclear magnetic resonance imaging (NMRI), NIRS, RS, electronic noses, electronic tongues, etc. are often applied in emerging technologies to realize non-destructive and rapid detection of tea quality.

As the raw material for tea production, the quality of tea leaves directly affects the quality of finished tea. The ratios of polyphenols to amino acids, polysaccharides, and caffeine content of tea leaves are one of the most important factors affecting the aroma, nutrition, and color of finished tea, while the fiber content determines the tenderness of tea leaves [10]. Non-destructive monitoring of the quality and material content of fresh tea leaves in situ can not only accurately grasp the growth of the tea tree but also assist in the decision-making process of tea-picking programs to ensure the quality of tea leaves [11]. Spectroscopic detection technology is widely used in rapid non-destructive testing of the quality and safety of agricultural products due to its advantages of rapidity, accuracy, and on-line real-time detection [12–14]. Spectral analysis is a qualitative and quantitative analysis of the composition of a sample using the unique absorption or emission spectral features of different substances in different spectral ranges. Due to its advantages of rapid, non-destructive, multiple simultaneous testing, and portability, spectral analysis finds wide applications in the quality testing of fresh tea leaves. At present, the most commonly used spectral analysis methods include HSI, NIRS, MIRS, Terahertz spectroscopy (THz), RS, and Fluorescence spectroscopy (FS).

NIRS obtains information by measuring the absorption and reflection of Near-infrared (NIR) light from a sample. NIR light is absorbed in the frequency band associated with molecular vibrations and chemical bonding and, therefore, provides information about the composition of the sample. MIRS focuses on the mid-infrared band and provides information on molecular vibrations and the rotation of matter. Different molecules and the bonds between them are uniquely characterized in the mid-infrared spectrum. The THz band is located between the microwave and infrared bands, which is highly penetrating. This is suitable for studying crystal structures, plant cell walls, moisture, and more. RS provides information about molecular vibrations and rotations based on the frequency shift of the light that is scattered from the sample. It has both high sensitivity and resolution. FS is based on the fluorescence signal emitted by the sample when exposed to excited light and is used to analyze fluorescently active substances. It is sensitive to biomolecules and pigments. These spectroscopic techniques help in the study of the chemical structure of fresh tea leaves' moisture, aroma composition, and pigment composition determination. Although these spectroscopic techniques have a wide range of applications in tea research, HSI is able to provide both rich spectral information and high-resolution spatial information. This grants HSI unique advantages in tea research in terms of quality assessment, authenticity identification, and growth environment monitoring. In addition, hyperspectral reflectance data, mid-infrared spectral data, Raman data, and terahertz data are all acquired by spectral techniques, and generally speaking, the steps of their data processing all include noise reduction, dimensionality reduction, feature extraction, and modeling. The data analysis of HSI includes image information analysis in addition to spectral information analysis. Therefore, in this paper, in order to keep readers abreast of the latest spectral technology at home and abroad in tea fresh leaves and the research and application progress, through China's knowledge network and the Web of Science literature database, this study employs the key words tea fresh leaves and spectral collation to review the last ten years of relevant literature. This study focuses on the principle of HSI technology, the analysis method, and its application in the non-destructive evaluation of the quality and safety of fresh tea leaves. At the same time, the principles and applications of other spectroscopic techniques are briefly introduced, including the application of MIRS, NIRS, RS, and other spectroscopic techniques in the nondestructive testing of the quality and safety of fresh tea leaves. Finally, the challenges and development trends of spectral analysis techniques in nondestructive testing of tea quality are discussed in terms of technical difficulties and practical applications.

2. Spectral Technology

2.1. Hyperspectral Imaging Technology

HSI is a combination of spectral detection technology and image technology. The difference between active and passive hyperspectral techniques is whether an active light source is required. Depending on the hyperspectral imaging method, the active hyperspectral imaging system is divided into four categories, namely swing-sweep, push-sweep, condensed acquisition, and snapshot [15]. The core devices of active hyperspectral imaging systems are generally light sources, spectroscopic elements, detectors, and data acquisition and processing systems [16]. Its working principle diagram is shown in Figure 1. The light source is an important part of an active hyperspectral imaging spectroscopy system. The three commonly used light sources are tungsten halogen lamps, quantum cascade lasers, and light-emitting diodes. The spectroscopic elements are mainly diffraction gratings and tunable filters. Detectors are key devices for converting optical signals into electrical signals in hyperspectral imaging systems. Currently, there are two main types of detectors used in hyperspectral imaging systems, namely line array detectors and surface array detectors. Optical signals can be converted into analog current signals, which are amplified, and the modulus to digital conversion of the current signals is used to acquire images. Data acquisition and processing systems are used to acquire spectral images collected from the camera and process and analyze these images.

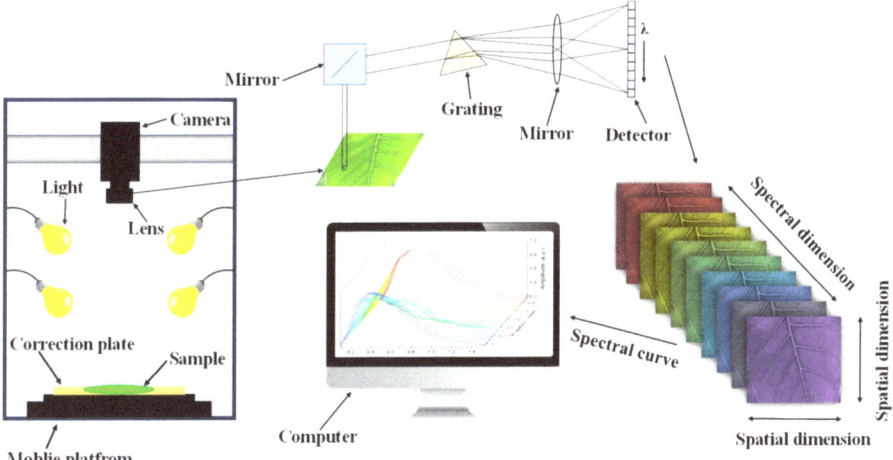

Figure 1. HSI working principle diagram.

While imaging the spatial features of the analyzed target, each spatial pixel is dispersed into dozens or even hundreds of narrow bands to achieve continuous spectral coverage [17]. Spectroscopic detection techniques utilize a series of spectral bands in a narrow wavelength range to capture spectral information reflected or emitted by an object. These bands typically include wavelengths in the visible, infrared, and ultraviolet ranges. Each band captures a different spectral signature of the object, thus providing detailed spectral data. Hyperspectral images are acquired through the use of hyperspectral cameras or sensors. These devices are capable of capturing images in a variety of wavelength ranges, often including hundreds to thousands of spectral channels [18]. Due to its benefits of high-spectrum resolution and the capacity to offer image and spectral information, HSI has steadily become a research hotspot and has been employed in a wide range of applications, including the quality inspection of fresh tea leaves. It mainly includes analyzing the chemical composition of tea, identifying the type and origin of tea, and detecting impurities.

2.2. Other Spectroscopic Technologies

The NIRS and MIRS components mainly include an optical system, a detector, signal acquisition, and a processing module [1]. The working principle of the infrared spectroscopy system is shown in Figure 2. NIRS is a technique used to determine which functional groups are contained in a molecule based on the characteristic frequencies of the infrared absorption spectra, thus identifying unknown classes of compounds for qualitative analysis [19]. MIRS is composed of molecules with vibrational fundamental frequencies, multiple and broad absorption bands, high absorption intensities, and significant absorption characteristics that provide more information about frequencies and intensities. Most of the characteristic vibrational peaks of typical functional groups are distributed in the mid-infrared region [2]. Compared with NIRS, it has the advantages of relatively easy modeling and stable results. The in situ RS test system mainly consists of a Raman spectrometer, a Raman optical system, and a sample detection chamber [3]. The working schematic of the RS system is shown in Figure 3. RS and infrared spectroscopy are complementary to each other. Infrared spectroscopy is suitable for studying the polar bonding vibrations of different atoms, while RS is suitable for studying the non-polar bonding vibrations of the same atom [20].

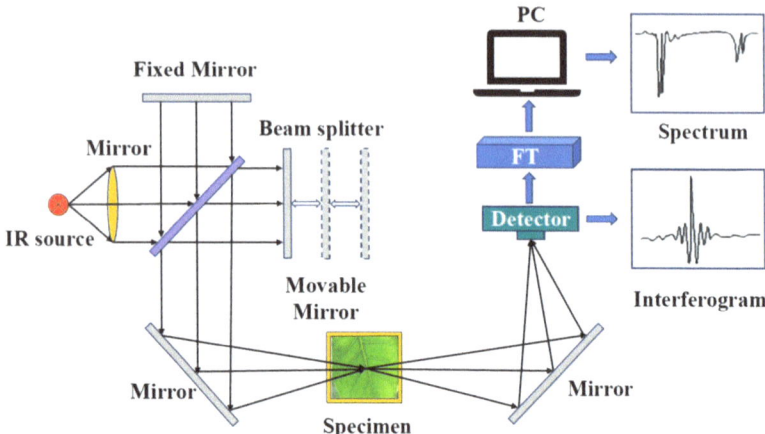

Figure 2. Infrared spectrometer working principle diagram.

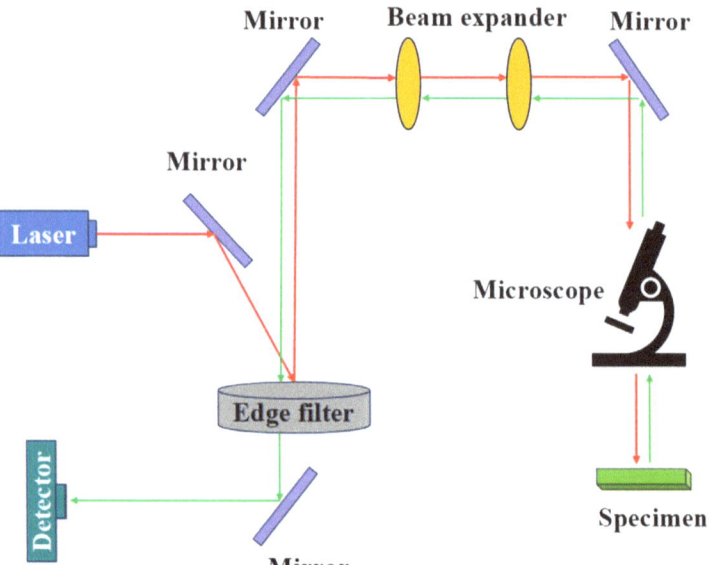

Figure 3. RS working principle diagram.

The THz system consists of a dual-laser-controlled intelligent electronic device, two distributed feedback lasers, and two fast scanning modes [4]. Its working schematic is shown in Figure 4. THz evaluates terahertz light using absorption, reflection, transmission, and other properties of a substance, which can be used for qualitative analysis of compounds [21]. The principle is to analyze the components of a mixture in the THz by using the absorption and transmission properties of a substance based on its absorption spectrum, refraction spectrum, dielectric coefficient, and other properties. The FS system consists of an excitation light source and a spectrometer [7]. Its working schematic is shown in Figure 5. FS is a method of quantitative and qualitative substance analysis based on the phenomenon of photoluminescence of substances and the investigation of fluorescence characteristics and intensity. [22]. Fluorescent compounds with different structures have unique excitation and emission spectra. Therefore, the shapes and peak positions of the excitation and emission spectra of fluorescent substances can be compared with the spectrograms of standard solutions for qualitative analysis. At low concentrations, the fluorescence intensity of a solution is proportional to the concentration of the fluorescent substance: $F = Kc$, where F is the fluorescence intensity, c is the concentration of the fluorescent substance, and K is the scale factor, which is the basis for the quantitative analysis of fluorescence spectra [23].

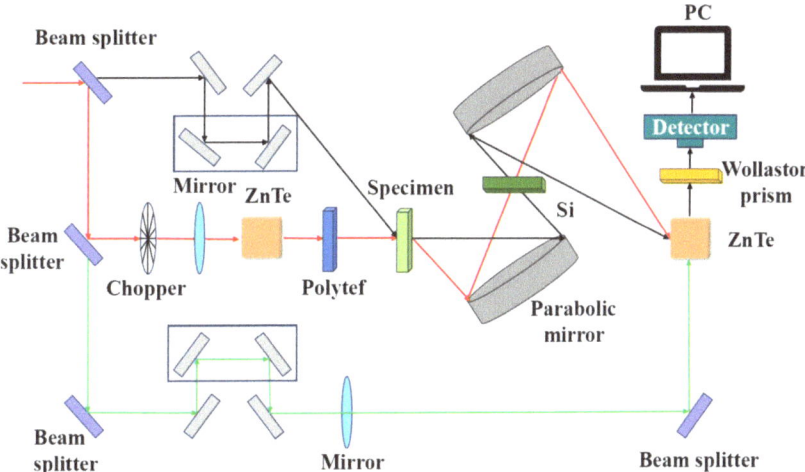

Figure 4. THz working principle diagram.

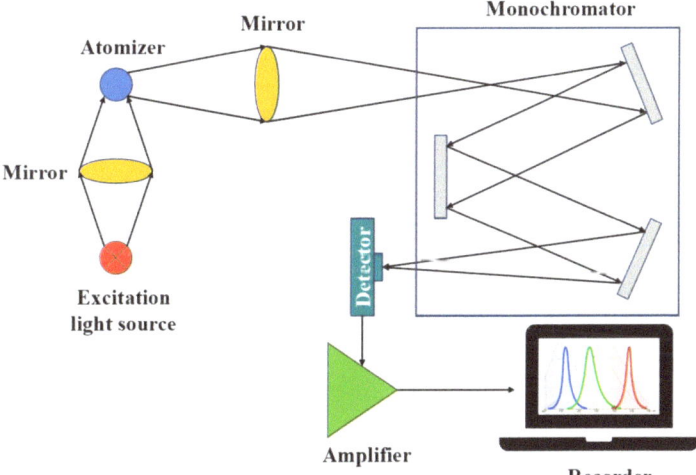

Figure 5. FS working principle diagram.

In Table 1, the advantages and disadvantages of several spectroscopic techniques are compared. In the analysis of tea fresh leaves, these spectroscopic techniques can be applied to study pigments, antioxidant substances, functional components, aroma substances, and the molecular structure of tea.

Table 1. Comparative analysis table of spectroscopic techniques.

Spectral Technology	Wavelength (nm)	Technical Principle	Benefits	Shortcomings
NIRS	780–2500	multiple- and combined-frequency absorption of vibrations of hydrogen-containing groups X-H (X = C, N, O) [24].	high penetration depth, weak background signal interference, high spatial, and temporal resolution [25].	spectral data processing is complex and susceptible to moisture interference [26].
MIRS	2500–25,000	absorption of functional groups in molecules that exhibit violent fundamental frequency vibrations in the mid-infrared band [27].	high absorption intensity, high sensitivity, no sample pretreatment required.	shallow penetration depth, susceptible to moisture interference.
THz	30,000–3,000,000	absorption of molecular vibrations and rotations in the terahertz band [28].	low photon energy, good penetration, wide frequency range, and high characterization capability.	time-consuming and expensive equipment [29].
RS	/	molecular vibration information is obtained by utilizing the frequency shift and intensity change of scattered light when the sample interacts with the laser light source [30].	efficient, non-destructive and moisture free.	susceptible to fluorescence, high background signal interference, weak signal [31].
FS	200–800	characterization of fluorescence and its intensity based on the phenomenon of photoluminescence of a substance.	high sensitivity, selectivity and ease of use [32].	not widely enough applied, environmentally sensitive [33].

3. Hyperspectral Information Analysis Method for Tea Fresh Leaf Quality Testing

Hyperspectral information includes one-dimensional spectral information and two-dimensional spatial (image) information [34]. Spectral information can reflect the internal structure of the sample such as the molecular composition and can be applied for the quantitative and qualitative analysis of tea fresh leaves. Image information can reflect the external quality characteristics such as size, shape, and defects of the sample, which can be made use of for a qualitative examination of tea fresh leaves. The fusion of spectral and image technologies can not only study the internal composition content of the analyzed object but also visualize and analyze its distribution, which can be employed to capture the spectral information and spatial distribution of the target object.

3.1. Spectral Information Analysis

Raw spectral data usually need to undergo some pre-processing and analysis before they can be used for specific research or applications. The main reason for this is that its acquisition may be affected by a variety of interfering factors such as noise, baseline drift, light scattering, etc. [35]. Therefore, the data need to be processed for noise reduction as well as baseline correction. In addition, the raw data may contain a large amount of redundant information or unnecessary details, and the key information needs to be extracted using the feature band selection method. Furthermore, the analysis phase requires modeling according to the research objectives in order to obtain the required information or conclusions from the data. The steps of spectral data parsing include data preprocessing, feature band extraction, modeling, and model evaluation.

3.1.1. Spectral Data Preprocessing

Spectral data preprocessing is a key step before analyzing spectral data, aiming at eliminating interference and improving data quality for subsequent analysis. Spectral data preprocessing mainly includes normalization, baseline correction, and noise reduction. The normalization method balances the distribution of variables and mean values by scaling the components of the data to a relatively consistent scale, which can attenuate the influence of factors such as light-range variation and sample sparsity on spectral information [36]. The normalization methods are Max-Min Normalization (MMN) and Vector Normalization (VN) [37,38]. MMN is a linear mapping of data to a specified range, usually [0, 1]. This process involves two key values: minimum (min) and maximum (max). By linearly transforming the data points, the min value is mapped to 0, the max value to 1, and the values in between will be distributed equiprimordially over this range. VN, on the other hand, distinguishes MMN, which, instead of mapping the data to a specific range, normalizes the data by changing its magnitude and direction. Its goal is to map data points to unit vectors.

Baseline correction is mainly used to correct the baseline shift problem in spectroscopy due to measurement variations of spectroscopic instruments or changes in measurement environment parameters [39]. Baseline correction methods include multiple scattering correction (MSC), standard normal variation (SNV), detrending (DT), orthogonal signal correction (OSC), and moving average (MA) [40–44]. The MSC method is used to correct the baseline translation and offset phenomena of spectral data by ideal spectra, which can effectively eliminate the scattering phenomena generated by uneven particle distribution and particle size, thus enhancing the correlation between spectra and data [45]. Similar to MSC, the SNV can also be used to correct the spectral errors caused by scattering between samples, but the algorithms are different. SNV is the process of subtracting the spectral value of each sample from the mean of the spectral value of that sample and dividing it by the standard deviation of the spectral value of that sample. This makes the processed spectral data conform to the standard normal distribution. It is mainly employed to eliminate the effects of diffuse reflections due to solid particle size, surface scattering, and variations in optical range [46]. Moreover, OSC is also used to eliminate errors arising from the surface scattering and baseline drift of spectral signals [47]. OSC is used to remove the information in the spectral matrix that is not related to the components to be measured by orthogonal projection and then carry out multivariate correction calculation. After achieving the purpose of simplifying the model, it then improves the predictive ability of the model [48]. MA is used to take the average of the data in a certain time period and use this average to represent the data in that time period, thus achieving the purpose of smoothing the data [49]. Spectral data contain information about the sample, but there may be some unrelated underlying trends in the data. These trends can be long-term variations in the data, usually related to time. They can also be trends due to other factors, such as temperature changes, instrument drift, etc. DT removes the trend or drift from the data [50]. DT usually involves fitting a trend model. Examples include linear regression or polynomial fitting, and then subtracting the estimates of this model from the raw data to obtain corrected data [51].

Noise reduction processing is performed by using various signal processing techniques and mathematical algorithms in order to remove or reduce the noise and retain the useful signal. Some of the methods for noise reduction are Savitzky–Golay smoothing (SG), first-order derivative (FD), second-order derivative (SD), Fourier Transform (FT), and Wavelet Transform (WT) [52–54]. SG smoothing reduces noise by smoothing the signal using a polynomial fit within a sliding window [55]. In addition, different window sizes and numbers of polynomials can be selected to balance the smoothing and noise suppression effects according to practical needs. The adaptability of SG smoothing methods to noise suppression and smoothing operations has led to their widespread use in spectral analysis. SG smoothing is often combined with FD and second-order derivatives for noise reduction in raw spectral data. The FD is the rate of change of the original signal and represents the slope or gradient in the signal. By calculating the FD, rapid changes or edges in the signal can be highlighted, thus helping to detect features and boundaries in the signal. The FD can help reduce high-frequency noise in a signal. The SD is the rate of change of the FD, which indicates the curvature in the signal. Calculating the SD helps to highlight features in the signal more strongly, especially spikes or troughs in the signal. This helps in identifying extreme points in the signal. SD can further reduce high-frequency noise and provide clearer information about features. The FT converts a signal from the time domain to the frequency domain, thereby breaking the signal into components of different frequencies. High- or low-frequency components can be selectively filtered out to extract the signal components of interest and reduce the effect of noise. Compared to FT, WT is a more flexible tool for signal analysis, as it is capable of local and multi-scale analysis of spectral data. The WT is used to effectively reduce noise and improve the signal-to-noise ratio of spectral data by decomposing the signal into wavelet functions at different scales and by analyzing and processing the different frequency components of the signal while retaining useful feature information. This makes spectral data easier to interpret and utilize. In Table 2, the characteristics and advantages and disadvantages of various pretreatment methods are summarized.

Table 2. Comparison table of different pretreatment methods.

Preprocessing	Methodologies	Specificities	Advantages	Disadvantages
normalization	MMN	linear scale	simple calculation	sensitivity to outliers
	VN	resizing vectors	maintaining spectral features	dependent on the selected spectral range
baseline correction	MSC	detection and correction of multiple scattering signals in spectra	eliminating the effect of multiple scattering on spectral data	computationally complex
	SNV	linear transformation	data standardized and easily interpretable	not applicable to non-normal distributions
	DT	eliminating trend	reducing the interference of trends in analysis	information loss
	OSC	orthogonal transform	elimination of cross-interference	higher real-time requirements
	MA	calculation of the average value	trend identification, noise reduction	produce lagged effect
noise reduction	SG	polynomial fitting	excellent fitting effect	computationally complex
	FD	calculating the rate of change	highlighting trends and changes in data	increased noise in the data
	SD	calculating curvature	highlighting curvature and variation in data	enhanced noise sensitivity
	FT	frequency and time domain transformation	ability to handle cyclical data	computationally complex
	WT	wavelet functions converted to different scales	capable of handling non-stationary and non-linear signals	complexity of processing

3.1.2. Characteristic Band Screening

Since raw data may contain a lot of irrelevant information, feature band selection can help identify and enhance task-relevant information [56]. This helps to improve the interpretability of the data. Also, feature band selection can reduce the dimensionality of the data, thus reducing the cost of data storage and processing. The selection of representative feature bands can reduce the size of the dataset without losing important information. The methods for feature band selection are stepwise discriminant analysis (SDA), the successive projection algorithm (SPA), the competitive adaptive reweighting algorithm (CARS), the genetic algorithm (GA), principal component analysis (PCA), random frog (RF), and Monte Carlo-uninformative variable elimination (MC-UVE) [57–63].

The goal of SDA is to improve classification accuracy by selecting the most relevant variables while reducing unnecessary dimensions. This helps to reduce the risk of overfitting and improve the generalization ability of the model. The SPA is a forward variable selection algorithm that eliminates redundant information in the original spectral matrix and minimizes the covariance of the variables in the spectrum [64]. CARS is a variable selection algorithm based on PLS and the Darwinian evolutionary principle of "survival of the fittest", which filters the wavelengths by the size of absolute regression coefficients and excludes the variable bands with small weights [65]. The GA is an optimization algorithm that simulates the biological evolution process and is applied to solve complex optimization problems. Through constant selection, crossover, and mutation operations, the GA can search for combinations of feature bands with high adaptation, thus realizing the extraction of feature bands of spectral data [66]. PCA is a commonly used dimensionality reduction technique, which transforms the original data into a new set of orthogonal variables called principal components by linear transformation [67]. In spectral data feature band extraction, PCA can be employed to find the principal components that contribute most to the variability of the data and use them as feature bands. The key to the RF is continuous iteration, where a subset of features is gradually improved through natural selection and randomness operations to find the optimal combination of feature bands for classification, regression, or other data analysis tasks. The MC-UVE method utilizes Monte Carlo sampling methods to estimate the informativeness of individual bands in spectral data, which helps to identify bands that are informative for a specific task, and then the uninformative variables are eliminated to extract the final set of feature bands [68]. In Table 3, the characteristics and advantages and disadvantages of each feature extraction method are listed.

Table 3. Comparison table of feature extraction methods.

Method	Specificities	Advantages	Disadvantages
SDA	stepwise selection and exclusion of variables	reduced data dimensions	data sensitivity
SPA	continuous-projection iterative computation	elimination of redundant information	noise sensitivity
CARS	dynamically adjusting feature weights	enhances image contrast and detail	sensitivity to noise and artifacts
GA	simulation of biological evolutionary processes	For high-dimensional data	higher computational costs, results dependent on parameterization
PCA	linear transformation	reduced data dimensions	loss of partial detail information
RF	simulating a frog jumping randomly to find an optimal solution	reduced computational complexity and risk of overfitting	unstable results
MC-UVE	simulation of Monte Carlo Sampling	no a priori information required	noise sensitivity

3.1.3. Model Building

Spectral data modeling typically includes categorical modeling and regression modeling. Both classification modeling and regression modeling use statistical and machine-learning techniques to process spectral data for different purposes. Classification modeling is used to classify data into different categories and can be applied in the qualitative analysis of fresh tea leaf quality testing. Regression modeling is used to predict continuous output values, which can be applied in the quantitative analysis of fresh tea leaf quality testing. The methods for classification modeling are the Random Forest Classifier (RF), the K Nearest Neighbor Classifier (KNN), the Linear Discriminant Classifier (LDC), Support Vector Machines (SVMs), Extreme Learning Machines (ELMs), and the Naive Bayes Classifier (NB) [69–73]. Methods for regression modeling are Partial Least Squares Regression (PLSR), Multiple Linear Regression (MLR), Support Vector Regression (SVR), Extreme Learning Machine Regression (ELMR), Gaussian Process Regression (GPR), Stochastic Gradient

Boosting (SGB), Kernel-based Extreme Learning Machines (KELM)s, and Random Forest Regression (RFR) [74–78].

The RF classifier is used to classify by integrating multiple decision tree models by voting or averaging. The KNN classifier makes classification decisions based on the neighbors of the data points. It is based on the assumption that the training samples that are close to a particular data point have similar category labels. Therefore, the KNN classifier decides the category of a new data point by summing the category labels of the K nearest neighbors weighted according to the distance [79]. The main goal of the LDC is to maximize the separation between different categories by maximizing the variance between categories and minimizing the variance within categories [80]. This makes it perform well in many classification problems, especially when the separation between categories is high. However, a limitation of the LDC is that it assumes that the data follow a multivariate normal distribution and are not applicable to nonlinear problems. For nonlinear problems, it is often necessary to use other classification methods such as SVM. The basic idea of SVM is to map the sample feature data into an n-dimensional space, where the size of n depends on the kernel function and the number of sample feature dimensions, and then construct the optimal classification hyperplane in the space [69]. A Naive Bayes Classifier uses Bayes' theorem to estimate the posterior probability of each category for a given feature case and then selects the category with the highest posterior probability as the final classification result [81,82]. ELM is a fast and simple machine learning algorithm that achieves classification or regression tasks by randomly initializing the weights of hidden layer neurons and then training a linear output layer.

PLSR is particularly suitable for high-dimensional datasets and situations where multicollinearity problems exist. It reduces the dimensionality of the data by finding the combination of independent variables that has the highest correlation with the dependent variable, which better captures the structure of the data and builds the regression model [74,83]. MLR is a statistical method widely employed to build regression models to analyze and predict the relationship between the dependent variable and one or more independent variables. SVMR maximizes the interval between the training samples and the hyperplane by finding the optimal hyperplane in the feature space for the prediction of continuous target variables [75,84]. ELMR achieves better performance with single training by random initialization and fixing the input layer weights. KELM is an extension of the traditional ELM that introduces the kernel trick, which enables the ELM to handle nonlinear problems. GPR is a nonparametric model that utilizes a Gaussian process prior to regression analysis of input data. SGB works by integrating multiple decision trees, each trained based on a randomly selected subset of data and a subset of features, and finally voting or averaging to obtain a combined result. RFR regresses by constructing multiple decision trees and averaging them [78]. In Table 4, this paper organizes the characteristics and advantages and disadvantages of each classification model and regression model.

3.1.4. Model Evaluation

The common evaluation criteria of model prediction performance are the prediction set correlation coefficient (R_P), the correction set correlation coefficient (R_C), the coefficient of determination (R^2), prediction standard deviation ($RMSEP$), correction standard deviation ($RESEC$), and residual prediction deviation (RPD). The R_P is a measure of the correlation between the model's predictions on the prediction set and the actual observations. The correlation coefficient can take values between -1 and 1, with closer to 1 indicating that the model's predictions are more correlated with the actual values. In some fields, a correlation coefficient of 0.7 or higher may be considered good predictive performance. In practice, it is usually desirable to be close to 1. The R_C is a measure of the correlation between the model's predictions on the correction set and the actual observations. Again, closer to 1 indicates better performance. However, an R_C that is too high may show signs of overfitting. In general, an R_C in the range of 0.7 to 0.9 may be a more appropriate range [85]. The R^2 is a measure of how well the model fits the observed data. It takes a value between

0 and 1 and indicates the proportion of variance of the target variable that is explained by the model. The closer the value is to 1, the better the model fits the observed data and is able to explain more of the variance. In some fields, a value above 0.7 may be considered a better fit. Higher values are required for applications where high precision is required. RMSEP is a measure of how discrete the model's prediction error is over the prediction set. It is usually asserted that the smaller this value is, the better, indicating that the model's predictions are more stable. The RESEC is a measure of how discrete the model's prediction error is on the calibration set [86]. Again, it is desired that this value be as small as possible. Residual prediction bias indicates how much the model's predictions in the prediction set deviate from the actual observations. A smaller bias indicates that the model is more accurate.

Table 4. Comparison table between each classification model and regression model.

Types	Method	Specificities	Advantages	Disadvantages
classification modeling	LD	finding linear decision boundaries	effective dimensionality reduction and categorization of data	sensitivity to outliers
	KNN	voting mechanism based on neighboring samples	for multi-category and non-linear problems	noise sensitivity
	RF	integration based on multiple decision trees	high accuracy and overfitting resistance	high memory and computing resource usage
	SVM	maximum margin criterion	ideal for handling high-dimensional data	computationally complex
	ELM	single hidden layer feed-forward neural network	fast training speed	handling nonlinear problems poorly
	NB	based on bayes theorem	simple and fast calculation	assumptions of independence of characteristics may not be realistic
regression Modeling	PLSR	minimizing the covariance	reducing dimensionality and multicollinearity	easily overfitted and sensitive to noise
	MLR	minimize the residual sum of squares	simple, highly interpretable	easily influenced by collinearity
	SVMR	maximum margin criterion	suitable for handling high-dimensional data	computationally complex
	ELM	single hidden layer feed-forward neural network	fast training speeds	handling nonlinear problems poorly
	KELM	single-layer neural networks combined with kernel tricks	efficient handling of non-linear problems	computationally complex
	GPR	based on Bayesian theory and statistical learning theory	suitable for dealing with high-dimensional data, nonlinear problems	computationally complex
	SGB	Integration based on several decision trees	efficient handling of large-scale data	noise sensitivity
	RFR	Integration based on multiple decision trees	high robustness	noise sensitivity

3.2. Image Information Parsing

Hyperspectral image information-parsing methods include region of interest selection, image correction, dimensionality reduction, and modeling. In the study of HSI features, it is usually necessary to select the region of interest (ROI) on the leaves of fresh tea. The selection of ROI can help to reduce the dimensionality of the data, reduce the amount of computation, and focus on a specific region for detailed analysis. Black and white correction of raw images is required to eliminate noise interference and other light source interference in the camera [87]. HSI has high dimensionality and redundant data, resulting in a time-consuming computational process. There is an urgent need for dimensionality reduction processing of hyperspectral data. The methods of dimensionality reduction processing mainly include feature selection and feature extraction. Feature selection is feature band selection [88]. In order to extract the spatial texture features of the image, feature extraction of the hyperspectral image is also required. Texture feature extraction methods include the Gray-Level Co-occurrence Matrix (GLCM), the Gray-Level Difference Matrix (GLDM), the Autocorrelation Function (AF), the Local Binary Pattern (LBP), and the Wavelet transform (WT) [85–87]. The GLCM is a statistical tool used to describe the texture of an image. It calculates the gray-level symbiosis between pixels in an image, including information such as the angle, the distance, and gray-level differences. The GLDM is used to measure the differences between gray levels in an image. The AF measures the correlation of gray values between pixels in an image. The LBP is a nonparametric method used for the analysis of image texture. It encodes image texture features by comparing the gray values of a pixel with its neighboring pixels and then LBP histograms or other statistical information can be computed. The WT can be used to capture multi-scale texture information in hyperspectral images. Image spatial texture feature extraction can capture the detailed information in the image, which helps to identify and distinguish different textures and improve the performance of image analysis and classification. After the image dimensionality reduction process, it then needs to be modeled and analyzed. The modeling method of image information is similar to Section 3.1.3 and will not be repeated here.

3.3. Information Analysis for Fusion of Image and Spectral

Fusion is the fitting of an image's spatial and spectral reflectance features into a single image. Thus, hyperspectral images integrate spectral and spatial texture features to optimize predictive capabilities. Typically, the fusion process can be performed at different levels, which can be categorized as signal level, pixel level, feature level, and decision level. Among them, signal-level image fusion is a problem of optimal concentration or distribution detection of signals and has the highest time and space requirements for alignment. Pixel-level fusion needs to process a large amount of data, which takes a relatively long time to process, is easily affected by noise, and cannot process data in real time. Decision-level fusion is the involvement of feature extraction of image data and some auxiliary information. This valuable information is combined to obtain a comprehensive decision-making result to improve recognition and interpretation. Feature-level fusion is used to extract the original information from the sensors, and then the feature information is comprehensively analyzed and processed, which can retain more original information [89]. Constructing a model after fusing features is similar to Section 3.1.3.

4. Application of Spectroscopic Techniques in Tea Fresh Leaf Quality Testing

4.1. Application of Hyperspectral Reflectance Information in Fresh Tea Leaf Quality Testing

4.1.1. Quantitative Analysis Applications

Based on hyperspectral reflectance information, many researchers have quantified the physicochemical constituents such as tea polyphenols, anthocyanins, carotenoids, and catechins of tea fresh leaves to evaluate the quality of tea fresh leaves. Zhang et al. selected SG, MA, and FTIR preprocessing methods for comparative analysis [75]. The PCA method was used to extract the characteristic bands. The estimation model of the relationship between spectral reflectance and tea polyphenol content of tea fresh leaves was established using MLR, ALR, and OLS. Among them, the least squares model had the highest accuracy, and the correlation coefficient of the prediction set was 0.99. It indicated that the prediction value of the tea polyphenol content in the test samples had a small error in the measured value, and it could be realized to estimate the tea polyphenol content of tea fresh leaves on-line by using hyperspectral technology. Anthocyanins are important chemical components of tea, which have a significant impact on the color, flavor, antioxidant properties, and medicinal value of tea. Therefore, the detection of anthocyanin content in tea fresh leaves is critical for assessing the quality and value of tea. Dai et al. applied four different pre-processing methods to eliminate the effects of unfavorable factors [76]. PLS models were established using the processed data. For total anthocyanins, the PLS model with MSC-S-G-FD treatment had the best Rp and RPD values and the lowest RMSEP, showing excellent predictive performance. Sonobe et al. and Wang et al. used the PROSPECT-D model and 2-Der-PLSR inversion to estimate the carotenoid content in tea fresh leaf blades, respectively [9,90]. The results showed that HSI combined with the variable selection method can be used as a fast and accurate method to predict carotenoid content. Kang et al. determined EC, EGC, ECG, and EGCG of catechins in green tea new shoots using hyperspectral imaging [40]. The PLSR model was used, and with few exceptions, hyperspectral reflectance explained more than 79% of each catechin in the new shoots. The moisture content of tea is an important indicator for the quality testing of fresh tea leaves and has a significant impact on both the quality and shelf life of tea. Dai et al. utilized four different algorithms (SG, MSC, SNV, and OSC) to preprocess the raw data, and used stepwise regression analysis to extract characteristic wavelengths from the preprocessed data. MLR and PLSR were used to establish the quantitative analysis model of the water content of tea fresh leaves [41]. The best prediction model was the SG-OSC-SW-PLSR model, and the correlation coefficients of the model correction set, cross-validation set, and prediction set were 0.8977, 0.8342, and 0.7749, respectively, and the minimum root-mean-square errors were 0.0091, 0.0311, and 0.0371, respectively. Both Wang et al. and Mao et al. used the SPA and competitive adaptive reweighted sampling selected feature wavelengths to establish a water content regression model [42,43]. The coefficients of determination of the models were all above 0.90, which can be used to evaluate the freshness of tea leaves and provide a basis for acquisition and tea withering. Sun et al. quantitatively assessed the water content of fresh tea leaves [91]. The most effective wavelengths were first extracted using four feature selection algorithms, SPA, CARS, SPA-sr, and CARS-sr. On this basis, a spectrum-based prediction model was established by using MLR after processing 20 different combinations of algorithms. The prediction coefficient of determination of the combined algorithms of SG-MSC and CARS-sr was 0.8631, and the $RMSE_P$ = 0.0163. The visualized distribution map of the tea leaves was able to more intuitively and comprehensively evaluate the water content of the tea leaves in each image element, which provided a new method for plant irrigation evaluation. It provides a new method for plant irrigation evaluation. It can be seen that hyperspectral technology can effectively realize the detection of water content in tea fresh leaves.

In addition, HSI data are widely used for the determination of nitrogen content and chlorophyll content of tea fresh leaves, which can provide a reference for the growth and fine management of tea plants. Nitrogen plays a pivotal role in the operation of tea plantations and has an important impact on the growth, productivity, and nutritional status of tea trees. Cao et al. proposed a method for estimating nitrogen content in tea tree fields based on the combination of a multispectral imaging system and hyperspectral data [92]. Firstly, 28 wavelengths were selected from hyperspectral data combined with 27 multispectral indices as raw data through competitive adaptive reweighted sampling. Subsequently, five variables were selected by variable combination. The results showed that the multispectral and hyperspectral data combined with SVR could effectively monitor soil nitrogen levels under field conditions, with R^2 and RMSE of 0.9186 and 0.0560, respectively. Wang et al. proposed the use of SNV to preprocess hyperspectral data of mature leaves of tea trees with different nitrogen applications [52]. PLSR was utilized to predict the nitrogen content. The results showed that the diagnostic accuracy of the LS-SVM model for different nitrogen applications and nitrogen status reached 82% and 92%, respectively, with a good prediction effect. Wang et al. proposed to estimate the nitrogen content by using wavelet coefficients extracted from the CWT technique with different decomposition layers of the CWT. Finally, the CWT (lscale)-VCPA method established the best model performance, and the R^2 of the model was 0.95 [53]. The accuracy was improved by 11% compared with the traditional spectral processing method. In situ determination of chlorophyll-b content as a marker for evaluating light stress and response to environmental changes in tea trees can be used to improve tea tree management. Sonobe et al. tested the performance of four machine learning algorithms, RF, SVM, Deep Belief Networks, and KELM, in evaluating tea data under different shade treatments [93]. The RMSE of KELM was 8.94 ± 3.05, showing the best performance. These results suggest that combining hyperspectral reflectance and KELM has the potential to track changes in the chlorophyll content of shaded tea leaves. Mao et al. determined the corresponding leaf physicochemical parameters and pre-processed the raw hyperspectral data collected using MSC, FD, and S-G algorithms [54]. After that, UVE and SPA were used to screen the pre-processed hyperspectral data for characteristic bands. Finally, CNN, SVM, and PLS were utilized to establish a quantitative prediction model for SPAD content. The best prediction model had an R^2 of 0.730.

The above study shows that for quantitative analysis of HSI reflectance data in fresh tea leaves, the commonly used data preprocessing methods are FD, SD, and SG smoothing, the feature selection is commonly used in CARS and SPA, and the models are PLSR and SVM. However, when measuring different indexes, it is necessary to screen out specific data preprocessing methods and estimation models in combination with the actual situation in order to ensure that rapid detection is realized.

4.1.2. Qualitative Analysis Applications

Qualitative studies on tea fresh leaves based on hyperspectral reflectance information have varietal classification and quality identification. Spectral information helps to capture small differences between varieties, thus giving unique spectral fingerprints to different tea varieties. Yan et al. used MSC and SNV for spectral preprocessing. The improved BP neural network, traditional BP neural network, and SVM fresh tea variety identification models were constructed. The results showed that the SVM model had the highest recognition accuracy of 96% [94]. Since different degrees of withering lead to changes in chemical composition and organizational structure in tea, these changes can be reflected in spectral data. Therefore, spectral information can help to realize the recognition of the degree of withering of tea leaves. Tu et al. collected hyperspectral data from the canopy of tea trees and classified tea varieties according to the spectral characteristics of the tea canopy [95]. Using appropriate spectral preprocessing methods, the overall accuracy of support vector machines for tea variety classification can reach more than 95%.

High-grade tea leaves have a high content of nutrients and low-grade tea leaves have relatively low content. Spectral analysis can be used to assess the quality and grade of tea by determining the content and proportion of chemical components in tea. Wang et al. combined hyperspectral technology with MBKA-Net for overall quality identification of tea leaves at different picking periods [17]. Firstly, the spectral information of six different tea-picking periods was obtained. Secondly, the MBKA method was proposed to realize the classification of tea leaves in different harvesting periods by effectively mining spectral features through multi-scale adaptive extraction. Ultimately, MBKA-Net obtained 96.18% correctness, 97.14% precision, and 97.18% recall. The study shows that the use of the variable screening method can effectively reduce the redundancy of hyperspectral information, simplify the model, and improve the model discrimination precision.

4.2. Application of Image and Spectral Information Fusion for Tea Fresh Leaf Quality Detection

HSI can provide detailed information on the surface microstructure and texture characteristics of tea leaves, but it has not been applied alone in the analysis of tea fresh leaf quality. It is often combined with hyperspectral reflectance information, and by fusing these two types of information, a more comprehensive and diverse set of tea leaf characteristics can be obtained. It is often applied for the qualitative analysis of tea leaves, including disease identification and variety classification.

Tea leaves usually have unique surface texture characteristics, and the change in hyperspectral image information after disease can distinguish healthy tea leaves from diseased ones and determine whether they are diseased or not. Lu et al. used hyperspectral images to identify white star disease and anthracnose in tea [96]. Preprocessing was first performed to select the best feature wavelengths for the spectral data using SPA. The diseases were then classified for prediction using SVM and ELM. The results showed that the prediction accuracy of the ELM model was higher than SVM with different kernel functions (RBF, Sigmod, and polynomial) in each disease category, and the recognition rate reached 90%. Yuan et al. proposed a new method for detecting anthracnose in tea trees based on hyperspectral imaging [97]. Two new disease indices, the tea anthracnose ratio index and the tea anthracnose normalized index, were first established based on sensitive bands. Based on the optimized spectral feature set, a disease scab detection strategy combining unsupervised classification and adaptive two-dimensional thresholding was proposed. The results showed that the overall accuracy of disease scab identification was 98% at the leaf level and 94% at the pixel level. Zhao proposed a multi-step plant adversity identification method based on HSI and CWT [98]. It was used to classify tea green leafhopper, anthracnose, and sunburn for anomaly detection. The method achieved an overall accuracy (OA) of 90.26~90.69%, with anthracnose having the highest OA (94.12~94.28%), followed by tea green leafhopper (93.99~94.20%), and sunburn having the lowest OA (82.50~83.91%).

Yan et al. used the fusion of image and spectral features as a tool for the recognition of Longjing fresh tea varieties [94]. The improved BP network was used to show the best performance, with a recognition accuracy of up to 100%, which was better than the results of analyzing with spectral features or images alone. Ning et al. used the data from the fusion of spectral and texture feature values as the input values of the LDA, SVM, and ELM models to establish a shriveling degree discriminative model [99]. When the fused data of combined spectral and textural eigenvalues were used as model inputs, the model was better than the model built based on a single eigenvalue. The overall discrimination rate reached 94.64%. The above studies have shown that the establishment of a characterization model for the integration of information is an important tool for the future use of hyperspectral "map-integrated" characterization.

4.3. Application of Other Spectroscopic Techniques in the Quality Testing of Fresh Tea Leaves

NIRS is widely used in quantitative and qualitative analyses of fresh tea leaves because of its sophisticated data processing methods, high accuracy, and reliability. In recent years, the effectiveness and accuracy of near-infrared spectroscopy have been fully verified in the detection of water content, catechins, caffeine, and other chemicals in tea, as well as the identification of tea varieties and the identification of tea quality. MIRS has a wide range of applications in chemical analysis and materials research, but relatively few applications in food and agriculture. Some studies have applied mid-infrared spectroscopy for the detection of dry matter, catechins, and caffeine content in tea, as well as the identification of tea varieties and the geographical origin of tea. However, due to the shallow penetration depth of the mid-infrared band, most of the studies on tea quality detection have been conducted in the near-infrared band. Compared with infrared spectroscopy, RS has the advantages of a wider determination range, convenient spectral analysis, favorable determination of aqueous solution, and simple preparation and processing of specimens. It is used to detect the carotenoid and chlorophyll content of fresh tea leaves. THz was characterized by low photon energy and good penetrability, and thus was used to detect the presence of tea stems, insects, and other foreign objects in tea. In recent years, FS has been widely used in the fields of tea grade evaluation, species differentiation, and heavy metal detection. Using FS at low concentrations, the fluorescence intensity of the solution is proportional to the concentration of the fluorescent substance. Therefore, FS was often used to detect the content of specific elements and important active ingredients in tea fresh leaves. This section summarizes the qualitative and quantitative studies of NIRS, MIRS, THz, RS, and FS in the quality detection of tea fresh leaves. It mainly includes variety identification, quality grading, disease discrimination, and the detection of tea polyphenols and other components' content, as shown in Table 5.

Table 5. Qualitative and quantitative studies of spectroscopic techniques in tea fresh leaf quality.

Spectroscopy	Quantitative Analysis	Qualitative Analysis
NIRS	moisture content [100,101], catechin, caffeine [102,103], theanine [104], nitrogen content [105], tea polyphenol [106], flavonoids [107], EGCG [108], Heavy metals [109].	Tea varieties [110], Tea quality grade [111,112], Tea maturity [113], Traceability of Tea Raw Materials [114], diseases [115], Tea tree growing environment [116].
MIRS	Dry Matter of Tea [117], Tea polyphenols, flavonoids [118]	Tea varieties identification [106,119]
THz	Tea tree cold injury detection [120].	Separation of tea leaves from foreign matter [121], Determination of the degree of oxidation of tea leaves [122].
RS	Carotenoid measurement [123,124], Chlorophyll measurement [125]	Quality Identification [126], Anthracnose Identification [127]
FS	Chlorophyll measurement [128]	Pesticide Residue Determination [129], Diagnosis of leaf spot disease [130].

5. Discussion

Based on the above literature, our discussion on the application of spectroscopic techniques in tea leaves mainly includes the rapid determination and prediction of tea leaf quality components such as tea polyphenols, carotenoids, and anthocyanins. We also included the classification of tea tree varieties, quality grading and quality identification of tea leaves, and the identification of tea tree pests and diseases. According to Table 6, we can see that in spectral data preprocessing, scholars mostly use SG, MSC, and SNV to smooth and correct spectral reflectance. In feature extraction, CARS and SPA are used extensively to reduce the dimensionality of spectral data for selecting effective wavelengths. Among the 21 papers listed in this paper applying hyperspectral analysis of fresh tea leaves, SG appeared nine times, MSC appeared nine times, and SNV appeared nine times. For feature extraction methods, CARS and SPA appeared six and seven times, respectively. The regression model PLSR is the most applied with a total of 10 occurrences. SVM in the classification model appeared a total of five times. Moreover, according to the final better results, PLSR, MLR, and SVM models were often used in quantitative analyses to predict the content of inbuilt components of tea fresh leaves, with the overall study showing that PLSR usually had better performances. In qualitative analyses, SVM models were mostly applied to classify and diagnose, which resulted in better discriminatory performance [76]. This may be due to the influence of light and the texture of the tea leaves themselves when collecting hyperspectral data of tea leaves. The SG and SNV can correct and eliminate this effect to some extent. Compared to spectral reflectance features, image features have not attracted much interest in fresh tea leaf quality assessment. This may be due to the fact that the information obtained when using only images to characterize the quality of tea leaves is similar to that of RGB images, whereas the cost of obtaining spectral images is much higher than that of obtaining RGB images. However, the information obtained from RGB images is limited, and scholars often fuse images with spectral data to analyze the quality of fresh tea leaves. The fused data show great feasibility in the quality assessment of tea fresh leaf quality due to the acquisition of more features, which improves the accuracy of quality assessment prediction. This is especially true for the assessment of the presence of diseases in tea leaves. Spectral reflectance features characterize the internal information of the material, which makes it possible to diagnose the disease in the early stages of the disease in tea leaves. Images are used as supplementary information to provide additional features for the pre-diagnosis of diseases, thus improving the disease diagnosis rate. After obtaining the phenotypic texture and color characteristics of tea leaves using images, an SVM or linear discriminant model was constructed to diagnose the disease by combining spectral reflectance. Generally, spectra can better characterize the component properties related to the quality of tea fresh leaves and characterize the internal properties of the lesions. Combined with image characterization of visible features such as color, damage, and texture, spectral techniques show great potential in non-destructive testing of tea fresh leaf quality.

Table 6. Application of HSI analysis in the study of the quality of fresh tea leaves.

Appliance	Pre-Process	Feature Extraction	Modeling	Best Result	Reference
Estimation of tea polyphenols	SG, FT, Polynomial smoothing, Neighbor average method, FD, SD	PCA	LSR, MLR, Polynomial regression	Neighbor average method-FD-PCA-LSR $R_c = 0.99$	[75]
Detection of anthocyanin content	MSC, SNV, SG, FD	CARS, VCPA, VCPA-IRIV	PLSR, SVR	MSC-SG-FD-VCPA-SVR $R_c = 0.96$	[76]
Prediction of chlorophylls and carotenoids content	MSC, SNV, FD	Second derivative and regression coefficient	PLSR	SNV-PLSR $R_p = 0.96, R_p = 0.93$	[9]
Detection of chlorophylls	Splice correction	Vegetation index	PROSPECT–D	Splice correction-Vegetation index-PROSPECT–D $R^2 = 0.83$	[90]
Estimating the catechin concentrations	/	/	PLSR, Mutual prediction	PLSR $R^2 = 0.87$	[40]
Estimation of water content	SG, MSC, SNV	SR	MLR, PLSR	SG-OSC-SW-PLSR $R_c = 0.83$	[41]
Prediction of tea polyphenols	SG, MSC, FD	CARS, SPA, UVE	SVM, PLSR, RF	MSC-FD-SG-CARS-PLSR $R^2 = 0.91$	[42]
Estimation of crude fiber contents	/	SPA, CARS	PLSR, MLR	SPA-MLR, $R^2 = 0.84$	[43]
Estimation of water content	SG, MSC, OSC	SPA, CARS, SPA-SR, CARS-SR	MLR	SG-MSC-CARS-SR-MLR $R^2 = 0.86$	[91]
Detection of nitrogen content	SNV	Vegetation index, VCPA, CARS	PLSR, SVM, RF	SNV-CARS-SVMR $R^2 = 0.91$	[92]
Prediction of nitrogen content	MSC, SNV, FD, SD	/	PLSR, PLS-DA, LS-VM	SNV-PLSR $R_c = 0.92$	[52]
Estimation of nitrogen content	SG, Detrending, FD, MSC, SNV, CWT	SPA, CARS, VCPA	PLSR	CWT-VCPA-PLSR $R^2 = 0.95$	[53]
Detection of chlorophyll content	FD	/	RF, SVM, DBN, KELM	KELM $RMSE = 8.94 \pm 3.05$	[93]
Detection of REC	MSC, SG, FD	SPA, UVE	PLSR, SVMR, CNN	MSC-FD-SG-UVE-SVMR $R^2 = 0.80$	[54]
Longjing fresh tea Variety identification	MSC, SNV, MSC+SNV	vegetation index, PCA	SVM, BP neural network	MSC+SNV-PCA-BP neural network Recognition accuracy = 98%	[94]
Identification of tea variety	MNF	PCA, ICA	MLC, MDC, ANN, SVM	MNF-SVM-PCA accuracy = 95%	[95]
Identification of tea quality	SNV, SG	/	MBKA-Net	SNV-MBKA-Net accuracy = 96.18%	[11]
Identification of white star disease	SG, SNV, SD, Semantic segmentation	SPA	PLS-DA, SVM, ELM	SG-SPA-ELM accuracy = 95.77%	[96]
Detection of anthracnose	color image extraction ROI	vegetation index	ISODATA, 2D thresholding	ISODATA Kappa = 0.91	[97]
Detection of anthracnose	extraction ROI, Continuum removal analysis, CWA	vegetation index	SVM, FLDA, RF	CWA- vegetation index-FLDA accuracy = 94.28%	[98]
Discriminant of withering quality	/	SPA, GLCM, PCA	LDA, SVM, ELM, PLS	PCA-LDA accuracy = 94.64%	[99]

Interestingly, based on this literature, we found that research scholars are not uniform or do not follow a certain method for selecting the region of interest (ROI) to obtain it. When doing quantitative analyses, some authors chose to use the whole leaf area as ROI, while some researchers avoided the main leaf veins to select ROI [41,42,76]. Since the ROI selection methods are different, the reflectance data obtained are different, which may also lead to inconsistent performance and bias in the final regression model. Of course, when performing qualitative analyses such as disease discrimination, scholars usually adopted semantic segmentation to separate the diseased region and used the diseased region as the ROI [11,96,97]. Simultaneously, a healthy part was selected as the ROI in order to obtain the reflectance data of the healthy and diseased regions. However, hyperspectral reflectance data are being used for non-destructive testing precisely because of their ability to reflect changes in the internal composition of tea leaves. The diseased area is segmented from the image as ROI when the leaf has already undergone qualitative changes visible to the naked eye, whereas the part of the leaf that is manually judged to be healthy may have changed in its internal composition. Such a result of ROI selection may also be the reason for inaccurate final classification results.

Tables 7–11 show the literature we have compiled on the application of NIRS, MIRS, THz, RS, and FS in tea fresh leaves. It is not difficult to find that NIRS is more widely used compared to several other spectrometers. This may be due to the fact that the band of NIRS is in the range of 780–2500 because the characteristic bands for observing and analyzing the intrinsic components of tea leaves such as tea polyphenols or caffeine are in the range of this band according to the results of existing literature. For several processing methods of spectral data, SNV in preprocessing was the most used with a total of 11 occurrences. PCA and PLSR were more frequently used for the screening and modeling of the characteristic bands, and according to the better results obtained, there was no one model that was universal. The preferred data processing methods chosen for different component quantitative analyses were inconsistent.

Table 7. Application of NIRS analysis in the study of quality of fresh tea leaves.

Appliance	Pre-Process	Feature Extraction	Modeling	Beat Result	Reference
Detection of Water content	SNV, Noise reduction, Normalization	RF, PCA, Pearson correlation analysis	SVR	RF-Pearson correlation analysis-SVR $R_p = 0.99$	[100]
Detection of catechin, caffeine	SG, SNV, MSC	CARS-SPA	MLR, LDA	SG-CARS-SPA-MLR $R_p = 0.97$	[102]
Determination of tea polyphenols	SG, SNV, Baseline	CARS, SPA, RF	PLS, MLR, LS-SVM	SNV-SPA-LS-SVM $R_p = 0.98$	[103]
Detection of nitrogen content	FD, External parameter orthogonalization	SPA, Ordered prediction selection, VCPA-IRIV	PLSR	EPO-VCPA-IRIV-PLSR $R_p = 0.97$	[105]
Estimation of total polyphenols	SNV, MSC, FD, SD	/	PLSR	MSC-PLSR $R^2 = 0.93$	[106]
Monitoring of flavonoid content	Remove noise and baseline, MA, SG, SNV, MSC, FD, SD	/	PLSR	SG-SD-PLSR $R_p = 0.95$	[107]
Prediction of EGCG	SG, SNV, VN, MSC, FD	CARS, RF	PLSR, LS-SVR	CARS-LS-SVR $R_p = 0.98$	[108]
Detection of heavy metals	/	correlation-based feature selection	PLS, RBFNN	CFS-PLS-RBFNN $R_p = 0.94$	[109]
Identification of tea varieties	MSC	CARS, SWR	GRNN, PNN	MSC-CARS-SWR-PNN Accuracy = 100%	[110]
Prediction of tea quality grade	SNV, SD, FD, SD, MSC	si-PLS, GA, PCA	BP-ANN	SNV-SD-si-PLS-GA-PCA-BP-ANN $R_p = 0.99$	[112]
Discrimination of tea maturity	FD, SD, Mean centering, SNV, MSC, SG	PCA	BPNN, GS-SVM, PSO-SVM	SG-PCA-PSO-SVM Accuracy = 98.92%	[113]
Traceability of Tea Raw Materials	Smoothing, MSC, FD, SD	/	PLS	MSC-PLS $R^2 = 0.82$	[114]
Discrimination of diseases	MSC, SNV, SG, KND, FD, SD	/	DPLS, DA	MSC-FD-SG-DA Accuracy = 100%	[115]
Identification of tea growing environment	Norris filter, SG, MSC, FD, Mean	/	SMLR, PCR, Si-PLS	Mean-Si-PLS $R_c = 0.96$	[116].

Table 8. Application of MIRS analysis in the study of quality of fresh tea leaves.

Appliance	Pre-Process	Feature Extraction	Modeling	Beat Result	Reference
Determination of dry matter content	Smoothing, MSC, SNV	KPCA, WPT–SA	LS-SVM, PLS	SNV-WPT-LS-SVM $R_p = 0.96$	[117]
Determination of polyphenols and flavonoids	/	PCA	PLS	PCA-PLS $R = 0.98$	[118]
Detection of tea stalk and insect foreign bodies	/	/	KNN	KNN Accuracy = 100%	[119]

Table 9. Application of THz analysis in the study of the quality of fresh tea leaves.

Appliance	Pre-Process	Feature Extraction	Modeling	Beat Result	Reference
Degrees of oxidation	/	PCA	Hierarchical cluster analysis	PCA-HCA	[120]
Detection of tea stalk and insect foreign bodies	/	/	KNN	KNN Accuracy = 100%	[121]
Assessment of cold injury	/	/	two-dimensional correlation spectroscopy-PLSR, average intensity-PLSR	2DCOS-PLSR $R = 0.91$	[122]

Table 10. Application of RS analysis in the study of the quality of fresh tea leaves.

Appliance	Pre-Process	Feature Extraction	Modeling	Beat Result	Reference
Detection of carotenoid content	Smooting, Normalization, MSC, Baseling, WT	SPA	PLSR	WT-SPA-PLS $R_p = 0.87$	[124]
Detection of photosynthetic pigments	MSC, WT, SNV, RCF, airPLS	CARS	PLSR	RCF-CARS-PLSR $R_p = 0.89$	[125]
Identification of tea Quality	Smoothing, Normalization	PCA	LDA	Smoothing-Normalization-PCA-LDA Accuracy = 100%	[126]
Anthracnose Identification	Baseline correction	PCA	/	Baseline correction-PCA Accuracy = 95%	[127]

Table 11. Application of FS analysis in the study of the quality of fresh tea leaves.

Appliance	Pre-Process	Feature Extraction	Modeling	Beat Result	Reference
Detection of chlorophyll content	SG	SPA, UVE	PLSR, BiPLS	SG-SPA-BiPLS $R_p = 0.96$	[128]
Determination of Pesticide Residue	Black and white correction	PCA	Spectral angle mappe	Black and white correction-PCA-SAM Accuracy = 100%	[129]
Diagnosis of leaf spot disease	SG	PCA	PLS-DA, SVM, LDA	SG-PCA-LDA Accuracy = 98.9%	[130]

Comparing the application of HSI with NIRS, MIRS, THz, RS, and FS in tea leaves, it can be found that although HSI can acquire reflectance information and spatial image information at the same time, the commonly used HSI band is often in the range of 400–1100. However, HSI with a wider range of wavebands is particularly costly, which makes it difficult to be widely used. Although water content and nitrogen can be screened out in the 400–1100 band and some of the built-in components of tea leaves can also be screened out in the band, similar to caffeine, gallic acid, etc., whose absorption peaks are in the 2000 band, they cannot be analyzed or the results of the analysis are poor [100,102,105]. In this regard, subsequent studies could move toward the simultaneous use of HSI and other spectrometers to obtain more comprehensive spectral information on tea leaves, and thus accurately analyze the quality of tea leaves. It is interesting to note that the number of sample sets for quantitative or qualitative analyses of tea leaves is usually between 100 and 300 [52,93]. Since spectral information is usually analyzed in conjunction with physicochemical measurements, the workload involved in obtaining samples is very high, which explains the small number of sample sets. However, due to this, it tends to make the final model suffer from overfitting and poor generalization. When dealing with spectral data, how to balance the spectral information signal-to-noise ratio is also a key factor in the subsequent construction of a stable and accurate model when using smoothing, correction, and other means. At the same time, when screening the feature band dimensionality reduction, determining how to preserve the complete information as much as possible and reduce the dimensionality of the operation is also particularly important. Only after dealing with these steps can we construct a stable and accurate model for tea leaf quality analysis.

6. Conclusions and Prospects

This review focuses on summarizing the principles of hyperspectral imaging technology and the progress of analytical methods and applications in the quality testing of fresh tea leaves. It also briefly introduces the principles and applications of infrared and Raman spectroscopic techniques in tea quality testing. According to the previous research results of scholars, hyperspectral imaging technology and infrared spectroscopic technology have been proven to be effective tools for detecting the quality of fresh tea leaves. Compared with traditional testing methods, they are fast, highly accurate, and non-destructive, and do not require chemical reagents. The application of hyperspectral imaging technology, infrared, and other spectroscopic techniques can be used to reliably and conveniently detect the water content and quality material content components of tea leaves, thus promoting the classification of tea raw materials and assisting in the harvesting of tea leaves. But, at the same time, based on the discussion section, there are some challenges in the application of spectroscopic technology for the quality detection of tea fresh leaves:

(1) First of all, due to the chromaticity and luminosity of the capture ability, field use of spectroscopy to collect samples reflectance, by the light conditions, will affect the final test results. At the same time, in determining how to detect the quality composition content of tea fresh leaves in the tree, there are also challenges of how to select the region of interest, obtain a more consistent reflectance of the sample, and then build a stable estimation model.

(2) Secondly, the visualization and prediction technique of hyperspectral imaging provides great convenience for the detection of tea fresh leaves quality, but its high cost, large amount of imaging data, and high redundancy usually require data preprocessing by extracting the feature wavelengths through a variety of effective algorithms for dimensionality reduction, as well as building a robust calibration model for extracting the depth features. Spectral techniques such as infrared and other spectral techniques are unable to obtain image phenotypic information, meaning some information is missing. It is especially important to obtain multi-spectral images of the characteristic bands of tea leaf quality substances and reduce the amount of data without losing the characteristic information of tea leaf quality substances.

(3) Finally, after constructing the quality classification model of tea leaves and the regression of component content detection, determining how to ensure the stability of the model and the subsequent generalization performance and reduce the data run-

ning memory are also important issues in spectral technology in the quality detection of tea leaves.

Author Contributions: Conceptualization, T.T. and C.L.; methodology, T.T.; software, L.Y.; validation, W.W.; formal analysis, C.G.; investigation, C.G.; resources, W.W. and C.L.; data curation, T.T. and Q.L.; writing—original draft preparation, T.T. and Q.L.; writing—review and editing, C.L.; funding acquisition, W.W. All authors have read and agreed to the published version of the manuscript.

Funding: This research was funded by the Guangdong Provincial Special Fund for Modern Agriculture Industry Technology Innovation Teams (Tea) (2023KJ120); Guangdong Digital Smart Agricultural Service Industrial Park (GDSCYY2022-046); Key Technology Research on Tea Shoot Recognition and Picking Robots (pdjh2022a0072); and Sichuan Provincial Natural Science Foundation Youth Fund (No.2023NSFSC1178).

Institutional Review Board Statement: Not applicable.

Informed Consent Statement: Not applicable.

Data Availability Statement: Data is contained within the article.

Conflicts of Interest: The authors declare no conflict of interest.

References

1. Lin, X.; Wu, Q.Y.; Yang, J.F. Research on the Effect Evaluation and Dynamic Mechanism of the Integrated Development of Tea and Tourism Industry. *J. Tea Sci.* **2023**, *43*, 718–732.
2. Zou, Y.; Hu, J.Q.; Wang, J.; Liu, S.; Wang, S. Studies of the Basic Components and Probiotic Properties of Tea Powder. *Food Res. Dev.* **2021**, *42*, 20–26.
3. He, L.; Chen, L.X.; Wang, N.; Zhang, F.J.; Chen, Y.N.; Jia, Z.; Han, B.; Chen, W.M.; Huang, Z.B. Medicinal property, taste, efficacy and prescriptions of tea from the perspective of TCM literature. *China J. Tradit. Chin. Med. Pharm.* **2021**, *36*, 5630–5634.
4. Ou, Y.L.; Zhang, Y.N.; Qin, L.; Miao, Y.C.; Xiao, L.Z. Research Advances on Quality Evaluation Methods of Tea Color, Aroma and Taste. *Sci. Technol. Food Ind.* **2019**, *40*, 342–347+360.
5. Liang, X.; Li, L.; Han, C.; Dong, Y.; Xu, F.; Lv, Z.; Zhang, Y.; Qu, Z.; Dong, W.; Sun, Y. Rapid Limit Test of Seven Pesticide Residues in Tea Based on the Combination of TLC and Raman Imaging Microscopy. *Molecules* **2022**, *27*, 5151. [CrossRef]
6. Wei, Y.Z.; Li, X.L.; He, Y. Generalisation of tea moisture content models based on VNIR spectra subjected to fractional differential treatment. *Biosyst. Eng.* **2021**, *205*, 174–186. [CrossRef]
7. Liu, Q.; Ouyang, J.; Liu, C.W.; Chen, H.Y.; Li, J.; Xiong, L.M.; Liu, Z.H.; Huang, J.A. Research Progress of Tea Quality Evaluation Technology. *J. Tea Sci.* **2022**, *42*, 316–330.
8. Romers, T.; Saurina, J.; Sentellas, S.; Núñez, O. Targeted HPLC-UV Polyphenolic Profiling to Detect and Quantify Adulterated Tea Samples by Chemometrics. *Foods* **2023**, *12*, 1501. [CrossRef]
9. Wang, Y.J.; Hu, X.; Jin, G.; Hou, Z.W.; Ning, J.M.; Zhang, Z.Z. Rapid prediction of chlorophylls and carotenoids content in tea leaves under different levels of nitrogen application based on hyperspectral imaging. *J. Sci. Food Agric.* **2019**, *99*, 1997–2004. [CrossRef]
10. Li, T.; He, C.L.; Cai, Y.L.; Li, M.H. Effects of Different Tenderness Materials on the Main Quality and Aroma of Tibetan Tea. *Sci. Technol. Food Ind.* **2019**, *40*, 76–81+321.
11. Wang, F.; Zhao, C.J.; Xu, B.; Xu, Z.; Li, Z.H.; Yang, H.B.; Duan, D.D.; Yang, G.J. Development of a portable detection device for the quality of fresh tea leaves using spectral technology. *Trans. Chin. Soc. Agric. Eng.* **2020**, *36*, 273–280.
12. Long, W.J.; Lei, G.H.; Guan, Y.T.; Chen, H.Y.; Hu, Z.K.; She, Y.B.; Fu, H.Y. Classification of Chinese traditional cereal vinegars and antioxidant property predication by fluorescence spectroscopy. *Food Chem.* **2023**, *424*, 136406. [CrossRef] [PubMed]
13. Prey, L.; Hanemann, A.; Ramgraber, L.; Seidl-Schulz, J.; Noack, P.O. UAV-Based Estimation of Grain Yield for Plant Breeding: Applied Strategies for Optimizing the Use of Sensors, Vegetation Indices, Growth Stages, and Machine Learning Algorithms. *Remote Sens.* **2022**, *14*, 6345. [CrossRef]
14. Wang, N.; Xing, K.W.; Zhang, W.; Jiang, L.Z.; Elfalleh, W.; Cheng, J.J.; Yu, D.Y. Combining multi–spectroscopy analysis and interfacial properties to research the effect of ultrasonic treatment on soybean protein isolate–tannic acid complexes. *Food Hydrocoll.* **2023**, *145*, 109136. [CrossRef]
15. Qian, L.Y.; Wu, D.C.; Liu, D.; Zhou, X.J.; Wei, W.; Zhong, L.J.; Wang, W.J.; Wang, Y.J.; Gong, W. Analysis and Design of Hyperspectral Imaging LiDAR Scanning Mirror. *Acta Opt. Sin.* **2021**, *41*, 232–238.
16. Zhang, Y.; Zhou, J.H.; Wang, S.M.; Wang, Y.Y.; Zhang, Y.H.; Zhao, S.; Liu, S.Y.; Yang, J. Identification of Xinhui Citri Reticulatae Pericarpium of Different AgingYears Based on Visible Near Infrared Hyperspectral Imaging. *Spectrosc. Spectral Anal.* **2023**, *43*, 3286–3292.
17. Wang, Y.W.; Ren, Y.Q.; Kang, S.Y.; Yin, C.B.; Shi, Y.; Men, H. Identification of tea quality at different picking periods: A hyperspectral system coupled with a multibranch kernel attention network. *Food Chem.* **2023**, *433*, 137307. [CrossRef]

18. Luo, X.L.; Sun, C.J.; He, Y.; Zhu, F.L.; Li, X.L. Cross-cultivar prediction of quality indicators of tea based on VIS-NIR hyperspectral imaging. *Ind. Crops Prod.* **2023**, *202*, 117009. [CrossRef]
19. Li, X.N.; Li, T.P.; Gao, X.B.; Cui, Y. Shielding performance evaluation of smoke screens and revision of the smoke screen mass extinction coefficient. *J. Ordnance Equip. Eng.* **2023**, *44*, 187–194.
20. Zhang, D.; Liang, P.; Ye, J.; Xia, J.; Zhou, Y.; Huang, J.; Ni, D.; Tang, L.; Jin, S.; Yu, Z. Detection of systemic pesticide residues in tea products at trace level based on SERS and verified by GC–MS. *Anal Bioanal Chem.* **2019**, *411*, 7187–7196. [CrossRef]
21. Cao, C.; Zhang, Z.H.; Zhao, X.Y.; Zhang, H.; Zhang, T.Y.; Yu, Y. Review of Terahertz Time Domain and Frequency Domain Spectroscopy. *Spectrosc. Spectral Anal.* **2019**, *46*, 118–137.
22. Zhang, L.H.; Iburaim, A. The Establishment of the Method of the Fiber Optic Chemical Sensor Synchronous Absorption-Fluorescence. *Spectrosc. Spectral Anal.* **2016**, *36*, 755–758.
23. Tang, J.L.; Ma, J. Synthesis and properties of thermo-sensitive and pH-sensitive poly(N-isopropyl acrylamide)/AAC. *J. Funct. Mater.* **2017**, *48*, 9157–9161+9166.
24. Li, Z.; Hu, H.M.; Zhang, W.; Pu, S.L.; Li, B. Spectrum Characteristics Preserved Visible and Near-Infrared Image Fusion Algorithm. *IEEE Trans. Multimed.* **2021**, *23*, 306–319. [CrossRef]
25. Tong, D.W.; Kong, M.; Xiang, Y.B. Synthesis, Photophysical Properties, Theoretical Calculation and Cell Imaging of a Tetraphenylethene Imidazole Compound with Methoxy Group. *Chin. J. Appl. Chem.* **2023**, *40*, 1322–1333.
26. Huang, X.Y.; Sun, Z.Y.; Tian, X.Y.; Yu, S.S.; Wang, P.C.; Joshua, H.A. Early Detection of Potato Rot Disease Caused by Fungal Based on Electronic Nose Technology. *Sci. Technol. Food Ind.* **2018**, *39*, 97–101.
27. Liu, X.S.; Zhang, S.Y.; Si, L.T.; Lin, Z.L.; Wu, C.Y.; Luan, L.J.; Wu, Y.J. A combination of near infrared and mid-infrared spectroscopy to improve the determination efficiency of active components in Radix Astragali. *J. Near Infrared Spectrosc.* **2020**, *28*, 10–17. [CrossRef]
28. Lu, X.J.; Ge, H.Y.; Jiang, Y.Y.; Zhang, Y. Application Progress of Terahertz Technology in Agriculture Detection. Spectrosc. Spectral Anal. *Spectrosc. Spectral Anal.* **2022**, *42*, 3330–3335.
29. Choi, G.C.; Lee, D.H.; Park, I.; Kang, D.; Lee, H.K.; Rhie, J.; Bahk, Y.M. Evaluation of moisturizing cream using terahertz time-domain spectroscopy. *Curr Appl Phys.* **2022**, *39*, 84–89. [CrossRef]
30. Xu, S.; Huang, X.; Lu, H. Advancements and Applications of Raman Spectroscopy in Rapid Quality and Safety Detection of Fruits and Vegetables. *Horticulturae* **2023**, *9*, 843. [CrossRef]
31. Baratto, C.; Ambrosio, G.; Faglia, G.; Turina, M. Early Detection of Esca Disease in Asymptomatic Vines by Raman Spectroscopy. *IEEE Sens. J.* **2022**, *22*, 23286–23292. [CrossRef]
32. Liu, D.P.; Gao, H.J.; Cui, B.; Yu, H.B.; Yang, F. Fluorescence spectra and multivariate statistical model characterization of DOM composition structure of Baitapu River sediment. *J. Environ. Eng. Technol.* **2021**, *11*, 249–257.
33. Zhang, Y.L.; Yan, K.T.; Wang, L.L.; Chen, P.C.; Han, X.F.; Lan, Y.B. Research Progress of Pesticide Residue Detection Based on FluorescenceSpectrum Analysis. *Spectrosc. Spectral Anal.* **2021**, *41*, 2364–2371.
34. Ye, W.; Xu, W.; Yan, T.; Yan, J.; Gao, P.; Zhang, C. Application of Near-Infrared Spectroscopy and Hyperspectral Imaging Combined with Machine Learning Algorithms for Quality Inspection of Grape: A Review. *Foods* **2023**, *12*, 132. [CrossRef] [PubMed]
35. Shu, S.; Yu, Z.; Zhang, J.; Chen, Z.; Liang, H.; Chen, J. An Improved Dual Asymmetric Penalized Least Squares Baseline Correction Method for High-Noise Spectral Data Analysis. *Nucl. Sci. Eng.* **2023**, *197*, 589–600. [CrossRef]
36. Liu, D.Y.; Sun, X.R.; Liu, C.L.; Du, X.; Ye, Z.S. Design of on-line detection system for wheat flour quality based on microNIR. *Food Sci. Technol.* **2019**, *44*, 333–337.
37. Dong, C.; Liu, Z.; Yang, C.; An, T.; Hu, B.; Luo, X.; Jin, J.; Li, Y. Rapid detection of exogenous sucrose in black tea samples based on near-infrared spectroscopy. *Infrared Phys. Technol.* **2021**, *119*, 103934. [CrossRef]
38. Sun, H.; Lv, G.; Mo, J.; Lv, X.; Du, G.; Liu, Y. Application of KPCA combined with SVM in Raman spectral discrimination. *Optik* **2019**, *184*, 214–219. [CrossRef]
39. Tan, B.; You, W.; Huang, C.; Xiao, T.; Tian, S.; Luo, L.; Xiong, N. An Intelligent Near-Infrared Diffuse Reflectance Spectroscopy Scheme for the Non-Destructive Testing of the Sugar Content in Cherry Tomato Fruit. *Electronics* **2022**, *11*, 3504. [CrossRef]
40. Kang, Y.S.; Ryu, C.; Suguri, M.; Park, S.B.; Kishino, S.; Onoyama, H. Estimating the catechin concentrations of new shoots in green tea fields using ground-based hyperspectral imagery. *Food Chem.* **2021**, *370*, 130987. [CrossRef]
41. Dai, C.X.; Liu, F.; Ge, X.F. Detection and Analysis of Moisture Content in Fresh Tea Leaves Based on Hyperspectral Technology. *J. Tea Sci.* **2018**, *38*, 281–286.
42. Mao, Y.L.; Li, H.; Wang, Y.; Fan, K.; Song, Y.J.; Han, X.; Zhang, J.; Ding, S.B.; Song, D.P.; Wang, H.; et al. Prediction of Tea Polyphenols, Free Amino Acids and Caffeine Content in Tea Leaves during Wilting and Fermentation Using Hyperspectral Imaging. *Foods* **2022**, *11*, 2537. [CrossRef] [PubMed]
43. Wang, Y.J.; Li, L.Q.; Shen, S.S.; Liu, Y.; Ning, J.M.; Zhang, Z.Z. Rapid detection of quality index of postharvest fresh tea leaves using hyperspectral imaging. *J. Sci. Food Agric.* **2020**, *100*, 3803–3811. [CrossRef] [PubMed]
44. Amneh, A.A. Application of Moving Average Filter for the Quantitative Analysis of the NIR Spectra. *J. Anal. Chem.* **2019**, *74*, 686–692. [CrossRef]
45. Xue, Y.W.; Wang, Y.; Wang, Y.; Ding, S.B.; Wang, Q.M.; Chen, S.Z.; Ding, Z.T.; Zhao, L.Q. Establishment of a Hyperspectral Spectroscopy-Based Biochemical Component Detection Model for Green Tea Processing Materials. *Sci. Technol. Food Ind.* **2023**, *44*, 280–289.

46. Li, H.D.; Li, J.Z.; Chen, Y.L.; Huang, Y.J.; Shen, X.T. Establishing Support Vector Machine SVM Recognition Model to IdentifyJadeite Origin. *Spectrosc. Spectral Anal.* **2023**, *43*, 2252–2257.
47. Yang, K.; An, C.Q.; Zhu, J.L.; Guo, W.C.; Lu, C.; Zhu, X.H. Comparison of near-infrared and dielectric spectra for quantitative identification of bovine colostrum adulterated with mature milk. *J. Dairy Sci.* **2022**, *105*, 8638–8649. [CrossRef] [PubMed]
48. Pu, H.B.; Wei, Q.Y.; Sun, D.W. Recent advances in muscle food safety evaluation: Hyperspectral imaging analyses and applications. *Crit. Rev. Food Sci. Nutr.* **2023**, *63*, 1297–1313. [CrossRef]
49. Kozinov, I.A.; Maltsev, G.N. Development and processing of hyperspectral images in optical–electronic remote sensing systems. *Opt. Spectrosc.* **2016**, *121*, 934–946. [CrossRef]
50. Ball, K.R.; Liu, H.; Brien, C.; Berger, B.; Power, S.A.; Pendall, E. Hyperspectral imaging predicts yield and nitrogen content in grass–legume polycultures. *Precision Agric.* **2022**, *23*, 2270–2288. [CrossRef]
51. Ge, X.; Ding, J.; Jin, X.; Wang, J.; Chen, X.; Li, X.; Liu, J.; Xie, B. Estimating Agricultural Soil Moisture Content through UAV-Based Hyperspectral Images in the Arid Region. *Remote Sens.* **2021**, *13*, 1562. [CrossRef]
52. Wang, Y.J.; Li, T.H.; Jin, G.; Wei, Y.M.; Li, L.Q.; Kalkhajeh, Y.K.; Ning, J.M.; Zhang, Z.Z. Qualitative and quantitative diagnosis of nitrogen nutrition of tea plants under field condition using hyperspectral imaging coupled with chemometrics. *J. Sci. Food Agric.* **2019**, *100*, 161–167. [CrossRef] [PubMed]
53. Wang, F.; Chen, L.Y.; Duan, D.D.; Cao, Q.; Zhao, Y.; Lan, W.R. Estimation of Total Nitrogen Content in Fresh Tea Leaves Based on Wavelet Analysis. *Spectrosc. Spectral Anal.* **2022**, *42*, 3235–3242.
54. Mao, Y.L.; Li, H.; Wang, Y.; Fan, K.; Sun, L.T.; Wang, H.; Song, D.P.; Shen, J.Z.; Ding, Z.T. Quantitative Judgment of Freezing Injury of Tea Leaves Based on Hyperspectral Imaging. *Spectrosc. Spectral Anal.* **2023**, *43*, 2266–2271.
55. Zhang, Y.; Xia, C.Z.; Zhang, X.Y.; Cheng, X.H.; Feng, G.Z.; Wang, Y.; Gao, Q. Estimating the maize biomass by crop height and narrowband vegetation indices derived from UAV-based hyperspectral images. *Ecol. Indic.* **2021**, *129*, 107985. [CrossRef]
56. Essa, A.; Sidike, P.; Asari, V. Volumetric Directional Pattern for Spatial Feature Extraction in Hyperspectral Imagery. *IEEE Geosci. Remote Sens. Lett.* **2017**, *14*, 1056–1060. [CrossRef]
57. Zhang, X.D.; Wang, P.; Wang, Y.F.; Hu, L.; Luo, X.W.; Mao, H.P.; Shen, B.G. Cucumber powdery mildew detection method based on hyperspectra-terahertz. *Front. Plant Sci.* **2022**, *13*, 488–498. [CrossRef]
58. Li, X.L.; Wei, Z.X.; Peng, F.F.; Liu, J.F.; Han, G.H. stimating the distribution of chlorophyll content in CYVCV infected lemon leaf using hyperspectral imaging. *Comput. Electron. Agric.* **2022**, *198*, 107036. [CrossRef]
59. Qin, F.L.; Wang, X.C.; Ding, S.R.; Li, G.S.; Hou, Z.C. Prediction of Peking duck intramuscle fat content by near-infrared spectroscopy. *Poult. Sci.* **2021**, *100*, 101281. [CrossRef]
60. Paul, A.; Bhattacharya, S.; Dutta, D.; Sharma, J.R.; Dadhwal, V.K. Band selection in hyperspectral imagery using spatial cluster mean and genetic algorithms. *GIsci Remote Sens.* **2015**, *52*, 643–659. [CrossRef]
61. Wang, Z.L.; Huang, W.Q.; Tian, X.; Long, Y.; Li, L.J.; Fan, S. Rapid and Non-destructive Classification of New and Aged Maize Seeds Using Hyperspectral Image and Chemometric Methods. *Front. Plant Sci.* **2022**, *13*, 849495. [CrossRef] [PubMed]
62. Bao, Y.; Mi, C.; Wu, N.; Liu, F.; He, Y. Rapid Classification of Wheat Grain Varieties Using Hyperspectral Imaging and Chemometrics. *Appl. Sci.* **2019**, *9*, 4119. [CrossRef]
63. Faqeerzada, M.A.; Lohumi, S.; Joshi, R.; Kim, M.S.; Baek, I.; Cho, B.-K. Non-Targeted Detection of Adulterants in Almond Powder Using Spectroscopic Techniques Combined with Chemometrics. *Foods* **2020**, *9*, 876. [CrossRef] [PubMed]
64. Huang, Y.K.; Wang, J.; Li, N.; Yang, J.; Ren, Z.H. Predicting soluble solids content in "Fuji" apples of different ripening stages based on multiple information fusion. *Pattern Recognit Lett.* **2021**, *151*, 76–84. [CrossRef]
65. Zhang, D.Y.; Xu, L.; Liang, D.; Xu, C.; Jin, X.L.; Weng, S.Z. Fast Prediction of Sugar Content in Dangshan Pear (*Pyrus* spp.) Using Hyperspectral Imagery Data. *Food Anal. Methods* **2018**, *11*, 2336–2345. [CrossRef]
66. Huang, X.D.; Wang, C.Y.; Fan, X.M.; Zhang, J.L.; Yang, C.; Wang, Z.D. Oil source recognition technology using concentration-synchronous-matrix-fluorescence spectroscopy combined with 2D wavelet packet and probabilistic neural network. *Sci. Total Environ.* **2018**, *616*, 632–638. [CrossRef] [PubMed]
67. Liu, Y.; Deng, C.; Lu, Y.Y.; Shen, Q.Y.; Zhao, H.F.; Tao, Y.T.; Pan, X.Z. Evaluating the characteristics of soil vis-NIR spectra after the removal of moisture effect using external parameter orthogonalization. *Geoderma* **2020**, *376*, 114568. [CrossRef]
68. Zhang, Z.Y.; Gui, D.D.; Sha, M.; Liu, J.; Wang, H.Y. Raman chemical feature extraction for quality control of dairy products. *J. Dairy Sci.* **2019**, *102*, 68–76. [CrossRef]
69. Abdolmaleki, M.; Consens, M.; Esmaeili, K. Ore-Waste Discrimination Using Supervised and Unsupervised Classification of Hyperspectral Images. *Remote Sens.* **2022**, *14*, 6386. [CrossRef]
70. Chen, F.; Tang, T.F.; Wang, K. Sparse smoothing preprocessing of hyperspectral images for improved classification performance. *Remote Sens Lett.* **2015**, *6*, 276–285. [CrossRef]
71. Munera, S.; Hernández, F.; Cubero, S.; Blasco, C. Maturity monitoring of intact fruit and arils of pomegranate cv. 'Mollar de Elche' using machine vision and chemometrics. *Postharvest Biol. Technol.* **2019**, *156*, 110936. [CrossRef]
72. Akbarzadeh, S.; Paap, A.; Ahderom, S.; Apopei, B.; Alameh, K. Plant discrimination by Support Vector Machine classifier based on spectral reflectance. *Comput. Electron. Agric.* **2018**, *148*, 250–258. [CrossRef]
73. Li, H.G.; Yu, Y.H.; Feng, Y.; Shen, X.F. Study on Near-Infrared Spectrum Acquisition Method of Non-UniformSolid Particles. *Spectrosc. Spectral Anal.* **2021**, *41*, 2748–2753.

74. Wang, F.; Qiong, C.; Zhao, C.J.; Duan, D.D.; Chen, L.Y.; Meng, X.Y. Non-destructive determination of taste-related substances in fresh tea using NIR spectra. *J. Food Meas. Charact.* **2023**, *17*, 5874–5885. [CrossRef]
75. Zhang, M.; Li, Y.H.; Yuan, Q.C.; Li, J.; Dai, S.H.; Liu, Z.H.; Li, M. Polyphenols inspecting method of living tea leaves based on hyperspectral reflection. *J. Hunan Agric. Univ.* **2015**, *41*, 450–454.
76. Dai, F.S.; Shi, J.; Yang, C.S.; Li, Y.; Zhao, Y.; Liu, Z.Y.; An, T.; Li, X.L.; Peng, Y.; Dong, C.W. Detection of anthocyanin content in fresh Zijuan tea leaves based on hyperspectral imaging. *Food Control* **2023**, *152*, 109839. [CrossRef]
77. Ong, P.L.; Chen, S.M.; Tsai, C.Y.; Chuang, Y.K. Prediction of tea theanine content using near-infrared spectroscopy and flower pollination algorithm. *Spectrochim. Acta Part A Mol. Biomol. Spectrosc.* **2021**, *255*, 119657. [CrossRef]
78. Yamashita, H.; Sonobe, R.; Hirono, Y.H.; Morita, A.; Ikka, T.S. Potential of spectroscopic analyses for non-destructive estimation of tea quality-related metabolites in fresh new leaves. *Sci. Rep.* **2021**, *11*, 4169. [CrossRef]
79. Hu, H.Q.; Wei, Y.P.; Xu, X.H.; Zhang, L.; Mao, X.B.; Zhao, Y.P. Identification of the Age of Puerariae Thomsonii Radix Based on Hyperspectral lmaging and Principal Component Analysis. *Spectrosc. Spectral Anal.* **2023**, *43*, 1953–1960.
80. Jiang, Y.P.; Chen, S.F.; Bian, B.; Li, Y.H.; Sun, Y.; Wang, X.C. Discrimination of Tomato Maturity Using Hyperspectral Imaging Combined with Graph-Based Semi-supervised Method Considering Class Probability Information. *Food Anal. Methods* **2021**, *14*, 968–983. [CrossRef]
81. Sendin, K.; Williams, P.J.; Manley, M. Near infrared hyperspectral imaging in quality and safety evaluation of cereals. *Crit Rev. Food Sci. Nutr.* **2018**, *58*, 575–590. [CrossRef] [PubMed]
82. Liu, B.; Yu, A.Z.; Zou, X.B.; Xue, Z.X.; Gao, K.L.; Guo, W.Y. Spatial-spectral feature classification of hyperspectral image using a pretrained deep convolutional neural network. *Eur. J. Remote Sens.* **2021**, *54*, 385–397. [CrossRef]
83. Feng, Z.; Liu, X.; Yang, S.; Zhang, K.; Jiao, L. Hierarchical Feature Fusion and Selection for Hyperspectral Image Classification. *IEEE Geosci. Remote Sens. Lett.* **2023**, *20*, 1–5.
84. Yang, B.H.; Gao, Y.; Li, H.M.; Ye, S.B.; He, H.X.; Xie, S.R. Rapid prediction of yellow tea free amino acids with hyperspectral images. *PLoS ONE* **2019**, *14*, 0210084. [CrossRef] [PubMed]
85. Yang, L.; Guo, Z.H.; Jin, Z.Y.; Bai, J.C.; Yu, F.H.; Xu, T.Y. Inversion Method Research of Phosphorus Content in Rice LeavesProduced in Northern Cold Region Based on WPA-BP. *Spectrosc. Spectral Anal.* **2023**, *43*, 1442–1449.
86. Hou, C.Y.; Wang, Y.; Li, F.; Yuan, X.H.; Yang, X.Z.; Zhang, Z.T.; Chen, J.Y.; Li, X.W. Hyperspectral inversion of water-soluble salt ion contents in frozen saline soil. *Chin. Soc. Agric. Eng.* **2023**, *39*, 100–107.
87. Ren, G.; Wang, Y.; Ning, J.; Zhang, Z. Using near-infrared hyperspectral imaging with multiple decision tree methods to delineate black tea quality. *Spectrochim. Acta Part A Mol. Biomol. Spectrosc.* **2020**, *237*, 118407. [CrossRef]
88. Feng, J.; Jiao, L.; Liu, F.; Sun, T.; Zhang, X. Unsupervised feature selection based on maximum information and minimum redundancy for hyperspectral images. *Pattern Recognit.* **2016**, *51*, 295–309. [CrossRef]
89. Liang, N.; Duan, P.; Xu, H.; Cui, L. Multi-View Structural Feature Extraction for Hyperspectral Image Classification. *Remote Sens.* **2022**, *14*, 1971. [CrossRef]
90. Sonobe, R.; Miura, Y.; Sano, T.; Horie, H. Estimating leaf carotenoid contents of shade-grown tea using hyperspectral indices and PROSPECT-D inversion. *Int. J. Remote Sens.* **2018**, *39*, 1306–1320. [CrossRef]
91. Sun, J.; Zhou, X.; Hu, Y.G.; Wu, X.H.; Zhang, X.D.; Wang, P. Visualizing distribution of moisture content in tea leaves using optimization algorithms and NIR hyperspectral imaging. *Comput. Electron. Agric.* **2019**, *160*, 153–159. [CrossRef]
92. Cao, Q.; Yang, G.J.; Duan, D.D.; Chen, L.Y.; Wang, F.; Xu, B.; Zhao, C.J.; Niu, F.F. Combining multispectral and hyperspectral data to estimate nitrogen status of tea plants (Camellia sinensis (L.) O. Kuntze) under field conditions. *Comput. Electron. Agric.* **2022**, *198*, 107084. [CrossRef]
93. Sonobe, R.; Hirono, Y.; Oi, A. Non-Destructive Detection of Tea Leaf Chlorophyll Content Using Hyperspectral Reflectance and Machine Learning Algorithms. *Plants* **2020**, *9*, 368. [CrossRef] [PubMed]
94. Yan, L.; Pang, L.; Wang, H.; Xiao, J. Recognition of different Longjing fresh tea varieties using hyperspectral imaging technology and chemometrics. *J. Food Process Eng.* **2020**, *43*, 13378. [CrossRef]
95. Tu, Y.X.; Bian, M.; Wan, Y.K.; Fei, T. Tea cultivar classification and biochemical parameter estimation from hyperspectral imagery obtained by UAV. *PeerJ.* **2018**, *6*, e4858. [CrossRef] [PubMed]
96. Lu, B.; Sun, J.; Yang, N.; Wu, X.H.; Zhou, X. Identification of tea white star disease and anthrax based on hyperspectral image information. *J. Food Process Eng.* **2021**, *44*, 13584. [CrossRef]
97. Yuan, L.; Yan, P.; Han, W.Y.; Huang, Y.B.; Wang, B.; Zhang, J.C.; Zhang, H.B.; Bao, Z.Y. Detection of anthracnose in tea plants based on hyperspectral imaging. *Comput. Electron. Agric.* **2019**, *167*, 105039. [CrossRef]
98. Zhao, X.H.; Zhang, J.C.; Huang, Y.B.; Tian, Y.Y.; Yuan, L. Detection and discrimination of disease and insect stress of tea plants using hyperspectral imaging combined with wavelet analysis. *Comput. Electron. Agric.* **2022**, *193*, 106717. [CrossRef]
99. Ning, J.M.; Sun, J.J.; Zhu, X.Y.; Li, S.H.; Zhang, Z.Z.; Huang, C.W. Discriminant of withering quality of Keemun black tea based on information fusion of image and spectrum. *Chin. Soc. Agric. Eng.* **2016**, *32*, 303–308.
100. Wang, S.; Wu, Z.; Cao, C.; An, M.; Luo, K.; Sun, L.; Wang, X. Design and Experiment of Online Detection System for Water Content of Fresh Tea Leaves after Harvesting Based on Near Infra-Red Spectroscopy. *Sensors* **2023**, *23*, 666. [CrossRef]
101. Chen, J.Y.; Yang, C.S.; Yuan, C.B.; Li, Y.; An, T.; Dong, C.W. Moisture content monitoring in withering leaves during black tea processing based on electronic eye and near infrared spectroscopy. *Sci. Rep.* **2022**, *12*, 20721. [CrossRef] [PubMed]

102. Huang, Y.F.; Dong, W.T.; Sanaeifar, A.; Wang, X.M.; Luo, W.; Zhan, B.S.; Liu, X.M.; Li, R.L.; Zhang, H.L.; Li, X.L. Development of simple identification models for four main catechins and caffeine in fresh green tea leaf based on visible and near-infrared spectroscopy. *Comput. Electron. Agric.* **2020**, *173*, 105388. [CrossRef]
103. Li, X.L.; Zhang, D.Y.; Dong, Y.L.; Jin, J.J.; He, Y. Spectral rapid detection of phytochemicals in tea (*Camellia sinensis*) based on convolutional neural network. *J. China Agric. Univ.* **2021**, *26*, 113–122.
104. Luo, W.; Tian, P.; Fan, G.Z.; Dong, W.T.; Zhang, H.L.; Liu, X.M. Non-destructive determination of four tea polyphenols in fresh tea using visible and near-infrared spectroscop. *Infrared Phys. Technol.* **2022**, *123*, 104037. [CrossRef]
105. Guo, J.M.; Huang, H.; He, X.L.; Cai, J.W.; Zeng, Z.X.; Ma, C.Y.; Lue, E.L.; Shen, Q.Y.; Liu, Y.H. Improving the detection accuracy of the nitrogen content of fresh tea leaves by combining FT-NIR with moisture removal method. *Food Chem.* **2023**, *405*, 134905. [CrossRef]
106. Hazarika, A.K.; Chanda, S.; Sabhapondit, S.; Sanyal, S.; Tamuly, P.; Tasrin, S.; Sing, D.; Tudu, B.; Bandyopadhyay, R. Quality assessment of fresh tea leaves by estimating total polyphenols using near infrared spectroscopy. *J. Food Sci. Technol.* **2018**, *55*, 4867–4876. [CrossRef] [PubMed]
107. Tian, Z.X.; Tan, Z.F.; Li, Y.J.; Yang, Z.L. Rapid monitoring of flavonoid content in sweet tea (*Lithocarpus litseifolius* (Hance) Chun) leaves using NIR spectroscopy. *Plant Methods.* **2022**, *18*, 44. [CrossRef]
108. Ye, S.; Weng, H.; Xiang, L.; Jia, L.; Xu, J. Synchronously Predicting Tea Polyphenol and Epigallocatechin Gallate in Tea Leaves Using Fourier Transform–Near-Infrared Spectroscopy and Machine Learning. *Molecules* **2023**, *28*, 5379. [CrossRef]
109. Sanaeifar, A.; Zhang, W.K.; Chen, H.T.; Zhang, D.Y.; Li, X.L.; He, Y. Study on effects of airborne Pb pollution on quality indicators and accumulation in tea plants using Vis-NIR spectroscopy coupled with radial basis function neural network. *Ecotoxicol. Environ. Saf.* **2022**, *229*, 113056. [CrossRef]
110. Liu, Y.; Peng, Q.W.; Yu, J.C.; Tang, Y.L. Identification of tea based on CARS-SWR variable optimization of visible/near-infrared spectrum. *J. Sci. Food Agric.* **2020**, *100*, 371–375.
111. Wang, S.; Feng, L.; Liu, P.; Gui, A.; Teng, J.; Ye, F.; Wang, X.; Xue, J.; Gao, S.; Zheng, P. Digital Prediction of the Purchase Price of Fresh Tea Leaves of Enshi Yulu Based on Near-Infrared Spectroscopy Combined with Multivariate Analysis. *Foods* **2023**, *12*, 3592. [CrossRef] [PubMed]
112. Sanaeifar, A.; Zhu, F.L.; Sha, J.J.; Li, X.L.; He, Y.; Zhan, Z.H. Rapid quantitative characterization of tea seedlings under lead-containing aerosol particles stress using Vis-NIR spectra. *Sci. Total Environ.* **2022**, *802*, 149824. [CrossRef]
113. Li, C.L.; Zong, B.Z.; Guo, H.W.; Luo, Z.; He, P.M.; Gong, S.Y.; Fan, F.Y. Discrimination of white teas produced from fresh leaves with different maturity by near-infrared spectroscopy. *Spectrochim. Acta Part A Mol. Biomol. Spectrosc.* **2020**, *227*, 117697. [CrossRef] [PubMed]
114. Zhou, J.; Cheng, H.; Zeng, J.M.; Wang, L.Y.; Wei, K.; He, W.; Wang, W.F.; Liu, X. Study on Identification and Traceability of Tea Material Cultivar byCombined Analysis of Multi-Partial Least Squares Models Based onNear Infrared Spectroscopy. *Spectrosc. Spectral Anal.* **2010**, *30*, 2650–2653.
115. Chen, Y.; Deng, J.; Wang, Y.X.; Liu, B.P.; Ding, J.; Mao, X.J.; Zhang, J.; Hu, H.T.; Li, J. Study on discrimination of white tea and albino tea based on near-infrared spectroscopy and chemometrics. *J. Sci. Food Agric.* **2014**, *94*, 1026–1033. [CrossRef] [PubMed]
116. Wang, S.P.; Zheng, P.C.; Gong, Z.M.; Zhang, Z.Z.; Teng, J.; Wang, X.P.; Lu, S.F. Establishment of discrimination model for different elevationfresh tea leaves based on near infrared spectroscopy. *J. Huazhong Agric. Univ.* **2018**, *37*, 89–94.
117. Li, X.L.; Luo, L.B.; He, Y.; Xu, N. Determination of dry matter content of tea by near and middle infrared spectroscopy coupled with wavelet-based data mining algorithms. *Comput. Electron. Agric.* **2013**, *98*, 46–53. [CrossRef]
118. Pielorz, S.; Fecka, I.; Bernacka, K.; Mazurek, S. Quantitative Determination of Polyphenols and Flavonoids in Cistus × incanus on the Basis of IR, NIR and Raman Spectra. *Molecules* **2023**, *28*, 161. [CrossRef]
119. Li, X.; Chen, Y.; Mei, W.J.; Wu, X.H.; Feng, Y.J.; Wu, B. Classification of Tea Varieties Using Fuzzy Covariance Learning Vector Quantization. *Spectrosc. Spectral Anal.* **2023**, *43*, 638–643.
120. Wu, D.M.; Guo, J.; Sun, M.M.; Zhang, Y. Infrared and Terahertz Spectra of Pu'er White Tea with Different Degrees of Oxidation. *J. Food Process. Preserv.* **2023**, *2023*, 3290917. [CrossRef]
121. Sun, X.D.; Xu, C.; Luo, C.G.; Xie, D.F.; Fu, W.; Gong, Z.Y.; Wang, X.P. Non-destructive detection of tea stalk and insect foreign bodies based on THz-TDS combination of electromagnetic vibration feeder. *Food Qual. Saf.* **2023**, *7*, fyad004. [CrossRef]
122. Lu, Y.; Asante, E.A.; Duan, H.; Hu, Y. Quantitative Assessment of Cold Injury in Tea Plants by Terahertz Spectroscopy Method. *Agronomy* **2023**, *13*, 1376. [CrossRef]
123. Zhang, Y.Y.; Gao, W.J.; Cui, C.J.; Zhang, Z.Z.; He, L.L.; Zheng, J.K.; Hou, R.Y. Development of a method to evaluate the tenderness of fresh tea leaves based on rapid, in-situ Raman spectroscopy scanning for carotenoids. *Food Chem.* **2020**, *308*, 125648. [CrossRef] [PubMed]
124. Li, X.L.; Xu, K.W.; He, Y. Determination of Carotenoids Contents in Tea Leaves Based on Raman Spectroscopy. *Spectrosc. Spectral Anal.* **2017**, *37*, 3465–3470.
125. Zeng, J.J.; Ping, W.; Sanaeifar, A.; Xu, X.; Luo, W.; Sha, J.J.; Huang, Z.X.; Huang, Y.F.; Liu, X.M.; Zhan, B.S.; et al. Quantitative visualization of photosynthetic pigments in tea leaves based on Raman spectroscopy and calibration model transfer. *Plant Methods* **2021**, *17*, 4. [CrossRef] [PubMed]
126. Chen, C.S.; Shi, X.Z.; Li, Q.; Liu, Z.W. Detection of fresh tea leaves of Zhuye by Raman spectroscopy. *Chin. J. Quantum Electron.* **2017**, *34*, 513–517.

127. Li, X.L.; Luo, L.B.; Hu, X.Q.; Lou, B.G.; He, Y. Revealing the Chemical Changes of Tea Cell Wall Induced by Anthracnose with Confocal Raman Microscopy. *Spectrosc. Spectral Anal.* **2014**, *34*, 1571–1576.
128. Liu, Y.D.; Lin, X.D.; Gao, H.G.; Gao, X.; Wang, S. Quantitative Analysis of Chlorophyll Content in Tea Leaves byFluorescence Spectroscopy. *Laser Optoelectron. Prog.* **2021**, *58*, 452–461.
129. Zheng, J.P.; Wu, R.M.; Xiong, J.F.; Wang, P.W.; Xiao, H.G.; Fan, Y.; Ai, S.R. Nondestructive Detection of Pesticide Residues on Fresh Tea Leave usingFluoresce Hyperspectral Imaging Combined with Spectral Angle Algorithm. *Laser J.* **2016**, *37*, 57–60.
130. Liu, Y.D.; Lin, X.D.; Gao, H.G.; Wang, S.; Gao, X. Research on Tea Cephaleuros Virescens Kunze Model Based onChlorophyll Fluorescence Spectroscopy. *Spectrosc. Spectral Anal.* **2021**, *41*, 2129–2134.

Disclaimer/Publisher's Note: The statements, opinions and data contained in all publications are solely those of the individual author(s) and contributor(s) and not of MDPI and/or the editor(s). MDPI and/or the editor(s) disclaim responsibility for any injury to people or property resulting from any ideas, methods, instructions or products referred to in the content.

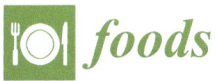

Review

Recent Advances Regarding Polyphenol Oxidase in *Camellia sinensis*: Extraction, Purification, Characterization, and Application

Chun Zou [1], Xin Zhang [1], Yongquan Xu [1,*] and Junfeng Yin [2,*]

1. Key Laboratory of Biology, Tea Research Institute, Chinese Academy of Agricultural Sciences, Ministry of Agriculture and Rural Affairs, Hangzhou 310008, China; zouchun@tricaas.com (C.Z.); xinzhang@tricaas.com (X.Z.)
2. National Engineering Research Center for Tea Processing, Hangzhou 310008, China
* Correspondence: yqx33@126.com (Y.X.); yinjf@tricaas.com (J.Y.); Tel.: +86-571-8601-7633 (Y.X.); +86-571-8665-0187 (J.Y.)

Abstract: Polyphenol oxidase (PPO) is an important metalloenzyme in the tea plant (*Camellia sinensis*). However, there has recently been a lack of comprehensive reviews on *Camellia sinensis* PPO. In this study, the methods for extracting PPO from *Camellia sinensis*, including acetone extraction, buffer extraction, and surfactant extraction, are compared in detail. The main purification methods for *Camellia sinensis* PPO, such as ammonium sulfate precipitation, three-phase partitioning, dialysis, ultrafiltration, ion exchange chromatography, gel filtration chromatography, and affinity chromatography, are summarized. PPOs from different sources of tea plants are characterized and systematically compared in terms of optimal pH, optimal temperature, molecular weight, substrate specificity, and activators and inhibitors. In addition, the applications of PPO in tea processing and the in vitro synthesis of theaflavins are outlined. In this review, detailed research regarding the extraction, purification, properties, and application of *Camellia sinensis* PPO is summarized to provide a reference for further research on PPO.

Keywords: polyphenol oxidase; *Camellia sinensis*; extraction; purification; characterization; application

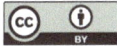

1. Introduction

Polyphenol oxidase (PPO) belongs to the category of oxidoreductases and is widely present in plants [1], animals [2], and fungi [3]. According to the different numbers of phenolic hydroxyl groups in the catalytic substrate, PPO can be divided into three categories [4,5]: monophenol oxidase (tyrosinase, EC 1.14.18.1), bisphenol oxidase (catechol oxidase, EC 1.10.3.1), and laccase (EC 1.10.3.2). PPO in plants mainly occurs in the form of catechol oxidase, which can catalyze the generation of its corresponding quinones from polyphenols under aerobic conditions [6,7].

PPO plays an important role in tea processing [8,9], and it determines the degree of tea oxidation. According to the degree of oxidation, tea can be divided into six categories: green tea [10] (non-oxidized), white tea [11] and yellow tea [12] (lightly oxidized), oolong tea [13] (semi-oxidized), black tea [14] (fully oxidized), and dark tea [15] (post-fermented with micro-organisms). By inhibiting or promoting the enzymatic oxidation of PPO, various categories of teas with distinct flavors are produced. Under the catalysis of enzymes such as PPO, the catechins in tea are oxidized to form catechin polymers [16], including theasinensins, theaflavins, and thearubigins.

Tea plant PPO is encoded and expressed by nuclear genes [17], which have multi-gene family characteristics [18]. Zeng et al. [19] obtained five coding genes of PPO from the tea plant genome database with a total length of 597–1839 bp in the CDS region and encoding 198–612 amino acids. Through real-time quantitative PCR, it was found that these genes exhibit different expression patterns among different tea plant varieties. Many PPO isoenzymes with significant differences in their properties were isolated from fresh tea leaves. PPO in fresh tea leaves mainly exists as low activity precursor enzymes, which bind to organelle membranes such as chloroplasts in an insoluble form [20], which is known as membrane-bound PPO (mPPO). In addition, there are small amounts of mature enzymes, known as soluble PPOs (sPPOs), which have been removed from their transfer peptides and are free in a soluble form within the cystic body. There are differences in the extraction and purification of different types of PPO; this poses a challenge to tea plant PPO research.

Due to the enzymatic browning caused by PPO [21], researchers have focused on studying how to inhibit PPO activity in other plants or fungi. However, the catalytic activity of PPO needs to be utilized in the processing of tea (except for unfermented tea) and the preparation of theaflavins. Therefore, it is necessary to elaborate in detail on the tea plant PPO. In this study, detailed research on the extraction, purification, properties, and application of *Camellia sinensis* PPO is summarized to provide a reference for further research on PPO.

2. Extraction of PPO

The methods for extracting PPO from fresh tea leaves include acetone extraction, buffer extraction, and surfactant extraction. The extraction solvents, as well as the advantages and disadvantages of the above three methods, are listed in Table 1.

Table 1. Comparison of extraction methods for *Camellia sinensis* PPO.

Method	Extract Solvent	Specific Enzyme Activity (U/mg)	Advantage	Disadvantage	References
Acetone extraction	Acetone	24,789	High enzyme activity, stable and easy to store	Low extraction rate of enzyme	[22,23]
Buffer extraction	Phosphate/citrate buffer	192	Easy operation, less impurity	Low enzyme activity and extraction rate	[24,25]
Surfactant extraction	Triton X-100	20,544	High extraction rate of enzyme	Surfactant needs to be removed	[26–28]

2.1. Acetone Extraction

The advantages of the acetone extraction method [29] are that it has high enzyme activity and can be directly applied; moreover, the enzyme is stable and easy to store. However, its disadvantage is that the enzyme extraction rate is too low, possibly due to acetone causing irreversible protein denaturation. To reduce this enzyme denaturation, acetone needs to be pre-cooled before use. Frozen tea leaves were homogenized in cold acetone (-25 °C), and the slurry was subjected to repeated filtration and cold acetone extraction to obtain a white crude enzyme powder [23]. The acetone extraction method has been applied to analyze the changes in PPO activity of different varieties of tea leaves during black tea processing [22]. In addition, this method has also been widely used for PPO extraction in other plants, including apple [29], *Physalis peruviana* L. [30], and *Cistanche deserticola* [31].

2.2. Buffer Extraction

The buffer extraction method is used to obtain PPO by mixing tea leaves with buffer and homogenizing them, then filtering them out. This method has the advantages of simple operation and low impurities in the enzyme solution. However, the PPO activity extracted by this method is relatively low, and the extraction solution needs to be further concentrated and purified before it can be applied. As shown in Table 1, the specific activity of PPO extracted by buffer is 192 U/mg, which is significantly lower than that extracted by acetone or surfactant. The types of buffers used in this method include phosphate buffer (pH 6.8) [24] and citric acid phosphate buffer (pH 5.6) [25]. In order to reduce the content of tea polyphenols in the extraction solution, polyvinyl pyrrolidone (PVP) and cross-linked polyvinylpyrrolidone (PVPP) are added to the buffer to adsorb polyphenols. It was found that the activity of PPO obtained by adding PVP was higher than that of PVPP, possibly due to the fact that PVP, with its good water solubility, can adsorb more tea polyphenols [25]. The buffer extraction method is widely used for the extraction of soluble PPO from different plants [32,33], but it cannot extract the membrane-bound PPO, resulting in a lower extraction rate.

2.3. Surfactant Extraction

Non-ionic surfactants mainly rely on hydrophobic interactions to dissolve membrane proteins, which are usually used for the extraction of membrane-bound PPO in plants [34–36]. The non-ionic surfactant used for extracting membrane-bound PPO from tea leaves is usually Triton X-100. The surfactant is dissolved in a buffer at a certain concentration (usually 50 mM) of salt ions, which contributes to stabilization of the enzyme protein. The fresh leaves of three tea tree varieties (Ningzhou population, Ningzhou 2, and Dayelong) were homogenized with phosphate buffer (pH 6.8) and centrifuged to obtain the supernatant containing soluble PPO. Then, the precipitate was extracted with 0.25% Triton X-100 to obtain membrane-bound PPO [26]. The surfactant extraction method can achieve a higher PPO extraction rate, but the addition of surfactants may interfere with the determination of enzyme properties.

3. Purification of PPO

The crude enzyme solution extracted from tea leaves contains not only nucleic acids, polyphenols, etc., but also other proteins in addition to PPO. As shown in Figure 1, the purification of PPO is generally divided into two major steps: crude purification and fine purification. The crude separation of PPO mainly includes ammonium sulfate precipitation [37], three-phase partitioning [38], dialysis [39], and ultrafiltration [40]. The fine purification of PPO is generally carried out via chromatography, including ion exchange chromatography [41], gel filtration chromatography [42], affinity chromatography [43], etc.

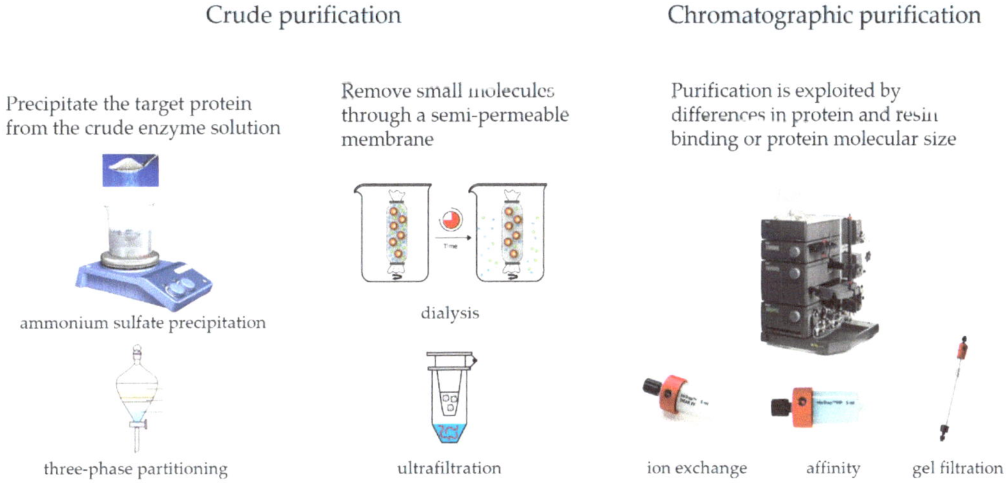

Figure 1. The main purification steps for *Camellia sinensis* PPO.

3.1. Crude Purification

3.1.1. Ammonium Sulfate Precipitation

The principle behind the ammonium sulfate precipitation method [44] is that high concentrations of salt ions can compete with proteins for water molecules, thereby destroying the hydration film on the surface of proteins, reducing their solubility, and allowing them to precipitate out of the solution. This method can remove a large amount of non-protein impurities and also concentrate the target protein. After a crude enzyme solution extracted from *Camellia sinensis* cv. Longjing 43 was precipitated with 80% ammonium sulfate, the specific activity of PPO was found to increase by 3.73-fold [45].

Graded ammonium sulfate precipitation is commonly used to remove some impurity proteins, and its principle is based on the difference in protein solubility in different ammonium sulfate concentrations. PPO crude enzyme was added with 10%, 20%, 30%, 70%, 80%, and 90% of ammonium sulfate in sequence and then left to stand at 4 °C to precipitate the proteins. While testing the enzymatic activities of the precipitated proteins mentioned above, it was found that the enzymatic activity of PPO proteins precipitated with 10–30% ammonium sulfate was very low (<3%), while that of proteins precipitated with 30–90% ammonium sulfate reached 65.26% of the total enzyme activity [46]. Therefore, it is important to select an appropriate concentration of ammonium sulfate to precipitate proteins during the crude separation of PPO.

3.1.2. Three-Phase Partitioning

Three-phase partitioning (TPP) is a method of crude purification of target proteins, which involves adding a certain proportion of salt and organic solvents to the crude extraction solution to create clear layering of the mixed solution [47]. This method promotes the aggregation of some of the proteins in the precipitation layer between the organic and aqueous phases, the dissolution of low-molecular-weight pigments, membrane lipids, etc., in the organic layer, and the dissolution of sugars and some proteins in the water layer. The sPPO and mPPO from tea leaves were purified via TPP, resulting in 2.80-fold and 2.32-fold increases in specific enzyme activity, respectively [26]. The activity yields of TPP to sPPO and mPPO were 73.8% and 79.8%, respectively. With its advantages of simple operation, wide applicability, and high activity yield, TPP has been widely used in the extraction of PPO from various plants, including *Rosmarinus officinalis* L. [47], *Lepiota procera* [48], and *Trachystemon orientalis* L. [38]. The PPO from *Trachystemon orientalis* L. was purified 3.59-fold with a 68.75% total recovery of activity using the TPP procedure twice in a row [38].

3.1.3. Dialysis

As a result of methods such as ammonium sulfate precipitation or three-phase partitioning, large amounts of salt ions are introduced into the enzyme solutions, requiring dialysis to remove them. Dialysis is a method of separating proteins and small molecules utilizing small molecules to penetrate through a semi-permeable membrane into a low salt buffer while large molecules, such as proteins, remain trapped within the semi-permeable membrane [49]. Usually, the sample is placed in a dialysis bag made of a semi-permeable membrane, and the dialysis bag is immersed in a low salt buffer solution. Salt and small-molecule substances are used to continuously diffuse and dialyze outside the bag, achieving purification [50]. To achieve good purification results, the low salt buffer needs to be replaced multiple times. Following ammonium sulfate precipitation, the PPO from fresh tea leaves was dialyzed in a cut-off with 8–12 kDa, and the purification factor was found to increase by 2.42 times [51].

3.1.4. Ultrafiltration

Ultrafiltration can achieve high concentration multiples, making it easy to concentrate and recover the target product from diluted and complex mixed samples [52]. It is necessary to select ultrafiltration tubes, which retain molecular weight based on the molecular weight of the target protein [53]. Rapidly reducing salt ions in samples can also be achieved through ultrafiltration. Following TPP treatment, sPPO and mPPO in fresh tea leaves were centrifuged through an ultrafiltration tube (molecular weight cut-off of 15 kDa) using centrifugal force of $4500 \times g$ at 4 °C, and their purification times were found to increase by 9.58-fold and 9.05-fold, respectively [27].

3.2. Chromatographic Purification

Chromatographic chromatography is generally used for fine purification of enzyme proteins after crude purification [54]. As shown in Table 2, the chromatographic methods used for PPO purification from tea sources mainly include ion chromatography, gel filtration chromatography, and affinity chromatography. In order to achieve good purification results, it is very important to choose the appropriate resin and elution buffer [55].

Table 2. Comparison of chromatographic chromatography for *Camellia sinensis* PPO.

Type of Chromatography	Chromatographic Matrix	Elution Buffer	Purification Fold	References
Anion exchange	DEAE-cellulose	A linear gradient of phosphate buffer (pH 6.8) concentration from 10 to 200 mM	3.32	[23]
Anion exchange	UNOsphere™ Q	A linear concentration gradient (0–1.0 M) of NaCl in 20 mM Tris-HCl (pH 9.0)	11.8	[56]
Gel filtration	Sephadex G-75	0.02 M Tris–HCl buffer (pH 7.5) containing 100 mL/L glycerol and 0.1 M NaCl	48.94	[51]
Affinity	Ni-NTA	Imidazole solution of 25–500 mM	Unknown	[57]
Affinity	Sepharose 4B-L-tyrosine-p-aminobenzoic acid	0.1 M Tris–HCl buffer (pH 8.5) containing 1 M NaCl	19.77	[28]

3.2.1. Ion Exchange Chromatography

The principle behind ion exchange chromatography is that the charge carried by the separated substance can combine with the opposite charge carried by the ion exchange agent [58]. The binding effect between the charged molecule and the stationary phase is reversible. When changing the pH or eluting with a buffer solution, which gradually increases the ion strength, the substance bound by the ion exchange agent can exchange with the ions in the eluent and be eluted into the solution [59]. Due to differences in the charges of different proteins, their binding abilities to ion exchangers also vary, resulting in different orders of elution into the solution [60]. The resins, which have been used for ion exchange chromatography in the purification of PPO, are DEAE-cellulose [61] and UNOsphere™ Q (BioRad, Hercules, CA, USA) [62]. The pH of the buffer solution for both DEAE and Q ion exchange chromatography needs to be at least one unit higher than the pI of the target protein to be bound, where the pH of the buffer solution for Q ion exchange chromatography is higher than that of DEAE. Based on the amino acid sequence of PPO published in the NCBI database, the pI of most tea tree PPOs is predicted to be about pH 6.4. PPO was separated by linearly increasing the buffer solution from a low salt ion concentration to a high salt ion concentration. The purification fold results of PPO purified using DEAE and Q ion exchange chromatography were found to be 3.32 [23] and 11.8 [56], respectively, which indicates that it is difficult to obtain high-purity PPO solely through ion exchange chromatography.

3.2.2. Gel Filtration Chromatography

Gel filtration chromatography [63], also known as steric exclusion chromatography and molecular sieves, is a method of separating the proteins based on their differences in molecular weight or shape. In order to obtain a good purification effect, it is necessary to select a chromatographic matrix with a pore size, which is suitable for the molecular weight of the target protein [64]. Sephadex G-75 was used as a chromatographic substrate for the purification of PPO from tea leaves, and a purification fold of 48.94 was achieved [51]. Therefore, the protein can be highly purified by gel filtration chromatography. Gel filtration chromatography is widely used for the purification of PPO from other sources, including *Coriandrum sativum* [65], *Musa acuminata* [66], and sweet potato [42]. Two sPPO and one mPPO from sweet potato peel [42] were purified by gel filtration chromatography with the purification fold of 69.03, 31.59, and 124.01, respectively.

3.2.3. Affinity Chromatography

Affinity chromatography is a protein purification method, which is designed based on the specific and reversible binding between proteins and matrices [43]. Nickel column affinity chromatography is a widely used method for purifying recombinant proteins [67]. Due to the competitive binding of Ni^{2+} ions in nickel columns to imidazole or proteins with His-Tag, increasing the concentration of imidazole in the elution buffer can elute the target protein to achieve protein purification. Two PPO isoenzymes with His-Tag expressed by *Escherichia coli* were purified via binding to an Ni IDA affinity chromatography column and eluting with different concentrations of imidazole (25–500 mM) [57]. PPO from tea leaf was purified 19.77-fold in one step using Sepharose 4B-L-tyrosine-p-aminobenzoic acid affinity chromatography [28]. Compared to other chromatography methods, affinity chromatography has the advantages of simplicity and speed. Sepharose 4B-L-tyrosine-p-aminobenzoic acid and Sepharose-6B-L-tyrosine-p-aminobenzoic acid were applied to the affinity chromatography of PPO from *Persea americana* [43], which obtained the purification fold of 147.73 and 154.00, respectively.

4. Characterizations of PPO

The characterizations of PPO from different sources of tea plants were systematically compared in terms of optimal pH, optimal temperature, molecular weight, substrate specificity, and activators and inhibitors. As shown in Table 3, PPO characterizations vary not only among different *Camellia sinensis* varieties but also among different isoenzymes derived from the same tea leaves.

Table 3. Comparison of *Camellia sinensis* PPO characterizations.

Source	pH	Temperature (°C)	Molecular Weight (kDa)	References
Two PPO isozymes from *Camellia sinensis* var. Zhenghedabai	5.5 and 6.0	33 and 38	85 and 42	[51]
PPO from *Camellia sinensis* var. Lapsang souchong	6.2	35	66	[56]
PPO from Turkish tea leaves	6.0	30	72	[23]
PPO from Turkish tea leaves	6.0	30	Unknown	[68]
PPO from Indian tea leaves	5.0	Unknown	72	[69]
Two recombinant PPO isozymes from Huangjinya tea	6.0 and 5.5	35 and 30	61.15 and 61.21	[57]

4.1. Optimal pH of PPO

In Table 3, the optimal pH values of PPO from different tea leaves are reported, varying between 5.0 and 6.2. The reason for the difference in the optimal pH of PPO from different tea plants may be its different structures, especially PPOs with large molecular weight differences. The optimum pH of PPO from tea leaves in Turkey was found to be 6.0 [23,68]. Different PPO isoenzymes isolated from tea leaves show differences at the optimal pH. Two PPO isozymes from *Camellia sinensis* var. Zhenghedabai were purified [51], with one PPO isozyme having an optimal pH of 6.0 and the other PPO isozyme having an optimal pH of 5.5. There are significant differences in the optimal pH of PPO from different plant sources [70]. The PPO from tea leaves with similar optimal pH levels includes *Vaccinium corymbosum* L. [71], Ataulfo mango [72], and *Solanum lycocarpum* [73].

4.2. Optimal Temperature of PPO

The optimal temperature of PPO from different tea leaves is mostly in the range of 30–38 °C. The catalytic activity of PPO is highest at the optimal temperature, and it decreases above or below the optimal temperature [74]. The optimal temperature for PPO varies among different tea varieties, as well as among the same variety of isoenzymes. The optimal temperature for one type of PPO isoenzyme from Huangjinya tea was determined to be 35 °C, while that for another type of PPO isoenzyme was 30 °C [57]. The optimal temperature for PPO in tea leaves is similar to that for some other plants, such as *Dioscorea alata* [75], *Terfezia arenaria* [76], and *Salacca zalacca* [77].

4.3. Molecular Weight of PPO

The molecular weight of PPO in tea leaves has been reported to range from 15 to 97 kDa [56,78]. Currently, there are 36 protein sequences of PPO from *Camellia sinensis*, which can be retrieved from the NCBI database, most of which have 599 amino acids. Based on the number of amino acids, it has been inferred that the molecular weight of most PPOs from *Camellia sinensis* is approximately 66 kDa. The PPO from *Camellia sinensis* var. Lapsang souchong was isolated from a black tea infusion, and its molecular weight was determined to be 66 kDa [56]. Five *ppo* genes from five cultivars of *Camellia sinensis* were expressed in *E. coli* BL21, and all of the five recombinant PPOs obtained exhibited molecular weights of 66 kDa [79].

Due to the presence of many PPO isoenzymes in tea plants, there are differences in the molecular weight of PPO reported in different studies. Two PPO isozymes were isolated from tea leaves [51], and their molecular weights were found to be 42 and 85 kDa, respectively. There are also differences in the molecular weight of PPOs derived from different plants. PPO in *Pueraria lobata* was purified [80], and its molecular weight was determined to be 21 kDa via SDS-PAGE. The molecular weight of PPO from Huaniu Apples [81] was determined to be 140 kDa using native-PAGE and SDS-PAGE, but on the basis of urea-SDS-PAGE, it was found to be 61 kDa, which indicates that it may be a dimer. The high abundance of the PPO homodimer suggests that it may be involved in proanthocyanidins polymerization, which leads to the formation of the dark-red skin of apples. However, it has not been reported whether PPO from *Camellia sinensis* is a polymer.

4.4. Substrate Specificity of PPO

The substrates used for PPO include catechol, 4-methyl catechol, catechins, pyrogallol, and gallic acid [6,7]. Among them, catechol is the most widely used substrate. Eight substances were used to test the substrate specificity of purified PPO [69]. Among them, three substances—p-quinol, p-cresol, and tyrosine—cannot be catalyzed by PPO; meanwhile, the other five substances—catechin, epicatechin, catechol, pyrogallol, and gallic acid—can be used as substrates for PPO. The Km value for catechin is the lowest, indicating that it has the highest affinity with PPO. Altunkaya [68] found that PPO not only had the highest affinity for catechin, but it also had the highest catalytic efficiency toward it, taking into account the highest Vmax/Km ratio. There is a significant difference in substrate specificity between PPO from tea leaves and other plants. PPO from *Irvingia gabonensis* [82] was found to show preference toward catechol, with a relative activity of 100%; on the other hand, it had lower catalytic activity toward catechin, with a relative activity of 77.1%.

4.5. Activators and Inhibitors of PPO

Due to the presence of two Cu^{2+} binding regions in the active center of PPO, Cu^{2+} is considered an activator of PPO [83]. Testing of the effect of different Cu^{2+} concentrations on the activity of *Camellia sinensis* PPO [78] showed that it had the highest catalytic activity when the Cu^{2+} concentration was 10^{-7} M. Although SDS, urea, and surfactants have been reported to activate some plant PPOs [5,84], they are considered to have no activating effect on *Camellia sinensis* PPO [69]. The purified PPO and crude enzyme extracts from tea leaves were treated with SDS (0.1–5 mM) and urea (0.5–2 M), but no activation effect was detected.

The inhibitors of *Camellia sinensis* PPO include sodium metabisulfite, sodium sulfite, ascorbic acid, EDTA, cysteine, citric acid, and oxalic acid [23,28]. However, there are differences in the inhibitory effects of inhibitors on PPO from different tea leaves. The inhibitory effect of cysteine on PPO from *Camellia sinensis* var. Lapsang souchong [56] was found to be stronger than that of ascorbic acid, while ascorbic acid was found to be the most effective inhibitor of PPO from Turkish tea leaves [68], followed by cysteine. Both cysteine and ascorbic acid have been determined as competitive inhibitors of PPO.

5. Application of PPO

Controlling the PPO activity in tea processing greatly affects its quality, especially in tea with high fermentation levels, such as black tea and dark tea. In addition, PPO is widely used in the in vitro synthesis of theaflavins.

5.1. The Role of PPO in Tea Processing

As shown in Table 4, there is a substantial difference between PPO in black tea processing and dark tea processing. In black tea processing, PPO comes from endogenous enzymes in fresh tea leaves. However, endogenous enzymes are inactivated in the first step in the processing of dark tea, while PPO is produced by micro-organisms in subsequent processes. The catalytic effect of PPO is present in the fermentation of black tea and in the pile fermentation of dark tea. In addition, the products of PPO oxidation are mainly theaflavins and thearubigins in black tea, but theabrownines in dark tea.

5.1.1. Black Tea

Black tea is fully fermented tea, and during its processing, it produces theaflavin pigments through enzymatic oxidation of catechins, forming its unique color and aroma [85]. PPO is a key enzyme in the enzymatic oxidation of black tea, and its enzyme activity dynamically changes during processing. In black tea processing, PPO activity increases during withering and rolling processes, while it decreases during fermentation and drying processes. PPO activity was found to increase with the prolongation of withering time during withering [86]; at the end of withering, PPO activity reached a level, which was 2.9 times that of fresh leaf PPO activity. Rolling can cause damage to the tea leaves through external forces, resulting in polyphenolic compounds, endogenous PPO, and other components leaking into the leaf epidermis and coming into full contact with oxygen and other substances. PPO activity was found to reach its highest level during the rolling process [87]. Fermentation is a key process in forming the quality characteristics of black tea, which is essentially a chemical change process, which occurs through enzymatic or non-enzymatic oxidation reactions with polyphenolic compounds. The fermentation process of black tea is influenced by various factors, such as oxygen [88], temperature [89], humidity [85], and fermentation time [90]. Oxygen [88] was found to be the key factor limiting the oxidation rate of polyphenols in regular black tea fermentation. A low fermentation temperature [89] was beneficial to promoting the accumulation of theaflavins and thearubigins. Under different temperature conditions, it was found that PPO activity in all samples decreased significantly with fermentation [91]. Drying rapidly deactivates various enzymes in tea due to the high temperature [92].

Enhancing PPO activity in black tea processing is an effective way of improving the quality of black tea. Comparing the processing of fresh tea leaves from different varieties, seasons, and regions for Congou Black Tea [93], it was found that the black tea obtained from processing fresh tea leaves with high PPO activity had a higher content of theaflavins. It was found that oxygen was consumed in large quantities during the processing of black tea [94]. Compared with traditional fermentation methods, a new dynamic fermentation method has been developed, which effectively improves PPO activity by increasing the oxygen content during the fermentation process [95], thereby promoting the formation of theaflavins and thearubigins and improving the quality of black tea. Moreover, oxygen-enriched fermentation [96] was found to improve the taste of black tea and promote the oxidation of catechins, flavonoid glycosides, and some phenolic acids. In addition, adding exogenous PPO [97,98] to black tea processing improves the color and aroma of its tea soup and also increases the content of theaflavins.

Table 4. Comparison of PPO in black and dark tea processing.

Tea Category	PPO Source	Enzyme-Catalyzed Process	Products	References
Black tea	Endogenous enzymes in fresh tea leaves	Fermentation	Theaflavins and thearubigins	[14,85]
Dark tea	Microbial secretion	Pile fermentation	Theabrownines	[99–101]

5.1.2. Dark Tea

Dark tea is a type of post-fermented tea [99]. As shown in Figure 2, the processing of black tea mainly includes fixation, primary rolling, pile fermentation, second rolling, and drying. During the fixation process, the endogenous enzymes in tea leaves are inactivated. The key process in dark tea processing is pile fermentation. In this process, micro-organisms proliferate in large numbers and secrete extracellular enzymes, such as PPO, protease, and cellulase, which form the unique flavor and quality of dark tea [100]. During the processing of Fuzhuan brick tea [101], there is a trend in PPO activity to initially increase and then decrease, which is significantly correlated with the growth curve of *Eurotium cristatum*. It was found that adding exogenous PPO to the pile fermentation of Pu-erh tea [102] can accelerate its fermentation, shorten the fermentation cycle, and improve its quality.

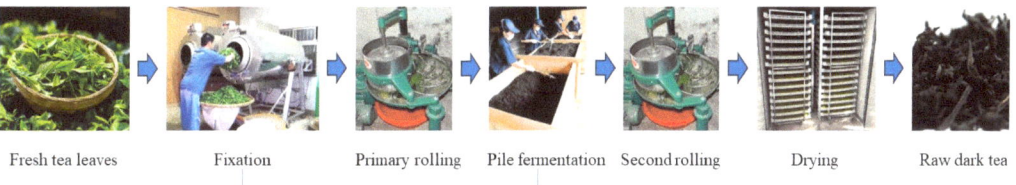

Figure 2. Primary processing of dark tea.

5.2. Synthesis of Theaflavins by PPO

Theaflavins are a type of plant pigment formed by the oxidation and condensation of catechins [103], which have various health benefits [104], such as anti-obesity, anti-inflammatory, and anti-cancer properties. Theaflavins are a key quality component of black tea and are mainly present in four forms (Figure 3): theaflavin (TF1), theaflavin-3-O-gallate (TF2a), theaflavin-3′-O-gallate (TF2b), and TF-3,3′-di-O-gallate (TF3) [104]. Catechins are first oxidized by PPO enzyme to form quinones, which are further oxidized to form theaflavins through non-enzymatic oxidation. However, TFs only account for about 1% of the dry weight of black tea, and the direct extraction cost is too high. Therefore, enzymatic oxidation through PPO in vitro is a more efficient and economical method for producing theaflavins [105,106]. Two types of PPO isoenzymes were isolated from fresh tea leaves and used for in vitro synthesis of theaflavins [51]. Among them, one PPO isoenzyme only resulted in the synthesis of simple TF, while the other isoenzyme could synthesize four types of TFs. Recombinant expression through micro-organisms is an important method for obtaining tea plant PPO [107]. Four tea plant PPO isoenzymes were prepared via recombinant expression in *E. coli* [108]. Although most of the recombinant enzymes exist as inclusion bodies, they can still efficiently catalyze the synthesis of TF3.

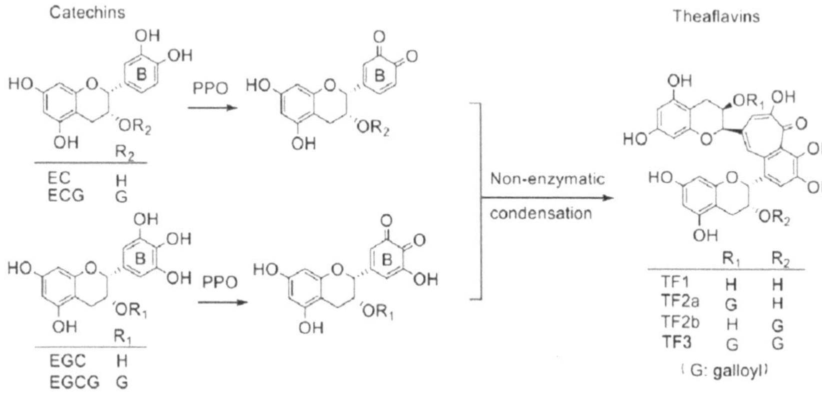

Figure 3. The formation of four theaflavins (TF1, TF2a, TF2b, and TF3) [104].

6. Conclusions and Perspectives

In this study, the isolation, purification, properties, and applications of tea plant PPO were systematically reviewed. The methods for extracting PPO from fresh tea leaves include acetone extraction, buffer extraction, and surfactant extraction, and their advantages and disadvantages were compared. The crude separation and fine purification methods of PPO and their purification effects were introduced in detail. The characterizations of PPO from different sources of tea plants were systematically compared in terms of optimal pH, optimal temperature, molecular weight, substrate specificity, and activators and inhibitors. The applications of PPO in tea processing and theaflavin synthesis were summarized.

Although significant achievements have been made in the research and application of tea plant PPO, there are still several aspects worth further investigation in the following areas: (1) the crystal structure of tea plant PPO protein needs to be detected. Currently, researchers have successfully purified PPO from multiple varieties of tea trees. If the protein structure of PPO can be further detected, this will help further explore its catalytic mechanism. (2) Further improvements are needed for the preparation of PPO through microbial recombinant expression. Currently, the main factor restricting widespread application of PPO is the difficulty in obtaining low-cost and highly active enzymes. The efficient recombinant expression of PPO through genetic engineering will greatly expand its application scope.

Author Contributions: Conceptualization, writing—original draft preparation, and funding acquisition, C.Z.; writing—review and editing, X.Z.; writing—review and editing, and project administration, Y.X. and J.Y. All authors have read and agreed to the published version of the manuscript.

Funding: This research was funded by the National Natural Science Foundation of China (32002094), the Key Research and Development Program of Zhejiang (2022C02033), the China Agriculture Research System of MOF and MARA (CARS-19), and the Innovation Project for Chinese Academy of Agricultural Sciences (CAAS-ASTIP-TRI).

Data Availability Statement: Data is contained within the article.

Conflicts of Interest: The authors declare no conflicts of interest.

References

1. Wei, X.M.; Shu, J.; Fahad, S.; Tao, K.L.; Zhang, J.W.; Chen, G.L.; Liang, Y.C.; Wang, M.Q.; Chen, S.Y.; Liao, J.G. Polyphenol oxidases regulate pollen development through modulating flavonoids homeostasis in tobacco. *Plant Physiol. Bioch.* **2023**, *198*, 107702. [CrossRef]
2. Hong, Q.; Chen, Y.L.; Lin, D.Q.; Yang, R.Q.; Cao, K.Y.; Zhang, L.J.; Liu, Y.M.; Sun, L.C.; Cao, M.J. Expression of polyphenol oxidase of *Litopenaeus vannamei* and its characterization. *Food Chem.* **2024**, *432*, 137258. [CrossRef] [PubMed]
3. Sarsenova, A.; Demir, D.; Caglayan, K.; Abiyev, S.; Darbayeva, T.; Eken, C. Purification and Properties of Polyphenol Oxidase of Dried *Volvariella bombycina*. *Biology* **2023**, *12*, 53. [CrossRef] [PubMed]

4. Tinello, F.; Lante, A. Recent advances in controlling polyphenol oxidase activity of fruit and vegetable products. *Innov. Food Sci. Emerg.* **2018**, *50*, 73–83. [CrossRef]
5. Mayer, A.M. Polyphenol oxidases in plants and fungi: Going places? A review. *Phytochemistry* **2006**, *67*, 2318–2331. [CrossRef] [PubMed]
6. McLarin, M.A.; Leung, I.K.H. Substrate specificity of polyphenol oxidase. *Crit. Rev. Biochem. Mol.* **2020**, *55*, 274–308. [CrossRef]
7. Li, J.F.; Deng, Z.Y.; Dong, H.H.; Tsao, R.; Liu, X.R. Substrate specificity of polyphenol oxidase and its selectivity towards polyphenols: Unlocking the browning mechanism of fresh lotus root (*Nelumbo nucifera* Gaertn.). *Food Chem.* **2023**, *424*, 136392. [CrossRef]
8. Hua, J.J.; Xu, Q.; Yuan, H.B.; Wang, J.J.; Wu, Z.Q.; Li, X.T.; Jiang, Y.W. Effects of novel fermentation method on the biochemical components change and quality formation of Congou black tea. *J. Food Compos. Anal.* **2021**, *96*, 103751. [CrossRef]
9. Zhang, G.Y.; Yang, J.H.; Cui, D.D.; Zhao, D.D.; Li, Y.Y.; Wan, X.C.; Zhao, J. Transcriptome and Metabolic Profiling Unveiled Roles of Peroxidases in Theaflavin Production in Black Tea Processing and Determination of Tea Processing Suitability. *J. Agric. Food Chem.* **2020**, *68*, 3528–3538. [CrossRef]
10. Song, F.H.; Zheng, Y.; Li, R.Y.; Li, Z.F.; Liu, B.Y.; Wu, X. Intelligent control of green tea fixation with Microwave Processing. *J. Food Eng.* **2023**, *349*, 111481. [CrossRef]
11. Zuo, H.; Si, X.Y.; Li, P.; Li, J.; Chen, Z.H.; Li, P.H.; Chen, C.S.; Liu, Z.H.; Zhao, J. Dynamic change of tea (*Camellia sinensis*) leaf cuticular wax in white tea processing for contribution to tea flavor formation. *Food Res. Int.* **2023**, *163*, 112182. [CrossRef]
12. Feng, X.Y.; Yang, S.Y.; Pan, Y.N.; Zhou, S.; Ma, S.C.; Ou, C.S.; Fan, F.Y.; Gong, S.Y.; Chen, P.; Chu, Q. Yellow tea: More than turning green leaves to yellow. *Crit. Rev. Food Sci.* **2023**, *3*, 1–18. [CrossRef]
13. He, C.; Zhou, J.T.; Li, Y.C.; Zhang, D.; Ntezimana, B.; Zhu, J.Y.; Wang, X.Y.; Xu, W.L.; Wen, X.J.; Chen, Y.Q.; et al. The aroma characteristics of oolong tea are jointly determined by processing mode and tea cultivars. *Food Chem. X* **2023**, *18*, 100730. [CrossRef]
14. Kaur, A.; Farooq, S.; Sehgal, A. A Comparative Study of Antioxidant Potential and Phenolic Content in White (Silver Needle), Green and Black Tea. *Curr. Nutr. Food Sci.* **2019**, *15*, 415–420. [CrossRef]
15. Liu, K.H.; Liu, W.T.; Ding, X.W.; Gao, X.; Lv, J.L.; Li, J.M. The key role of LeuRS in the development of the cleistothecium and the metabolization of the flavor during the fermentation of dark tea with *Aspergillus montevidensis*. *LWT Food Sci. Technol.* **2023**, *185*, 115188. [CrossRef]
16. Long, P.P.; Rakariyatham, K.; Ho, C.T.; Zhang, L. Thearubigins: Formation, structure, health benefit and sensory property. *Trends Food Sci. Technol.* **2023**, *133*, 37–48. [CrossRef]
17. Ramkumar, S.; Perumal, P.C.; Gandhi, P.S.; Mandal, A.K.A.; Padmanabhan, M.; Kumar, P.S.; Gopalakrishnan, V.K. Computational structure analysis of PPO enzyme from UPASI selected clone of *Camellia sinensis* (L.) O. Kuntze. *J. Young Pharm.* **2015**, *7*, 118–121. [CrossRef]
18. Huang, X.X.; Ou, S.Q.; Li, Q.; Luo, Y.; Lin, H.Y.; Li, J.; Zhu, M.Z.; Wang, K.B. The R2R3 Transcription Factor CsMYB59 Regulates Polyphenol Oxidase Gene in Tea Plants (*Camellia sinensis*). *Front. Plant Sci.* **2021**, *12*, 739951. [CrossRef] [PubMed]
19. Zeng, Z.; Luo, Y.; Zheng, C.; Li, J.; Li, Q.; Lin, H.; Wang, K. The identification and analysis of polyphenol oxidase gene family in tea plant (*Camellia sinensis*). *J. Tea Sci.* **2018**, *38*, 385–395.
20. Gregory, R.P.F.; Bendall, D.S.J.B.J. The purification and some properties of the polyphenol oxidase from tea (*Camellia sinensis*). *Biochem. J.* **1967**, *101*, 569–581. [CrossRef] [PubMed]
21. Sui, X.; Meng, Z.; Dong, T.T.; Fan, X.T.; Wang, Q.G. Enzymatic browning and polyphenol oxidase control strategies. *Curr. Opin. Biotech.* **2023**, *81*, 102921. [CrossRef]
22. Ravichandran, R.; Parthiban, R. Changes in enzyme activities (polyphenol oxidase and phenylalanine ammonia lyase) with type of tea leaf and during black tea manufacture and the effect of enzyme supplementation of dhool on black tea quality. *Food Chem.* **1998**, *62*, 277–281. [CrossRef]
23. Ünal, M.Ü.; Yabacı, S.N.; Şener, A. Extraction, partial purification and characterisation of polyphenol oxidase from tea leaf (*Camellia sinensis*). *Gida* **2011**, *36*, 137–144.
24. Takeo, T. Tea Leaf Polyphenol Oxidase: Part IV. The Localization of Polyphenol Oxidase in Tea Leaf Cell. *Agric. Biol. Chem.* **1966**, *30*, 931–934. [CrossRef]
25. Xu, L.; Zhang, S.Q.; Xu, X.Y.; Chen, S.H.; Yao, Y.N.; Huang, Y.Y. Optimization of the extraction method of polyphenol oxidase from *Camellia sinensis* var. Longjing. *J. Food Saf. Qual.* **2015**, *6*, 1237–1242.
26. Zhan, K.; Yang, Z.; Xu, Z.; Lai, Z.; Zhou, S.; Gan, Y.; Li, M.; Li, J.; Chen, L. Comparison of soluble and membrane-bound polyphenol oxidase from cultivars suitable to Ninghong tea production. *J. Tea Sci.* **2023**, *43*, 356–366.
27. Liu, Y.; Chen, Q.; Liu, D.; Yang, L.; Hu, W.; Kuang, L.; Teng, J.; Liu, Y. Comparison of the biochemical properties and enzymatic synthesis of theaflavins by soluble and membrane-bound polyphenol oxidases from tea (*Camellia sinensis*) leaves. *Food Sci. Technol.* **2022**, *42*, 117321. [CrossRef]
28. Öztürk, C.; Aksoy, M.; Küfrevioğlu, Ö.İ. Purification of tea leaf (*Camellia sinensis*) polyphenol oxidase by using affinity chromatography and investigation of its kinetic properties. *J. Food Meas. Charact.* **2020**, *14*, 31–38. [CrossRef]
29. Villamil-Galindo, E.; Van de Velde, F.; Piagentini, A.M. Extracts from strawberry by-products rich in phenolic compounds reduce the activity of apple polyphenol oxidase. *LWT Food Sci. Technol.* **2020**, *133*, 110097. [CrossRef]

30. Bravo, K.; Osorio, E. Characterization of polyphenol oxidase from Cape gooseberry (*Physalis peruviana* L.) fruit. *Food Chem.* **2016**, *197*, 185–190. [CrossRef]
31. Huang, J.; Gao, X.; Su, L.; Liu, X.; Guo, L.; Zhang, Z.; Zhao, D.; Hao, J. Purification, characterization and inactivation kinetics of polyphenol oxidase extracted from *Cistanche deserticola*. *Planta* **2023**, *257*, 85. [CrossRef]
32. Agunbiade, O.J.; Adewale, I.O. Studies on latent and soluble polyphenol oxidase from *Moringa oleifera* Lam. leaves. *Biocatal. Agric. Biotechnol.* **2022**, *45*, 102515. [CrossRef]
33. Jia, S.; Jiang, S.; Chen, Y.; Wei, Y.; Shao, X. Comparison of Inhibitory Effects of Cinnamic Acid, β-Cyclodextrin, L-Cysteine, and Ascorbic Acid on Soluble and Membrane-Bound Polyphenol Oxidase in Peach Fruit. *Foods* **2022**, *12*, 167. [CrossRef] [PubMed]
34. Liu, H.; Pan, M.; Lu, Y.; Wang, M.; Huang, S.; Li, J.; Luo, K.; Luo, L.; Yao, M.; Hua, D. Purification and comparison of soluble and membrane-bound polyphenol oxidase from potato (*Solanum tuberosum*) tubers. *Protein Expr. Purif.* **2023**, *202*, 106195. [CrossRef]
35. Zhou, H.; Bie, S.; Li, Z.; Zhou, L. Comparing the Effect of HPP on the Structure and Stability of Soluble and Membrane-Bound Polyphenol Oxidase from 'Lijiang Snow' Peach: Multispectroscopic and Molecular Dynamics Simulation. *Foods* **2023**, *12*, 1820. [CrossRef] [PubMed]
36. Han, Q.-Y.; Liu, F.; Li, M.; Wang, K.-L.; Ni, Y.-Y. Comparison of biochemical properties of membrane-bound and soluble polyphenol oxidase from Granny Smith apple (*Malus* × *domestica* Borkh.). *Food Chem.* **2019**, *289*, 657–663. [CrossRef] [PubMed]
37. Ioniţă, E.; Gurgu, L.; Aprodu, I.; Stănciuc, N.; Dalmadi, I.; Bahrim, G.; Râpeanu, G. Characterization, purification, and temperature/pressure stability of polyphenol oxidase extracted from plums (*Prunus domestica*). *Process Biochem.* **2017**, *56*, 177–185. [CrossRef]
38. Alici, E.H.; Arabaci, G. Purification of polyphenol oxidase from borage (*Trachystemon orientalis* L.) by using three-phase partitioning and investigation of kinetic properties. *Int. J. Biol. Macromol.* **2016**, *93*, 1051–1056. [CrossRef] [PubMed]
39. Adeseko, C.J.; Fatoki, T.H. Isolation and partial purification of polyphenol oxidase from seed of melon (*Cucumeropsis edulis*). *Biointerface Res. Appl. Chem.* **2021**, *11*, 9085–9096.
40. Schmidt, J.M.; Greve-Poulsen, M.; Damgaard, H.; Hammershøj, M.; Larsen, L.B. Effect of membrane material on the separation of proteins and polyphenol oxidase in ultrafiltration of potato fruit juice. *Food Bioprocess. Technol.* **2016**, *9*, 822–829. [CrossRef]
41. Çınar, F.; Aksay, S. Purification and characterization of polyphenol oxidase from myrtle berries (*Myrtus communis* L.). *J. Food Meas. Charact.* **2022**, *16*, 2282–2291. [CrossRef]
42. Li, F. Purification, kinetic parameters, and isoforms of polyphenol oxidase from "Xushu 22" sweet potato skin. *J. Food Biochem.* **2020**, *44*, e13452. [CrossRef]
43. Alishah, M.M.; Yıldız, S.; Bilen, Ç.; Karakuş, E. Purification and characterization of avocado (*Persea americana*) polyphenol oxidase by affinity chromatography. *Prep. Biochem. Biotechnol.* **2023**, *53*, 40–53. [CrossRef]
44. Burgess, R.R. Protein precipitation techniques. *Methods Enzymol.* **2009**, *463*, 331–342. [PubMed]
45. Zhang, S.Q.; Xu, L.; Chen, S.H.; Xu, X.Y.; Huang, Y.J.; Yao, Y.N.; Huang, Y.Y. Study on the Characterization of Polyphenol Oxidase Isoenzyme Isolated from *Camellia sinensis* cv. Longjing 43. *Hubei Agric. Sci.* **2016**, *55*, 1487–1491. [CrossRef]
46. Xu, L.; Zhang, S.Q.; Chen, S.H.; Xu, X.Y.; Yao, Y.N.; Huang, Y.Y. Isolation and purification of polyphenol oxidase isoenzyme from *Camellia sinensis* var. *J. Huazhong Agric. Univ.* **2015**, *34*, 114–118.
47. Yuzugullu Karakus, Y.; Kahveci, B.; Acemi, A.; Kocak, G. Application of three-phase partitioning to the purification and characterization of polyphenol oxidase from antioxidant rosemary (*Rosmarinus officinalis* L.). *Int. J. Food Eng.* **2020**, *16*, 20200118. [CrossRef]
48. Saki, N.; Akin, M.; Alici, E.H.; Arabaci, G. Partial purification and characterization of polyphenol oxidase from the wild edible mushroom *Lepiota procera* using three-phase partitioning. *Int. J. Food Eng.* **2018**, *14*, 20170208. [CrossRef]
49. Zawada, A.M.; Lang, T.; Ottillinger, B.; Kircelli, F.; Stauss-Grabo, M.; Kennedy, J.P. Impact of Hydrophilic Modification of Synthetic Dialysis Membranes on Hemocompatibility and Performance. *Membranes* **2022**, *12*, 932. [CrossRef]
50. Krediet, R.T.; Barreto, D.L.; van Diepen, A.T.N. Assessment of the size selectivity of peritoneal permeability by the restriction coefficient to protein transport. *Periton Dial. Int.* **2022**, *42*, 335–343. [CrossRef]
51. Teng, J.; Gong, Z.H.; Deng, Y.L.; Chen, L.; Li, Q.; Shao, Y.Y.; Lin, L.; Xiao, W.J. Purification, characterization and enzymatic synthesis of theaflavins of polyphenol oxidase isozymes from tea leaf (*Camellia sinensis*). *LWT Food Sci. Technol.* **2017**, *84*, 263–270. [CrossRef]
52. Zhao, Y.; Tian, R.; Xu, Z.J.; Jiang, L.Z.; Sui, X.A. Recent advances in soy protein extraction technology. *J. Am. Oil Chem. Soc.* **2023**, *100*, 187–195. [CrossRef]
53. Schuster, B.; Sleytr, U.B. S-Layer Ultrafiltration Membranes. *Membranes* **2021**, *11*, 275. [CrossRef] [PubMed]
54. Haas, A.; Vaz, C.; Kempka, A.P. Extraction and Purification of Vegetable Peroxidase: A Review. *Period. Tche Quim.* **2019**, *16*, 692–703. [CrossRef]
55. Sánchez-Trasviña, C.; Flores-Gatica, M.; Enriquez-Ochoa, D.; Rito-Palomares, M.; Mayolo-Deloisa, K. Purification of Modified Therapeutic Proteins Available on the Market: An Analysis of Chromatography-Based Strategies. *Front. Bioeng. Biotech.* **2021**, *9*, 717326. [CrossRef] [PubMed]
56. Ke, L.J.; Xu, W.; Gao, J.N.; Gao, G.Z.; Wang, H.Q.; Zhou, J.W.; Liu, J.; Rao, P.F.; Xu, Y.Q. Isolation and characterization of thermo-tolerant polyphenol oxidases in a black tea infusion. *Food Control* **2021**, *119*, 107465. [CrossRef]

57. Cai, H.L.; Zhong, Z.H.; Chen, Y.R.; Zhang, S.Y.; Ling, H.; Fu, H.W.; Zhang, L. Genes cloning, sequencing and function identification of recombinant polyphenol oxidase isozymes for production of monomeric theaflavins from *Camellia sinensis*. *Int. J. Biol. Macromol.* **2023**, *240*, 124353. [CrossRef]
58. Cummins, P.M.; Rochfort, K.D.; O'Connor, B.F. Ion-Exchange Chromatography: Basic Principles and Application. *Methods Mol. Biol.* **2017**, *1485*, 209–223. [CrossRef]
59. Agustoni, E.; Teixeira, R.D.; Huber, M.; Flister, S.; Hiller, S.; Schirmer, T. Acquisition of enzymatic progress curves in real time by quenching-free ion exchange chromatography. *Anal. Biochem.* **2022**, *639*, 114523. [CrossRef]
60. Taddia, A.; Rito-Palomares, M.; Mayolo-Deloisa, K.; Tubio, G. Purification of xylanase from NRRL3 extract by an integrated strategy based on aqueous two-phase systems followed by ion exchange chromatography. *Sep. Purif. Technol.* **2021**, *255*, 117699. [CrossRef]
61. Ma, Y.; Luo, M.; Xu, Y.P.; Liu, Y.J.; Liu, X.C.; Bi, X.F.; Yuan, Y.P.; Su, F.; Yin, X.C. Purification and characterization of a thaumatin-like protein-1 with polyphenol oxidase activity found in *Prunus mume*. *RSC Adv.* **2020**, *10*, 28746–28754. [CrossRef] [PubMed]
62. Vishwasrao, C.; Chakraborty, S.; Ananthanarayan, L. Partial purification, characterisation and thermal inactivation kinetics of peroxidase and polyphenol oxidase isolated from Kalipatti sapota (*Manilkara zapota*). *J. Sci. Food Agric.* **2017**, *97*, 3568–3575. [CrossRef]
63. Mogilnaya, O.; Ronzhin, N.; Posokhina, E.; Bondar, V. Extracellular Oxidase from the Fungus as a Promising Enzyme for Analytical Applications. *Protein J.* **2021**, *40*, 731–740. [CrossRef]
64. Benaceur, F.; Gouzi, H.; Meddah, B.; Neifar, A.; Guergouri, A. Purification and characterization of catechol oxidase from Tadela (*Phoenix dactylifera* L.) date fruit. *Int. J. Biol. Macromol.* **2019**, *125*, 1248–1256. [CrossRef]
65. Lin, H.B.; Ng, A.W.R.; Wong, C.W. Partial purification and characterization of polyphenol oxidase from Chinese parsley (*Coriandrum sativum*). *Food Sci. Biotechnol.* **2016**, *25*, 91–96. [CrossRef] [PubMed]
66. Sajjad, N.; Naqvi, S.M.S.; Asad, M.J.; Raja, N.I.; Pusztai-Carey, M.; Ahmad, M.S. Biochemical, Purification, Sequencing and Alignment Studies of the Novel Polyphenol Oxidase Isoforms from *Musa acuminata* Fruit Pulp. *J. Anim. Plant Sci.* **2021**, *31*, 542–555. [CrossRef]
67. Popovic, G.; Kirby, N.C.; Dement, T.C.; Peterson, K.M.; Daub, C.E.; Belcher, H.A.; Guthold, M.; Offenbacher, A.R.; Hudson, N.E. Development of Transient Recombinant Expression and Affinity Chromatography Systems for Human Fibrinogen. *Int. J. Mol. Sci.* **2022**, *23*, 1054. [CrossRef] [PubMed]
68. Altunkaya, A. Partial Purification and Characterization of Polyphenoloxidase from Turkish Tea Leaf (*Camellia sinensis* L.). *Int. J. Food Prop.* **2014**, *17*, 1490–1497. [CrossRef]
69. Halder, J.; Tamuli, P.; Bhaduri, A.N. Isolation and characterization of polyphenol oxidase from Indian tea leaf (*Camellia sinensis*). *J. Nutr. Biochem.* **1998**, *9*, 75–80. [CrossRef]
70. Zhang, S. Recent Advances of Polyphenol Oxidases in Plants. *Molecules* **2023**, *28*, 2158. [CrossRef]
71. Siddiq, M.; Dolan, K.D. Characterization of polyphenol oxidase from blueberry (*Vaccinium corymbosum* L.). *Food Chem.* **2017**, *218*, 216–220. [CrossRef] [PubMed]
72. Cheema, S.; Sommerhalter, M. Characterization of polyphenol oxidase activity in Ataulfo mango. *Food Chem.* **2015**, *171*, 382–387. [CrossRef] [PubMed]
73. Batista, K.A.; Batista, G.L.A.; Alves, G.L.; Fernandes, K.F. Extraction, partial purification and characterization of polyphenol oxidase from *Solanum lycocarpum* fruits. *J. Mol. Catal. B Enzym.* **2014**, *102*, 211–217. [CrossRef]
74. Laad, S.; Premakshi, H.G.; Mirjankar, M.; Mulla, S.; Pujari, N.; Kamanavalli, C. Partial Purification, Characterization and Investigation of Inhibitory Effects of Organic Compounds on *Cinnamomum verum* Polyphenoloxidase Enzymes. *Appl. Food Biotechnol.* **2020**, *7*, 183–193. [CrossRef]
75. Peng, X.Y.; Du, C.; Yu, H.Y.; Zhao, X.Y.; Zhang, X.Y.; Wang, X.Y. Purification and characterization of polyphenol oxidase (PPO) from water yam (*Dioscorea alata*). *CyTA J. Food* **2019**, *17*, 676–684. [CrossRef]
76. Benaceur, F.; Chaibi, R.; Berrabah, F.; Neifar, A.; Leboukh, M.; Benaceur, K.; Nouioua, W.; Rezzoug, A.; Bouazzara, H.; Gouzi, H.; et al. Purification and characterization of latent polyphenol oxidase from truffles (*Terfezia arenaria*). *Int. J. Biol. Macromol.* **2020**, *145*, 885–893. [CrossRef]
77. Zaini, N.A.M.; Osman, A.; Hamid, A.A.; Ebrahimpour, A.; Saari, N. Purification and characterization of membrane-bound polyphenoloxidase (mPPO) from Snake fruit [*Salacca zalacca* (Gaertn.) Voss]. *Food Chem.* **2013**, *136*, 407–414. [CrossRef]
78. Liu, J.W.; Huang, Y.Y.; Ding, J.A.; Liu, C.; Xiao, X.D.; Ni, D.J. Prokaryotic expression and purification of *Camellia sinensis* polyphenol oxidase. *J. Sci. Food Agric.* **2010**, *90*, 2490–2494. [CrossRef]
79. Wu, Y.L.; Pan, L.P.; Yu, S.L.; Li, H.H. Cloning, microbial expression and structure-activity relationship of polyphenol oxidases from *Camellia sinensis*. *J. Biotechnol.* **2010**, *145*, 66–72. [CrossRef]
80. Liu, J.P.; Zhang, J.Y.; Liao, T.; Zhou, L.; Zou, L.Q.; Liu, Y.F.; Zhang, L.; Liu, W. Thermal Inactivation Kinetics of Kudzu (*Pueraria lobata*) Polyphenol Oxidase and the Influence of Food Constituents. *Foods* **2021**, *10*, 1320. [CrossRef]
81. Liu, B.; Zhou, X.F.; Guan, H.Y.; Pang, X.Q.; Zhang, Z.Q. Purification and Characterization of a Dark Red Skin Related Dimeric Polyphenol Oxidase from Huaniu Apples. *Foods* **2022**, *11*, 1790. [CrossRef] [PubMed]
82. Adeseko, C.J.; Sanni, D.M.; Salawu, S.O.; Kade, I.J.; Bamidele, S.O.; Lawal, O.T. Purification and biochemical characterization of polyphenol oxidase of African bush mango (*Irvingia gabonensis*) fruit peel. *Biocatal. Agric. Biotech.* **2021**, *36*, 102119. [CrossRef]

83. Gorshkov, V.; Tarasova, N.; Gogoleva, N.; Osipova, E.; Petrova, O.; Kovtunov, E.; Gogolev, Y. Polyphenol oxidase from *Pectobacterium atrosepticum*: Identification and cloning of gene and characteristics of the enzyme. *J. Basic. Microb.* **2017**, *57*, 998–1009. [CrossRef] [PubMed]
84. Kampatsikas, I.; Bijelic, A.; Rompel, A. Biochemical and structural characterization of tomato polyphenol oxidases provide novel insights into their substrate specificity. *Sci. Rep.* **2019**, *9*, 4022. [CrossRef] [PubMed]
85. Zhang, S.R.; Jiang, X.F.; Li, C.; Qiu, L.; Chen, Y.Q.; Yu, Z.; Ni, D.J. Effect of Fermentation Humidity on Quality of Congou Black Tea. *Foods* **2023**, *12*, 1726. [CrossRef] [PubMed]
86. Feng, J.Y.; Liu, K.Y.; Yu, Q.; Shuo, X.; Li, D.Y.; Hua, G.Z.; Jun, X.W. Activity Changes of Polyphenol Oxidase, Peroxidase and β-Glycosidase in Black Tea Processing. *J. Agric.* **2014**, *4*, 96–99+113.
87. Mahanta, P.K.; Boruah, S.K.; Boruah, H.K.; Kalita, J.N. Changes of polyphenol oxidase and peroxidase activities and pigment composition of some manufactured black teas (*Camellia sinensis* L.). *J. Agric. Food Chem.* **1993**, *41*, 272–276. [CrossRef]
88. Chen, L.; Wang, H.J.; Ye, Y.; Wang, Y.F.; Xu, P. Structural insight into polyphenol oxidation during black tea fermentation. *Food Chem. X* **2023**, *17*, 100615. [CrossRef]
89. Zhu, J.Y.; Wang, J.J.; Yuan, H.B.; Ouyang, W.; Li, J.; Hua, J.J.; Jiang, Y.W. Effects of Fermentation Temperature and Time on the Color Attributes and Tea Pigments of Yunnan Congou Black Tea. *Foods* **2022**, *11*, 1845. [CrossRef]
90. Wang, H.J.; Shen, S.; Wang, J.J.; Jiang, Y.W.; Li, J.; Yang, Y.Q.; Hua, J.J.; Yuan, H.B. Novel insight into the effect of fermentation time on quality of Yunnan Congou black tea. *LWT Food Sci. Technol.* **2022**, *155*, 112939. [CrossRef]
91. Samanta, T.; Cheeni, V.; Das, S.; Roy, A.B.; Ghosh, B.C.; Mitra, A. Assessing biochemical changes during standardization of fermentation time and temperature for manufacturing quality black tea. *J. Food Sci. Technol.* **2015**, *52*, 2387–2393. [CrossRef] [PubMed]
92. Wang, L.L.; Xie, J.L.; Deng, Y.L.; Jiang, Y.W.; Tong, H.R.; Yuan, H.B.; Yang, Y.Q. Volatile profile characterization during the drying process of black tea by integrated volatolomics analysis. *LWT Food Sci. Technol.* **2023**, *184*, 115039. [CrossRef]
93. Jiang, Y.W.; Hua, J.J.; Wang, B.; Yuan, H.B.; Ma, H.L. Effects of Variety, Season, and Region on Theaflavins Content of Fermented Chinese Congou Black Tea. *J. Food Qual.* **2018**, *2018*, 5427302. [CrossRef]
94. Das, S.; Datta, A.K. Mass transfer coefficient and mass diffusivity of O_2 and CO_2 during oxidation of macerated CTC and rolled orthodox leaves in black tea manufacturing. *J. Food Process Eng.* **2018**, *41*, 12875. [CrossRef]
95. Hua, J.J.; Wang, H.J.; Yuan, H.B.; Yin, P.; Wang, J.J.; Guo, G.Y.; Jiang, Y.W. New insights into the effect of fermentation temperature and duration on catechins conversion and formation of tea pigments and theasinensins in black tea. *J. Sci. Food Agric.* **2022**, *102*, 2750–2760. [CrossRef] [PubMed]
96. Chen, L.; Liu, F.; Yang, Y.F.; Tu, Z.; Lin, J.Z.; Ye, Y.; Xu, P. Oxygen-enriched fermentation improves the taste of black tea by reducing the bitter and astringent metabolites. *Food Res. Int.* **2021**, *148*, 110613. [CrossRef]
97. Ye, F.; Gao, S.W.; Gong, Z.M. Effects of Pyrus pyrifolia Nakai Polyphenol Oxidase Treatment on the Quality of Black Tea in Summer and Autumn. *Food Sci.* **2013**, *34*, 92–95.
98. Chiang, S.H.; Yang, K.M.; Wang, S.Y.; Chen, C.W. Enzymatic treatment in black tea manufacturing processing: Impact on bioactive compounds, quality, and bioactivities of black tea. *LWT Food Sci. Technol.* **2022**, *163*, 113560. [CrossRef]
99. Zhu, M.Z.; Li, N.; Zhou, F.; Ouyang, J.; Lu, D.M.; Xu, W.; Li, J.; Lin, H.Y.; Zhang, Z.; Xiao, J.B.; et al. Microbial bioconversion of the chemical components in dark tea. *Food Chem.* **2020**, *312*, 126043. [CrossRef]
100. Hu, Z.Y.; Liu, S.C.; Xu, Z.G.; Liu, S.Q.; Li, T.T.; Yu, S.L.; Zhao, W.P. Comparison of and related species in dark tea at different aspects: Morphology, enzyme activity and mitochondrial genome. *J. Food Process Pres.* **2021**, *45*, 15903. [CrossRef]
101. Liu, L.; Shi, J.J.; Yuan, Y.H.; Yue, T.L. Changes in the metabolite composition and enzyme activity of fermented tea during processing. *Food Res. Int.* **2022**, *158*, 111428. [CrossRef]
102. Fu, Y.X.; Xun, L.T. The Effect of Polyphenol Oxidase on the Pile-fermentation Process and Quality of Pu-erh Tea. *Mod. Food Sci. Technol.* **2015**, *31*, 197–201. [CrossRef]
103. He, H.F. Research progress on theaflavins: Efficacy, formation, and preparation. *Food Nutr. Res.* **2017**, *61*, 1344521. [CrossRef]
104. Takemoto, M.; Takemoto, H. Synthesis of Theaflavins and Their Functions. *Molecules* **2018**, *23*, 918. [CrossRef] [PubMed]
105. Liu, K.Y.; Chen, Q.Y.; Luo, H.; Li, R.Y.; Chen, L.J.; Jiang, B.; Liang, Z.W.; Wang, T.; Ma, Y.; Zhao, M. An In Vitro Catalysis of Tea Polyphenols by Polyphenol Oxidase. *Molecules* **2023**, *28*, 1722. [CrossRef] [PubMed]
106. Teng, J.; Liu, Y.; Zeng, W.; Zhou, M.Z.; Liu, Y.F.; Huang, Y.H.; Chen, Q.C. In vitro enzymatic synthesis of a monomeric theaflavin using a polyphenol oxidase isozyme from tea (*Camellia sinensis*) leaf. *Int. J. Food Sci. Technol.* **2022**, *57*, 5621–5631. [CrossRef]
107. Singh, S.; Singh, D.; Kumar, S. Expression and biochemical analysis of codon-optimized polyphenol oxidase from *Camellia sinensis* (L.) O. Kuntze in *E. coli*. *Process Biochem.* **2017**, *59*, 180–186. [CrossRef]
108. Liu, C.W.; Zhou, J.H.; Huang, J.A.; Xu, W.; Liu, Z.H. Study on the Synthesis of Theaflavin-3,3′-Digallate Catalyzed by Expressing Tea Tree Polyphenol Oxidase Isozymes and Its Enzymatic Solution. *Fermentation* **2023**, *9*, 770. [CrossRef]

Disclaimer/Publisher's Note: The statements, opinions and data contained in all publications are solely those of the individual author(s) and contributor(s) and not of MDPI and/or the editor(s). MDPI and/or the editor(s) disclaim responsibility for any injury to people or property resulting from any ideas, methods, instructions or products referred to in the content.

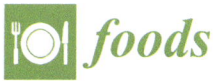

Article

Distinct Changes in Metabolic Profile and Sensory Quality with Different Varieties of *Chrysanthemum* (Juhua) Tea Measured by LC-MS-Based Untargeted Metabolomics and Electronic Tongue

Xing Tian [1,2,3], Haodong Wang [1], Liang Chen [1], Hanwen Yuan [1,3], Caiyun Peng [1,4] and Wei Wang [1,*]

1. TCM and Ethnomedicine Innovation & Development International Laboratory, Innovative Material Medical Research Institute, School of Pharmacy, Hunan University of Chinese Medicine, Changsha 410208, China; acctianxing@hotmail.com (X.T.); whd9974@163.com (H.W.); chenliang_201230@163.com (L.C.); hanwyuan@hnucm.edu.cn (H.Y.); caiyunpeng@hnucm.edu.cn (C.P.)
2. Department of Food and Drug Engineering, School of Pharmacy, Hunan University of Chinese Medicine, Changsha 410208, China
3. Engineering Technology Research Center of Hunan Province Xiangnan Area Authentic Chinese Medicinal Materials, Yongzhou 425600, China
4. Confucius Institute, Wonkwang University, 460 Iksandae-ro, Iksan 54538, Republic of Korea
* Correspondence: wangwei402@hotmail.com; Tel.: +86-73188458240; Fax: +86-73188458240

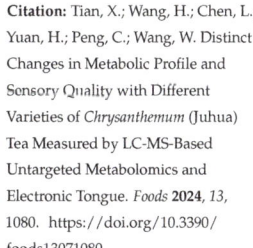

Abstract: *Chrysanthemum* tea, a typical health tea with the same origin as medicine and food, is famous for its unique health benefits and flavor. The taste and sensory quality of *chrysanthemum* (Juhua) tea are mainly determined by secondary metabolites. Therefore, the present research adopted untargeted metabolomics combined with an electronic tongue system to analyze the correlation between the metabolite profiles and taste characteristics of different varieties of *chrysanthemum* tea. The results of sensory evaluation showed that there were significant differences in the sensory qualities of five different varieties of *chrysanthemum* tea, especially bitterness and astringency. The results of principal component analysis (PCA) indicated that there were significant metabolic differences among the five *chrysanthemum* teas. A total of 1775 metabolites were identified by using untargeted metabolomics based on UPLC-Q-TOF/MS analysis. According to the variable importance in projection (VIP) values of the orthogonal projections to latent structures discriminant analysis (OPLS-DA), 143 VIP metabolites were found to be responsible for metabolic changes between Huangju and Jinsi Huangju tea; among them, 13 metabolites were identified as the key metabolites of the differences in sensory quality between them. Kaempferol, luteolin, genistein, and some quinic acid derivatives were correlated with the "astringency" attributes. In contrast, l-(-)-3 phenyllactic acid and L-malic acid were found to be responsible for the "bitterness" and "umami" attributes in *chrysanthemum* tea. Kyoto Encyclopedia of Genes and Genomes pathway enrichment analysis showed that the flavonoid and flavonol biosynthesis pathways had important effects on the sensory quality of *chrysanthemum* tea. These findings provide the theoretical basis for understanding the characteristic metabolites that contribute to the distinctive sensory qualities of *chrysanthemum* tea.

Keywords: *chrysanthemum* (Juhua); tea; metabolomics; sensory quality; LC-MS; electronic tongue

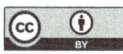

1. Introduction

Dietary herbal teas, defined as water-based immersions or decoctions prepared with herbal ingredients, have been used in healthcare and as part of a healthy diet [1]. As a traditional medicine- and food-homologous plant, *Chrysanthemum morifolium* Ramat. (Juhua) has been used for over 3000 years as a herbal tea-based drink, the third-most widely consumed drink after tea and coffee [2]. Notably, drinking *chrysanthemum* tea or beverages was thought to have similar preventive or therapeutic effects on high blood pressure, sore throat, and eye diseases [3]. Modern pharmacological studies have shown that flavonoids, anthocyanins, alkaloids, phenolic acids, and other phytochemicals in *chrysanthemum*, which have antimicrobial, antioxidant, anti-inflammatory, anti-cancer, anti-obesity, nerve-protective, and other functions, provide a theoretical basis for the development of *chrysanthemum* tea and its deeply processed products [4]. However, the literature on *chrysanthemums* mainly focuses on the biological activity, vegetative propagation, and cultivation technology of medicinal *chrysanthemum* [5]. In contrast, there are few reports on edible *chrysanthemum*'s flavor and sensory qualities in dietary herbal teas.

The taste and sensory qualities of *chrysanthemum* (Juhua) tea are mainly determined by secondary metabolites, such as flavonols, anthocyanins, amino acids, alkaloids, and organic acids [6]. Generally, the variety, region, climate, soil type, and production process of *chrysanthemum* tea determine its sensory qualities, related to its chemical composition [7]. At present, many researchers have systematically analyzed the flavor components of edible *chrysanthemum* using GC-MS, HS-GC-IMS, GC-O, HPLC, sensory evaluation, and other methods [8–10]. However, to the best of our knowledge, numerous studies on the sensory qualities and flavor substances of edible chrysanthemum have some problems, such as a single method and lack of multi-omics research [11]. In addition, few studies have been conducted on the core metabolites that influence the sensory qualities of *chrysanthemum* tea.

Metabolomics, as a method of omics, is the science of studying the species, quantity, and changes of metabolites (endogenous metabolites) with molecular weights less than 1500 Da caused by the response of organisms to external stimuli, pathophysiological changes, and gene mutations [12]. Through plant metabolomics, a variety of analysis platforms can be used to study the metabolites of different plant samples after physical or chemical treatment and obtain different meanings, including geographical traceability, food processing, biological activity, etc. [1,13]. In addition, as an intelligent instrument to simulate human taste, electronic tongue systems have been reported to be able to quantitatively and qualitatively analyze the taste of different foods and Chinese herbs [14–16]. Thus, the combined analysis of untargeted metabolomics and food flavomics based on LC-MS/MS and an electronic tongue is an excellent method to establish the relationship between *chrysanthemum* tea's chemical constituents and sensory qualities. However, as far as we know, this multi-omics analysis has not been applied to reveal the key flavor metabolites of different varieties of *chrysanthemum* tea.

The chemical composition, metabolites, and taste of *chrysanthemum* (Juhua) tea may vary somewhat depending on its variety [17]. The objective of this study builds on previous studies [15]. It aims to compare the metabolites and sensory qualities of five different varieties of *chrysanthemum* tea by using LC-MS-based untargeted metabolomics combined with electronic tongue analysis, investigating key differential metabolites associated with sensory quality differences in *chrysanthemum* tea. Importantly, the implementation of this study offers a high-resolution marker for the sensory quality evaluation of *chrysanthemum* tea. This study will provide insight into ascertaining the characteristic metabolites in different varieties of *chrysanthemum* tea.

2. Materials and Methods

2.1. Chrysanthemum Tea Samples

The 5 varieties of *chrysanthemum* tea selected in this study were selected from local producers in Hunan, Anhui, and Hangzhou Provinces, and the 6 biological replicates were found for each variety of *chrysanthemum* tea in the metabolomics study. "JinshihuangJu" (J) and "HuangJu" (X) were selected from local producers in Yongzhou, Hunan Province; "BaoJu" (B) and "GongJu" (G) were collected in the region of Bozhou, Anhui Province; and "HanbaiJu"(H) was collected from Hangzhou, Zhejiang Province. Detailed information on the *chrysanthemum* tea samples is provided in Figure 1.

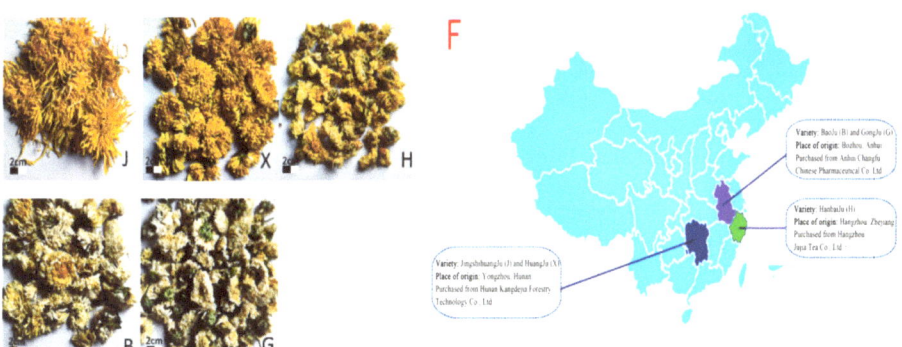

Figure 1. Appearance and origin of five different species of chrysanthemum. Notes: (J) JinshihuangJu; (X) HuangJu; (H) HanbaiJu; (B) BaoJu; (G) GongJu; (F) diagram of the source of five different varieties of *chrysanthemum* tea.

2.2. Sensory Evaluation for Chrysanthemum Tea Samples

Ten study participants ($n = 10$, 3 males and 7 females, 18–21 years of age) were recruited from the Hunan University of Chinese Medicine's internal student panel without any exclusion parameters aside from being in good health, nonsmoking, and not currently taking medication. In order to eliminate the influence of environmental factors on the sensory evaluation results, sensory testing experiments were conducted in a single room at 20–25 °C and were performed in the morning (9:00 to 11:00 a.m.). According to the National Standards of China (GB/T23776-2018) [18], all subjects were trained 4 times in 2 weeks, and the sensory attributes used for the sensory quality evaluation of *chrysanthemum* tea samples were screened and identified. Briefly, the different varieties of *chrysanthemum* tea were weighed (2.00 ± 0.05 g), brewed with 150 mL of boiling water for 30 min, and then filtered out with gauze to prepare samples to be immediately evaluated by the panel. Each *chrysanthemum* tea sample was triplicated and randomly coded at room temperature, and each sensory participant tasted a total of 15 tea samples. Each sensory participant scored the *chrysanthemum* tea samples for aroma, astringent sensation, and three taste characteristics (bitterness, umami, and sweetness). The intensity of the sensory attributes was scored on a six-point scale from "0" (unobservable) to "5" (the strongest observable) [19,20]. Still pure water was used as a neutralizer between the *chrysanthemum* tea samples. All participants signed a written informed consent form to participate in this study before the evaluation, and the sensory panels did not communicate with each other during the whole sensory evaluation.

2.3. Electronic Tongue Analysis for Chrysanthemum Tea Samples

The taste attributes of the five different varieties of *chrysanthemum* tea were determined using a TS-sa402b electronic tongue system (Intelligent Sensor Technology Co., Ltd., Atsugi, Japan) with wide-area selection-specific artificial lipid membrane sensors. The changes in the membrane potential caused by electrostatic interactions or hydrophobic interactions between various flavor substances and artificial lipid membranes were detected to evaluate the eight sensory attributes (saltiness, bitterness, sourness, umami, umami aftertaste, astringency, bitter aftertaste, and astringency aftertaste) of each sample. The taste sensory index data in the samples to be tested were calculated according to the absolute value of the lipid membrane potential of each artificial sensor on the basis of the potential of the solution, in which the output value of the reference solution is called the tasteless point. In this study, as shown by the tasteless blank sample, the tasteless points for different taste components were 0, and values higher than these tasteless points were considered to be meaningful. Specifically, the (2.00 ± 0.05 g) *chrysanthemum* tea sample was accurately weighed and brewed with 150 mL of boiling water for 30 min. Then, the tea broth was filtered through 3 layers of gauze to obtain the sample to be cooled to room temperature before being detected by the TS-sa402b electronic tongue system. In this study, each sample was cycled 4 times, and the mean values of the last three cycles were used for the statistical analysis and analyzed using TS-sa402b library search software (Intelligent Sensor Technology Co., Ltd., Atsugi, Japan). Data collected by the electronic tongue were calculated according to the formula as described. In order to ensure that the sensors were working in the correct mV range, each sensor was checked before measurement, according to the manufacturer's instructions.

2.4. HPLC Analysis for Chrysanthemum Tea Samples

All *chrysanthemum* tea samples were ground separately into 100-mesh-size fine powders. A 25 ± 0.01 mg sample of each *chrysanthemum* tea was extracted using ultrasonic extraction (power: 300 W, frequency: 45 kHz) (SB-5200DTD; Scientz, Ningbo, China) with 25 mL of ultrapure water at room temperature for 40 min. The available range for extraction temperature was from 0 to 80 °C. After ultrasonic extraction, the sample was centrifuged at 3000 rpm for 10 min to collect the supernatant. Subsequently, the sample was shaken and filtered to obtain the filtrate through a 0.22 μm microfiltration membrane before HPLC analysis.

The contents of chlorogenic acid, luteolin, and 3,5-O-dicaffeyl quinin acid in the *chrysanthemum* tea samples were analyzed using a high-performance liquid chromatography (HPLC) analytical method, following the *Pharmacopoeia of the People's Republic of China*. The HPLC system had pumps and an autosampler (Agilent 1260 Infinity II Prime liquid chromatography system, Agilent Technologies, Inc., Palo Alto, CA, USA). An HPLC column (250 × 4.6 mm, 5 μm particle size, Welch Technologies, Shanghai, China) was used. An auto-injector injected 10 μL of the test solution into the HPLC system, and the flow rate was 1.0 mL/min. The mobile phase consisted of mobile phase A [H_2O containing 0.05% (v/v) phosphoric acid] and mobile phase B [0.1% (v/v) acetonitrile]. Additionally, the gradient elution was as follows: 0–11 min, the gradient of phase B increased from 10% to 18%, 11–30 min, the gradient of phase B increased to 20%, 30–40 min, the gradient of phase B was maintained at 20% for 10 min, 40–45 min, the gradient of phase B continued to rise to 95%, 45–60 min, and the gradient of phase B was maintained at 90% for 15 min. Furthermore, samples (10 μL) were eluted at 0.8–1.0 mL/min, and the column oven was kept at 30 °C. The HPLC chromatograms of the five different varieties of *chrysanthemum* tea can be found in the Supplementary Materials (Figure S1).

2.5. Measurement of Total Polyphenols and Total Flavonoids in Chrysanthemum Tea

To determine total polyphenols and total flavonoids, 3.0 ± 0.01 g of each *chrysanthemum* tea powder sample was mixed with 120 mL of distilled water in a 250 mL round-bottomed flask and extracted at 90 °C for 40 min in a water bath. After extraction, each extracted solution was centrifuged at 5000 r/min for 5 min, concentrated at 65 °C under reduced pressure for 1 h, and then freeze-dried. After drying, the extracted powder was stored immediately at −20 °C for future analysis. The total polyphenol contents of the *chrysanthemum* tea samples were measured according to the Folin-Denis method. Briefly, 0.01 g of each extracted *chrysanthemum* tea powder was mixed with 1.0 mL of Folin-Ciocâlteu reagent (1.0 mol/L) and reacted at room temperature for 1 min. Then, 8 mL of 10% sodium carbonate (100 g/L) was mixed well, and the mixture was left in a dark place for 2 h. The absorbance was measured at 760 nm using a spectrophotometer (UV-1700, Shimadzu, Kyoto, Japan). The results were expressed as milligrams of gallic acid equivalents per gram of dry matter (mg GAE/g), using gallic acid as a reference standard. The total flavonoid contents of the *chrysanthemum* tea samples were determined according to the aluminum chloride complex formation method and expressed as milligrams of rutin equivalents per gram of extracted *chrysanthemum* tea powder in dry weight (mg RE/g).

2.6. LC-MS/MS-Based Untargeted Metabolomics Analysis

The *chrysanthemum* tea samples (80 ± 0.1 mg) were immediately frozen in liquid nitrogen and ground into fine powder with a mortar and pestle. Then, 1000 μL of methanol/acetonitrile/H$_2$O (2:2:1, $v/v/v$) was added to the homogenized solution for metabolite extraction. The mixture was centrifuged for 20 min (14,000× g, 4 °C). The supernatant was dried in a vacuum centrifuge. For LC-MS analysis, the samples were re-dissolved in 100 μL of acetonitrile/water (1:1, v/v) as a solvent and centrifuged at 14,000× g and 4 °C for 15 min, after which the supernatant was injected. The untargeted metabolomics analysis of the *chrysanthemum* tea samples was performed using a UHPLC system (1290 Infinity LC, Agilent Technologies, Santa Clara, CA, USA) equipped with a binary pump and a C18 column (2.1 mm × 100 mm, i.d., 1.8 μm, Agilent) operated at 40 °C. Mobile phase A consisted of 25 mmol L ammonium acetate and 0.5% formic acid in water, and mobile phase B was methanol. Additionally, the gradient elution was as follows: 0–0.5 min, 5% B; then B changed to 100% linearly from 0.5 to 10 min; 10–12.0 min, B was maintained at 100%; from 12.0 to 12.1 min, B changed linearly from 100% to 5%; 12.1–16 min, B was maintained at 5%. The sample was placed in an automatic sampler at 4 °C during the analysis. The separated components were then detected with a quadrupole time-of-flight device (AB Sciex TripleTOF 6600, Shanghai Applied Protein Technology Co., Ltd., Shanghai, China). To avoid the effects of instrument fluctuations, a random sequence was used to analyze the samples. QC samples were inserted into the sample queue to monitor and evaluate the stability and reliability of the data.

The ESI source parameters were set as follows: ion source gas 1 (Gas1) as 60, ion source gas 2 (Gas2) as 60, curtain gas (CUR) as 30, source temperature 600 °C, ion spray voltage floating (ISVF) ± 5500 V. In MS-only acquisition, the instrument was set to acquire over the m/z range 60–1000 Da, and the accumulation time for the TOF MS scan was set to 0.20 s/spectrum. In auto MS/MS acquisition, the instrument was set to acquire over the m/z range 25–1000 Da, and the accumulation time for the product ion scan was set to 0.05 s/spectrum. Moreover, the product ion scan was acquired using information-dependent acquisition (IDA), with high-sensitivity mode selected. The parameters were set as follows: the collision energy (CE) was fixed at 35 V with ± 15 eV; the declustering potential (DP) was 60 V (+) and −60 V (−); we excluded isotopes within 4 Da; 10 candidate ions were monitored per cycle.

2.7. Metabolomics Data Acquisition and Analysis

The TIC diagram in the ESI-positive and -negative modes for the five different varieties of *chrysanthemum* tea is shown in Figure S2. The raw MS data were converted to MzXML files using ProteoWizard MSConvert before importing them into the freely available XCMS ^{plus} software (https://sciex.com/cl/products/software/xcms-plus-software, accessed on 12 March 2024) (Sciex, Framingham, MA, USA). For peak picking, the following parameters were used: centWave m/z = 10 ppm, peak width = c (10, 60), prefilter = c (10, 100). For peak grouping, bw = 5, mzwid = 0.025, minfrac = 0.5 were used. The R-package CAMERA (Collection of Algorithms for MEtabolite pRofile Annotation) was used for annotating isotopes and adducts. In the extracted ion features, only the variables with more than 50% of the nonzero measurement values in at least one group were kept. Compound identification of metabolites was performed by comparing the accuracy of m/z values (<10 ppm) and MS/MS spectra with an in-house database established with available authentic standards.

After normalizing to total peak intensity, the processed data were analyzed using an R package (ropls), where they were subjected to multivariate data analysis, including Pareto-scaled principal component analysis (PCA) and orthogonal partial least squares discriminant analysis (OPLS-DA). The 7-fold cross-validation and response permutation testing were used to evaluate the robustness of the model. Furthermore, the variable importance in projection (VIP) value of each variable in the OPLS-DA model was calculated to indicate its contribution to the classification. In this study, metabolites with VIP values > 1.0

were further subjected to Student's t-test (p-value < 0.05) at the univariate level to measure the significance of each metabolite.

2.8. Bioinformatics Analysis

The statistically significant differences in metabolites among the varieties of *chrysanthemum* tea (VIP values > 1 in the OPLS-DA model and $p < 0.05$) were screened for bioinformatics analysis, including hierarchical clustering analysis, correlation analysis and pathway analysis. The hierarchical clustering analysis was also carried out using TBtools software V2.2030 (TBtools, Guangzhou, China). Moreover, the differentially expressed metabolites were matched against the Kyoto Encyclopedia of Genes and Genomes (KEGG) database by the KEGG Automatic Annotation Server (KAAS; website: https://www.genome.jp/tools/kaas/, accessed on 30 July 2023). Values of $p < 0.05$ in Fisher's exact test were considered statistically significant.

2.9. Statistical Analysis

Each experiment was conducted in triplicate, and the results are presented as the mean ± standard deviation. The multiple comparisons of the five varieties of *chrysanthemum* tea groups were calculated by one-way analysis of variance (ANOVA) with Duncan's test for Statistics 25.0 software (IBM, Chicago, IL, USA). The hierarchical clustering analysis was carried out using TBtools software (TBtools, Guangzhou, China). SIMCA-P 14.1 multivariate statistical software (Umetrics, Umea, Sweden) was specifically used for radar plot generation, PCA, OPLS-DA, and other graphical presentations.

3. Results and Discussion

3.1. Sensory Quality of the Five Different Varieties of Chrysanthemum Tea

The differences in sensory attributes of the five different varieties of *chrysanthemum* tea were detected by the electronic tongue system. As shown in Table 1, the astringency, bitterness, and umami of the five different varieties of *chrysanthemum* tea were significantly higher than the tasteless point ($p < 0.05$). Therefore, the astringency, bitterness, and umami indices could be used as effective sensory indices for the five *chrysanthemum* tea varieties. As a unique-scented tea health drink, *chrysanthemum* tea has gradually entered the field of view of more consumers. However, *chrysanthemum* tea has astringency, which cannot provide some consumers with oral pleasure, resulting in the low market recognition of simple *chrysanthemum* tea products [15]. It is worth noting that astringent sensation is an important sensory perception of *chrysanthemum* tea, with hydrolyzed and concentrated tannins responsible for this property [21]. Moreover, astringent sensation, one of the most complex oral sensations, is an important essential affecting the sensory quality of food, tea, and other beverages [22]. The astringency index of the HuangJu sample (X) was significantly higher than that of the other three species except for the BaoJu sample (B) ($p < 0.05$). Meanwhile, the umami aftertaste of the HuangJu sample (X) was also significantly higher than that of the other four varieties of *chrysanthemum* tea ($p < 0.05$). In fact, astringent sensation is not a basic taste but, rather, a feeling of convergence caused by the coagulation of proteins in the oral mucosa, which is the result of stimulating the oral nerve endings [22]. Notably, this dry, wrinkled taste occurs when drinking tea or consuming g other foods containing polyphenols.

In addition, the three taste qualities (including bitterness, umami, and sweetness), astringency, and aroma intensity of the five different varieties of *chrysanthemum* tea were quantified using a sensory evaluation panel consisting of ten trained individuals (Table 2). The results showed no significant differences in umami taste among the five different varieties of *chrysanthemum* tea ($p < 0.05$), while the astringency, bitterness, and aroma of "HuangJu" (X) were significantly ($p < 0.05$) higher than those of the other four species of *chrysanthemum*. Additionally, the results of sensory evaluation also showed that astringency and bitterness could be used as effective sensory attributes of *chrysanthemum* tea. The astringent sensation is mainly caused by the precipitation or aggregation of polyphenols associated with proteins in saliva. In fact, chlorogenic acid and other phenolic acids are easily soluble in *chrysanthemum* tea brewing, thus enhancing acidity and influencing the tasting process of other polyphenols [16]. Therefore, further analysis of the main active compounds and untargeted metabolomics analysis of the five different varieties of *chrysanthemum* tea were carried out.

Table 1. Determination of taste characteristics of different varieties of *chrysanthemum* tea by electronic tongue.

Taste Characteristics	*Chrysanthemum* Varieties				
	JinshihuangJu (J)	HuangJu (X)	HanbaiJu (H)	BaoJu (B)	GongJu (G)
Sourness	−25.02 ± 0.00 [d]	−21.36 ± 0.09 [a]	−24.06 ± 0.09 [c]	−21.38 ± 0.08 [a]	−23.36 ± 0.05 [b]
Bitterness	11.11 ± 0.00 [b]	7.36 ± 0.01 [e]	11.34 ± 0.01 [a]	9.33 ± 0.01 [d]	9.63 ± 0.02 [c]
Astringency	13.60 ± 0.00 [d]	15.79 ± 0.07 [b]	14.89 ± 0.05 [c]	16.79 ± 0.04 [a]	14.96 ± 0.03 [c]
Bitter Aftertaste	1.89 ± 0.00 [a]	0.58 ± 0.03 [e]	0.90 ± 0.05 [c]	1.03 ± 0.05 [b]	0.69 ± 0.02 [d]
Astringency Aftertaste	2.79 ± 0.00 [c]	3.36 ± 0.02 [a]	2.03 ± 0.06 [e]	3.00 ± 0.07 [b]	2.60 ± 0.02 [d]
Umami	11.88 ± 0.00 [a]	11.79 ± 0.02 [a]	9.55 ± 0.02 [e]	10.25 ± 0.01 [d]	10.30 ± 0.02 [c]
Umami Aftertaste	2.17 ± 0.00 [c]	3.19 ± 0.06 [a]	1.54 ± 0.06 [e]	2.33 ± 0.09 [b]	1.87 ± 0.01 [d]
Saltiness	−7.32 ± 0.00 [b]	−2.97 ± 0.03 [a]	−13.25 ± 0.01 [e]	−7.74 ± 0.01 [c]	−9.82 ± 0.06 [d]

Standard error of means ($n = 3$). [a–e] Means within the same row with different superscripts differ significantly ($p < 0.05$).

Table 2. Traditional sensory evaluation of different varieties of *chrysanthemum* tea.

Sensory Attributes	*Chrysanthemum* Varieties				
	JinshihuangJu (J)	HuangJu (X)	HanbaiJu (H)	BaoJu (B)	GongJu (G)
Bitterness	2.90 ± 0.72 [b]	4.13 ± 0.53 [a]	2.70 ± 0.60 [bc]	3.13 ± 0.67 [b]	2.23 ± 0.65 [c]
Astringent	2.47 ± 0.69 [b]	3.37 ± 0.95 [a]	2.33 ± 0.50 [b]	2.50 ± 0.45 [b]	2.27 ± 0.68 [b]
Umami	1.93 ± 0.75 [a]	1.47 ± 0.85 [a]	2.06 ± 0.93 [a]	1.57 ± 0.39 [a]	2.10 ± 0.75 [a]
Sweetness	1.60 ± 0.54 [ab]	1.07 ± 0.14 [c]	1.77 ± 0.57 [a]	1.23 ± 0.42 [bc]	1.93 ± 0.66 [a]
Aroma	2.17 ± 0.57 [c]	3.43 ± 0.83 [a]	3.07 ± 0.72 [ab]	2.23 ± 0.72 [c]	2.43 ± 0.97 [bc]

Each value is expressed as the mean ± SD ($n = 10$). [a–c] Different letters within a column indicate a significant difference ($p < 0.05$). The taste strength of each sample was evaluated using a standard scale (0, no taste; 1 to 2, slightly strong; 3 to 4, strong; 5, very strong).

3.2. Comparison of the Contents of Main Active Compounds

Flavonoids are phenolic compounds that are widely present in *chrysanthemum* tea. As shown in Table 3, among the five different varieties of *chrysanthemum* tea, both total polyphenols and total flavonoids had the highest concentrations in HuangJu (X), which were 58.91 ± 0.02 mg GAE/g dw and 201.07 ± 0.05 mg RE/g dw, respectively, significantly higher than in the other four kinds of *chrysanthemum* tea ($p < 0.05$). In contrast, the lowest content of phenolic acids was found in BaoJu (B), which was significantly lower than that of the other four *chrysanthemum* teas ($p < 0.05$). According to Tables 2 and 3, the results also confirmed that the contents of flavonoids and polyphenols were positively correlated with bitterness and astringent sensation. In fact, chlorogenic acid, luteolin, isochlorogenic acid, and other phenolic acids are the major components of *chrysanthemum* tea [23]. Phenolic acids are responsible for *chrysanthemum* tea's distinctive color and taste, and the bioactive components contribute to its antibacterial, antiviral, antioxidant, antihypertension, and hypolipidemic activities [24]. Notably, the astringent sensation produced by drinking *chrysanthemum* tea is caused by the polyphenol–protein complex reaction [25]. HuangJu (X) had the highest contents of three phenolic acids and astringent sensation, indicating that the major bioactive substances in the five varieties of *chrysanthemum* tea showed highly comparable curves with the sensory quality data. In fact, due to these differences in variety and origin, HuangJu (X) may be quite different from other types of *chrysanthemum* tea in terms of chemical compounds and sensory characteristics. Hence, follow-up untargeted metabolomics analysis was conducted to provide in-depth information regarding the relationships between the characteristic metabolites and sensory qualities of *chrysanthemum* tea by identifying metabolites in five different varieties.

Table 3. Contents of main bioactive substances of different varieties of *chrysanthemum* tea.

Chrysanthemum Varieties	Detection Index				
	Chlorogenic Acid (%)	Galuteolin (%)	Isochlorogenic Acid (%)	Total Flavonoid Content (mg GAE/g)	Total Polyphenol (mg RE/g)
JinshihuangJu (J)	1.23 ± 0.03 [c]	1.82 ± 0.01 [b]	2.13 ± 0.04 [d]	116.95 ± 0.59 [a]	53.88 ± 0.08 [b]
HuangJu (X)	2.11 ± 0.01 [a]	2.62 ± 0.01 [a]	0.18 ± 0.01 [e]	201.07 ± 0.05 [c]	58.91 ± 0.02 [a]
HanbaiJu (H)	1.55 ± 0.02 [b]	0.18 ± 0.01 [e]	4.01 ± 0.10 [b]	106.76 ± 0.42 [d]	38.39 ± 0.08 [d]
BaoJu (B)	0.66 ± 0.05 [e]	0.67 ± 0.05 [d]	5.93 ± 0.02 [a]	100.56 ± 0.05 [b]	29.69 ± 0.05 [a]
GongJu (G)	1.01 ± 0.01 [d]	0.83 ± 0.02 [c]	4.01 ± 0.10 [b]	106.49 ± 0.18 [d]	44.37 ± 0.03 [c]

Standard error of means ($n = 3$), [a–e] Means within the same row with different superscripts differ significantly ($p < 0.05$).

3.3. Untargeted Metabolomics Analysis

Untargeted metabolomics combined with multivariate analysis was applied to investigate the differences in metabolites between the five varieties of *chrysanthemum* tea, and to identify critical metabolites responsible for metabolomic variations caused by different varieties of *chrysanthemum* tea. This study identified metabolites in *chrysanthemum* tea samples according to the in-house database (Shanghai Applied Protein Technology, Shanghai, China) [26]. After pre-treatment and data normalization, 1105 and 670 metabolites were identified from the total ion chromatogram of UPLC-QTOF-MS in positive and negative ion modes, respectively. According to their chemical taxonomy, all metabolites (identified by combining positive and negative ions) were classified and performed on the attribution information. The proportions of the various metabolites are shown in Figure 2, including 473 lipids and lipid-like molecules (25.918%), 361 phenylpropanoids and polyketides (19.781%), 184 organoheterocyclic compounds (10.082%), 173 benzenoids (9.479%), 148 organic oxygen compounds (8.11%), 109 organic acids and derivatives (5.973%), 40 alkaloids and derivatives (2.192%), 32 nucleosides and analogs (1.753%), 26 lignans, neolignans, and related compounds (1.425%), 21 organic nitrogen compounds (1.151%), 1 hydrocarbon derivative (0.055%), and 257 other undefined compounds (14.082%).

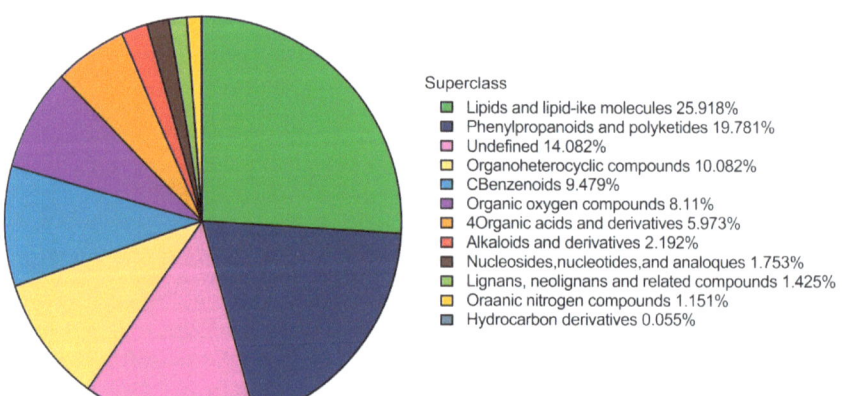

Figure 2. The proportions of the various metabolites in *chrysanthemum* tea samples. Notes: Different color blocks represent items belonging to different chemical classifications, and the percentage represents

the items belonging to each chemical classification. The number of metabolites is given as a percentage of all identified metabolites. Metabolites that have no chemical classification are defined as undefined.

The principal component analysis (PCA), partial least squares discriminant analysis (PLS-DA), and orthogonal projections to latent structures discriminant analysis (OPLS-DA) methods have been used to identify combinations of metabolites accounting for the most variance, and to visualize sample cluster trends in tea [27]. All metabolites were subjected to multivariate analysis using SIMCA-P 14.1 multivariate statistical software. As an unsupervised data analysis method, the PCA can reflect variability between and within sample groups. As shown in Figure 3A, when using all of the data on the metabolite ion features of five *chrysanthemum* tea samples, the QCs were clustered together on the PCA score plots, which revealed that the data variability was small. It is noteworthy that the X ("HuangJu") and J ("JinshihuangJu") *chrysanthemum* tea samples were similar in the PCA but were separated in PLS-DA (Figure 3A,B). In addition, these two kinds of *chrysanthemum* tea samples are from the same origin in Yongzhou, Hunan Province. Therefore, to obtain a higher level of population separation and better understand the differences between different varieties of *chrysanthemum* tea, OPLS-DA was used for classification and to confirm the separation between the "JinshihuangJu" (J) and "HuangJu" (X) tea samples in terms of the various significant parameters. Based on OPLS-DA, the separation trends between J and X samples showed more obvious variations (Figure 3C), and the cross-validation with 200 permutation tests indicated that this OPLS-DA model was reliable, with the intercepts of R^2 and Q^2 being 0.5555 and -0.6665, respectively (Figure 3D). Differential metabolites of J and X samples were found by OPLS-DA, and variable importance in projection (VIP > 1, $p < 0.01$) and |log2 (fold change)| values > 1.5 were used for screening. In both positive and negative ion modes, 143 VIP metabolites were responsible for metabolic changes between the J and X samples, including 13 metabolites, 40 flavonoids and flavone glycosides, 31 acids, 22 ketones, 8 esters, 7 amino acids, 7 glycosides, 6 alkaloids, 6 alcohols, and 16 other metabolites. (Table S1).

A multiple analysis was applied to visualize the differences in these critical metabolites between the "JingshihuangJu" (J) and "HuangJu" (X) samples (Figure 4). The x-coordinate represents the log2 FC value of the differential metabolite, and each row represents a critical metabolite. The red and green bar charts correspond to differential metabolites up and down, visually showing the changes in the multiple metabolic differences identified as significant.

Polyphenols are phytonutrients, the most abundant contents in *chrysanthemum* tea, containing flavonoids, phenolic acids, lignans, and stilbenes [3]. Isochlorogenic acid C, luteolin, apigenin-7-glucoside, chlorogenic acid, apigenin, and cryptochlorogenic acid play important roles in distinguishing different chrysanthemum varieties [11]. According to Figure 4, the most abundant marker metabolites in J and X samples were flavonoids and flavone glycosides. For example, the abundance of thunalbene, isoschaftoside, delphinidin 3-glucoside, primeverin, genistein, astragalin, bracteatin, maritimein, apigenin, kaempferol, luteolin, naringenin-7-O-glucoside, apigenin-7-O-glucoside, apigenin-7-O-glucuronide, naringenin, orientin, luteolin-7-O-glucoside, baicalinEriodictyol-7-O-glucoside, and quercetin 3-O-sophoroside was upregulated, while the contents of kaempferol-3,7-O-bis-alpha-L-rhamnoside, rutarensin, violanthin, luteolin 7-O-rutinoside,3′,5-dneohesperidoside, chrysosplenetin, acacetin-7-O-rutinoside, jaceidin, 5,7,3′,4′-tetrahydroxy-6,8-dimethoxyflavone, vitexin, cirsimaritin, and eupatilin were downregulated. In fact, flavonoids and flavonoid glycosides play a central role in all aspects of plant life, particularly in the interactions between the plant and the environment, and determine taste and biological activity [13]. The flavonoid glycoside is an important astringency compound in *chrysanthemum* teas, with a velvety taste and an oral coating sensation [16]. In this study, the data of untargeted metabolomics analysis showed a correlation with the taste index of the electronic tongue analysis, where the luteolin and apigenin had the highest contributions to the differences between these *chrysanthemum* teas, as indicated by high VIP values, which were responsible for tea infusion's bitterness and astringency [28]. Moreover, the abundance of luteolin and apigenin in X ("HuangJu") samples was significantly different that in J ("JinshihuangJu") samples (Figure 4, $p < 0.01$). Thus, the degradation of flavonols and flavonoids in different *chrysanthemum* varieties may play a crucial role in forming *chrysanthemum* tea's flavor. In practice, *chrysanthemum* tea contains extraordinarily high levels of flavonoids that contribute to the tea's health benefits and flavor characteristics [29]. In fact, phenolic compounds, such as flavonoids and isoflavonoids, are the focus of health research. However, many flavonoids and xenoflavones have bitterness and astringency, which are undesirable and unavoidable to consumers, hindering their use as bioactive substances in foods and beverages [30]. Understanding edible *chrysanthemum*'s "bitterness and astringency motif" might prevent the introduction of bitter taste and astringent sensation in the design of functional foods enriched in bioactive (iso)flavonoids. Therefore, improving the bioavailability and reducing the bitterness and astringency of *chrysanthemum* tea by modifying its flavonoids without affecting its sensory quality will be one of the directions of in-depth, comprehensive research in the future.

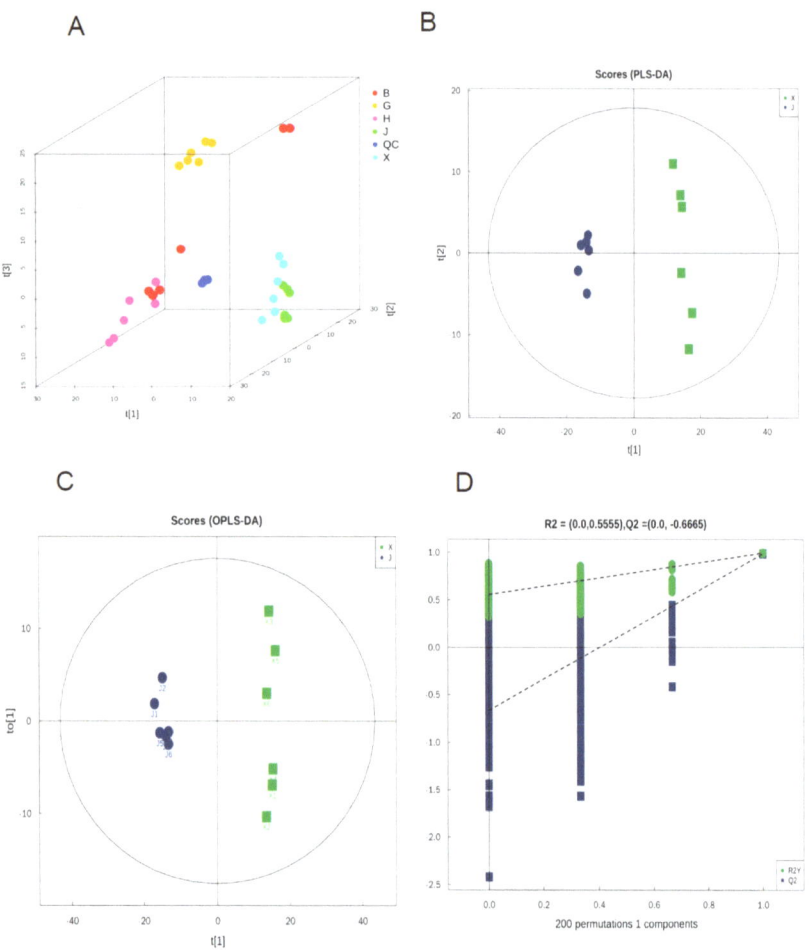

Figure 3. Multivariate analysis of *chrysanthemum* tea samples: (**A**) The 3D PCA of five different species of chrysanthemum. (**B**) The PLS-DA plot (X vs. J), R2X = 0.751, R2Y = 0.994, Q2 = 0.979. (**C**) The OPLS-DA score plot (X vs. J), R2X = 0.753, R2Y = 0.994, Q2 = 0.987. (**D**) Permutation plot of OPLS-DA, R2 = (0.0, 0.5555), Q2 = (0.0, − 0.6665). Notes: (J) JinshihuangJu; (X) HuangJu; (H) HanbaiJu; (B) BaoJu; (G) GongJu.

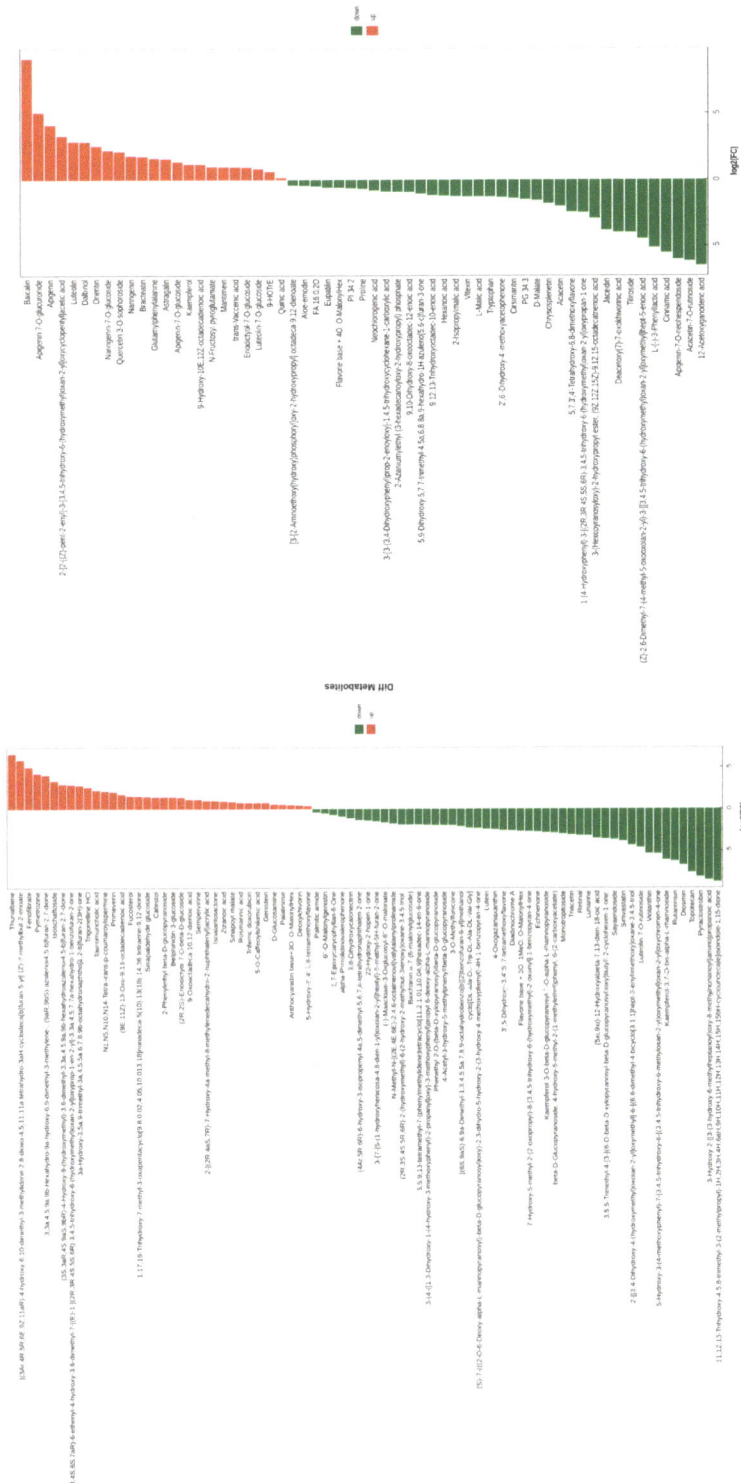

Figure 4. Multiple analysis of significant differences in metabolite expression between X and J samples (VIP > 1, $p < 0.01$): (**A**) In positive ion mode. (**B**) In negative ion mode. Notes: the x-coordinate represents the log2 FC value of the differential metabolite, that is, the logarithmic value of the differential multiple of the differential metabolite is taken as the base 2, and the ordinate axis represents significant differential metabolites. The red indicates upregulated differential metabolites, while green indicates downregulated differential metabolites.

3.4. Identifying the Core Metabolites

Since different metabolites coordinate their biological functions, the KEGG pathway-based analysis would be helpful to further understand their biological function [31]. A KEGG analysis was conducted to correlate the core metabolites identified between X and J samples (Kyoto Encyclopedia of Genes and Genomes, http://www.kegg.jp/, accessed on 30 July 2023). The KEGG pathway enrichment analysis is based on the KEGG pathway as the unit and the metabolic pathways involved in this species or closely related species as the background. Fisher's exact test was used to analyze and calculate the significance level of metabolite enrichment in each pathway to identify the metabolic and signal transduction pathways that were significantly affected. Additionally, the KEGG enrichment pathway map between X and J samples is shown in Figure 5A. Most of the identified metabolites were mainly related to flavone and flavonol biosynthesis, flavonoid biosynthesis, isoflavonoid biosynthesis, and other pathways identified by the KEGG enrichment analysis ($p < 0.05$). The important secondary metabolites, flavones, and flavonols were also detected in all *chrysanthemum* cultivars.

The flavonoid biosynthesis pathway has been extensively investigated in different *chrysanthemum* species [32]. Flavonols belong to polyphenols, which mainly exist as glycosides in *chrysanthemum* tea, contributing to the tea's bioactivities, bitterness, and astringency [33]. Considering the detection of flavonoids in *chrysanthemum* and previous studies on flavonoid biosynthesis pathways [34], a hypothesized *chrysanthemum* biosynthesis pathway was detected for flavonoids and flavonols (Figure 5B). As shown in Figure 5B, this pathway includes the mutual synthesis and transformation of apigenin, luteolin, two flavonoid components (glycosides), and their derivatives, along with the mutual synthesis and transformation of kaempferol, quercetin, myricetin, three flavonol components, and their derivatives. At the same time, apigenin and kaempferol can also be synthesized and transformed through the flavonoid biosynthesis pathway. To facilitate the observation of the expression of different metabolites annotated in the KEGG metabolic pathway, heatmaps of the different metabolites in the flavone and flavonol biosynthesis pathways were plotted, as shown in Figure 5C. Furthermore, quinic acid, genistein, 5-O-caffeoylshikimic acid, luteolin, apigenin, kaempferol, and naringenin were found to be the top marker metabolites for X ("HuangJu") samples, where they were significantly more abundant than in J ("Jingshihuangju") samples. D-malate, tryptophan, L-(-)-3-phenyllactic acid, L-malic acid, and proline were found to be the top marker metabolites for J ("JinshihuangJu") samples, where they were significantly abundant than in X ("HuangJu") samples.

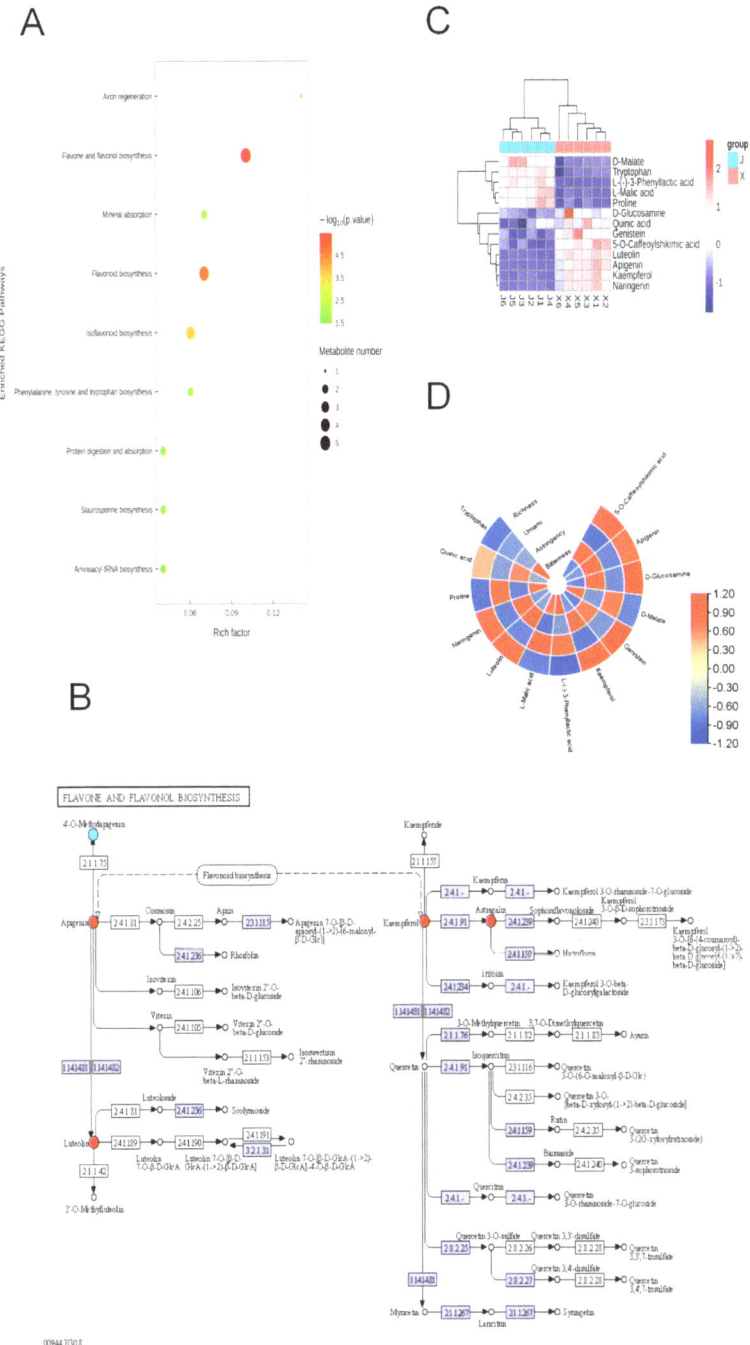

Figure 5. Identifying the core metabolites: (**A**) The KEGG enrichment pathway bubble map between X and J samples. (**B**) The flavone and flavonol biosynthesis pathways. (**C**) Heatmap analysis of critical metabolites in the flavone and flavonol biosynthesis pathways. (**D**) Associations between taste characteristics and metabolite data. Note: (**A**) Each bubble in the figure represents a metabolic

pathway (the top 20 with the highest significance were selected according to *p*-value). The horizontal coordinate where the bubble is located and the bubble size represent the influence factor size of the path in the topology analysis, and the larger the size, the larger the influence factor. The vertical coordinate where the bubble is located and the bubble color represent the *p*-value of enrichment analysis (take the negative common logarithm, i.e., $-\log 10$ *p*-value); the darker the color, the smaller the *p*-value, and the more significant the enrichment degree; the enrichment factor represents the proportion of the number of differential metabolites in this pathway in the total number of annotated metabolites in this pathway. (**B**) The small circular nodes in the metabolic pathway diagram represent metabolites; the metabolites labeled in red are the significantly upregulated differential metabolites detected in the experiment (VIP > 1, $p < 0.05$, fold change > 1), while the metabolites labeled in blue are the significantly downregulated differential metabolites detected experimentally (VIP > 1, $p < 0.05$, fold change > 1). The depth of the color indicates the degree of downward adjustment.

Numerous studies have shown that flavonols and flavones are key contributors to tea infusions' astringency and bitterness and can also significantly enhance the bitterness of caffeine [35,36]. Therefore, to statistically calculate the relationship between core metabolite compounds and taste intensity, Spearman's correlation analysis coefficient was utilized, as shown in Figure 5D. There was a significant correlation between sensory characteristics (astringency and bitterness) and some core metabolites. According to Figure 5D, 13 core metabolites were found for the first time that could be used as quick markers for the difference in taste between the X ("HuangJu") and J ("JinshihuangJu") chrysanthemum teas, including 5-O-caffeoylshikimic acid, apigenin, D-glucosamine, D-malate, genistein, kaempferol, L-(-)-3-phenyllactic acid, L-malic acid, luteolin, naringenin, proline, quinic acid, and tryptophan. The main astringency contributors with tight correlations were kaempferol, luteolin, genistein, and some quinic acid derivatives. As the more common taste characteristics of *chrysanthemum* tea, these key metabolites can form various flavonol glycosides with various sugar groups to bring an astringent and convergent taste to the tea [16]. Most noteworthy, astringency is a tactile sensation caused by the interaction of astringent substances (such as polyphenols) with salivary proteins, resulting in protein precipitation and decreased lubrication in the mouth. Saliva was proven to be an oxidative agent that leads to the formation of corresponding phenolic acids [37,38]. As important bitter and astringent compounds, phenolic acid derivatives dissolve easily during oral processing, thus enhancing acidity and affecting the taste of other polyphenols. Therefore, studies on the flavonol metabolism of *chrysanthemum* tea should take into consideration that the decomposition of flavonols starts in the oral cavity. Furthermore, L-(-)-3 phenyllactic acid and L-malic acid were found to be bitter compounds in *chrysanthemum* tea. Interestingly, these compounds are also associated with the umami flavor of *chrysanthemum* tea. Umami substances have been proposed in human sensory evaluation to inhibit the bitter taste of various chemicals [39]. However, bitterness and astringency are generally undesirable; still, they are important for providing the complex sensory perceptions of *chrysanthemum* teas. Therefore, all of these are essential tasting elements of a delicious drink. According to Tables 1 and 2 there was no significant difference in umami taste between J ("JinshihuangJu") samples and X ("HuangJu") samples ($p > 0.05$). In contrast, they obviously differed in bitterness and astringency ($p < 0.05$). Metabolic pathway analysis (Figure 5A,B) showed significant differences in flavonoid metabolism levels between the two varieties of *chrysanthemum* tea, which may be the reason for the difference in taste quality between the two varieties. In fact, the taste of *chrysanthemum* tea is closely related to some core chemical constituents, as shown in Figure 5D, and forms sensory qualities. Therefore, this study advances our understanding of metabolic changes, bitter taste, and astringent sensation in different varieties of *chrysanthemum* tea, and these data provide a theoretical basis for the control of sensory qualities.

4. Conclusions

Chrysanthemum tea is rich in many secondary metabolites related to its sensory qualities. This study used an untargeted metabolomics and sensory evaluation method based on UPLC-QTOF-MS and an electronic tongue to investigate key differential metabolites associated with sensory quality differences among five *chrysanthemum* (Juhua) tea varieties. A total of 1775 metabolites were identified in five varieties of *Chrysanthemum* tea by using UPLC-Q-TOF/MS analysis. The PCA, PLS-DA, and OPLS-DA results indicated significant differences in metabolome between X ("HuangJu") samples and J ("JinshihuangJu") samples.

To the best of our knowledge, this is the first report to reveal key taste metabolites of *chrysanthemum* tea. Of these metabolites, the contents of 13 key taste metabolites could be used for the first time as quick markers of the differences in taste between the X ("HuangJu") and J ("JinshihuangJu") *chrysanthemum* teas. Kaempferol, luteolin, genistein, and some quinic acid derivatives were correlated with the "astringent" attributes, while l-(-)-3 phenyl-lactic acid and L-malic acid were found to be responsible for the "bitterness" and "umami" in *chrysanthemum* tea. Additionally, KEGG pathway enrichment analysis showed that there were significant differences in flavonoids' metabolism levels between X ("HuangJu") and J ("JinshihuangJu") *chrysanthemum* tea samples, and the pathways involved in flavonoid metabolism had important effects on the sensory qualities of different *chrysanthemum* tea varieties. Notably, this study enriches our understanding of the relationships between the key metabolites and the bitterness and astringency of *chrysanthemum* tea varieties. Untargeted metabolomics combined with electronic tongue analysis based on LC-MS can be effectively used to evaluate the differences in the sensory qualities of different varieties of *chrysanthemum* tea cultivars, which is essential for improving the quality of the finished *chrysanthemum* tea and the effective utilization of edible *chrysanthemum*. Further studies are ongoing in the authors' lab, focusing on the formation mechanism of the key flavor components and the functional components in *chrysanthemum* tea during oral processing. We hope to report more about these advancements in the future.

Supplementary Materials: The following supporting information can be downloaded at: https://www.mdpi.com/article/10.3390/foods13071080/s1, Figure S1: The HPLC chromatogram of the five different varieties of *chrysanthemum* tea; Figure S2: The TIC diagram in the ESI positive and negative modes for the five different varieties of *chrysanthemum* tea; Table S1: Contents of main bioactive substances of five different varieties of *chrysanthemum* tea; Table S2: Critical Compounds Metabolites Responsible for the Metabolomics Variation Caused between X and J Samples (VIP > 1, $p < 0.01$).

Author Contributions: X.T.: conceptualization, methodology, formal analysis, investigation, writing—original draft, writing—review and editing. H.W.: formal analysis, investigation, writing—original draft. W.W.: supervision, writing—review and editing, funding acquisition. H.Y.: methodology, conceptualization, data curation. L.C.: visualization, data curation. C.P.: supervision, writing—review and editing. All authors have read and agreed to the published version of the manuscript.

Funding: This study was supported by the "Project of Hunan Province Enterprise Science and Technology Commissioner Plan (2021–2022)" (Project No. 2021GK5087), "Hunan Natural Science Foundation Program" (Project No. 2023JJ30445), "Hunan Provincial Department of Education Outstanding Youth Project" (Project No. 22B0378), "The Central Government Guides Local Funds for Science and Technology Development Program" Project No. 2022ZYT029), and "Hunan University of Chinese Medicine 'double first-class' Construction Discipline open ranking" Program (Project No. 22JB2053). The authors thank Hunan Kangdejia Forestry Technology Co., Ltd. for providing the *chrysanthemum* raw materials.

Data Availability Statement: The original contributions presented in the study are included in the article/supplementary material, further inquiries can be directed to the corresponding author.

Conflicts of Interest: The authors declare no conflicts of interest.

Abbreviations

Liquid Chromatography-tandem Mass Spectrometry (LC-MS/MS); Mass Spectrometry (MS); High-Performance Liquid Chromatography (HPLC); False Discovery Rate (FDR); Principal Component Analysis (PCA); Kyoto Encyclopedia of Genes and Genomes (KEGG); Traditional Chinese medicine (TCM); Gas Chromatography-Mass Spectrography (GC-MS); Headspace-gas Chromatography-ion Mobility Spectrometry (HS-GC-IMS); Gas chromatography olfactometry (GC-O); Electron Spray Ionization (ESI).

References

1. Li, Y.; Quan, H.; Liang, L.; Yang, T.; Feng, L.; Mao, X.; Wang, Y. Nontargeted metabolomics reveals the discrimination of *Cyclocarya paliurus* leaves brewed by different methods. *Food Res. Int.* **2021**, *142*, 110221. [CrossRef]
2. Yuan, H.; Jiang, S.; Liu, Y.; Daniyal, M.; Jian, Y.; Peng, C.; Shen, J.; Liu, S.; Wang, W. The flower head of *Chrysanthemum morifolium* Ramat. (Juhua): A paradigm of flowers serving as Chinese dietary herbal medicine. *J. Ethnopharmacol.* **2020**, *261*, 113043. [CrossRef]
3. Han, A.R.; Nam, B.; Kim, B.R.; Lee, K.C.; Song, B.S.; Kim, S.H.; Kim, J.B.; Jin, C.H. Phytochemical Composition and Antioxidant Activities of Two Different Color *Chrysanthemum* Flower Teas. *Molecules* **2019**, *24*, 329. [CrossRef] [PubMed]
4. Jiang, S.; Wang, M.; Jiang, Z.; Zafar, S.; Xie, Q.; Yang, Y.; Liu, Y.; Yuan, H.; Jian, Y.; Wang, W. Chemistry and Pharmacological Activity of Sesquiterpenoids from the *Chrysanthemum* Genus. *Molecules* **2021**, *26*, 3038. [CrossRef] [PubMed]
5. Xiang-Wei, C.; Dan-Dan, W.; Dong-Jie, C.; Hui, Y.; Xiao-Dong, S.; Wen-Bin, Z.; Jin-Ao, D. Historical Origin and Development of Medicinal and Tea *Chrysanthemum morifolium* Resources. *Mod. Chin. Med.* **2019**, *1*, 116–123. [CrossRef]
6. Liao, Y.; Zhou, X.; Zeng, L. How does tea (*Camellia sinensis*) produce specialized metabolites which determine its unique quality and function: A review. *Crit. Rev. Food Sci. Nutr.* **2022**, *62*, 3751–3767. [CrossRef] [PubMed]
7. Yang, L.; Cheng, P.; Wang, J.H.; Li, H. Analysis of Floral Volatile Components and Antioxidant Activity of Different Varieties of *Chrysanthemum morifolium*. *Molecules* **2017**, *22*, 1790. [CrossRef]
8. Choi, H.; Kim, G. Volatile flavor composition of gamguk (*Chrysanthemum indicum*) flower essential oils. *Food Sci. Biotechnol.* **2011**, *20*, 319–325. [CrossRef]
9. Wang, Z.; Yuan, Y.; Hong, B.; Zhao, X.; Gu, Z. Characteristic Volatile Fingerprints of Four *Chrysanthemum* Teas Determined by HS-GC-IMS. *Molecules* **2021**, *26*, 7113. [CrossRef]
10. Kaneko, S.; Chen, J.; Wu, J.; Suzuki, Y.; Ma, L.; Kumazawa, K. Potent Odorants of Characteristic Floral/Sweet Odor in Chinese *Chrysanthemum* Flower Tea Infusion. *J. Agric. Food Chem.* **2017**, *65*, 10058–10063. [CrossRef]
11. Wang, X.; Zhang, J.; Liu, Z.; Wang, S.; Huang, B.; Hu, Z.; Liu, Y. Comparative transcriptome analysis of three *chrysanthemums* provides insights into flavonoid and terpenoid biosynthesis. *J. Plant Biol.* **2021**, *64*, 389–401. [CrossRef]
12. Sumner, L.W.; Mendes, P.; Dixon, R.A. Plant metabolomics: Large-scale phytochemistry in the functional genomics era. *Phytochemistry* **2003**, *62*, 817–836. [CrossRef] [PubMed]
13. Zhao, J.; Liu, W.; Chen, Y.; Zhang, X.; Wang, X.; Wang, F.; Qian, Y.; Qiu, J. Identification of markers for tea authenticity assessment: Non-targeted metabolomics of highly similar oolong tea cultivars (*Camellia sinensis var. sinensis*). *Food Control* **2022**, *142*, 109223. [CrossRef]
14. Phat, C.; Moon, B.; Lee, C. Evaluation of umami taste in mushroom extracts by chemical analysis, sensory evaluation, and an electronic tongue system. *Food Chem.* **2016**, *192*, 1068–1077. [CrossRef] [PubMed]
15. Xing, T.; Hui-jie, Y.E.; Shi-feng, L.; Yao-li, O. Study on the interaction between the astringent constituents of different varieties of *Chrysanthemum* and saliva. *Food Mach.* **2022**, *4*, 42–46. [CrossRef]
16. Zhang, L.; Cao, Q.; Granato, D.; Xu, Y.; Ho, C. Association between chemistry and taste of tea: A review. *Trends Food Sci. Technol.* **2020**, *101*, 139–149. [CrossRef]
17. Li, J.; Wang, J.; Yao, Y.; Hua, J.; Zhou, Q.; Jiang, Y.; Deng, Y.; Yang, Y.; Wang, J.; Yuan, H.; et al. Phytochemical comparison of different tea (*Camellia sinensis*) cultivars and its association with sensory quality of finished tea. *LWT* **2020**, *117*, 108595. [CrossRef]
18. GB/T 23776-2018; Methodology for Sensory Evaluation of Tea. Standardization Administration of China: Beijing, China, 2018. Available online: http://down.foodmate.net/standard/sort/3/52614.html (accessed on 2 February 2024).
19. Cheng, L.; Yang, Q.; Chen, Z.; Zhang, J.; Chen, Q.; Wang, Y.; Wei, X. Distinct Changes of Metabolic Profile and Sensory Quality during Qingzhuan Tea Processing Revealed by LC-MS-Based Metabolomics. *J. Agric. Food Chem.* **2020**, *68*, 4955–4965. [CrossRef] [PubMed]
20. Cheng, L.; Yang, Q.; Peng, L.; Xu, L.; Chen, C.J.; Zhu, Y.; Wei, X. Exploring core functional fungi driving the metabolic conversion in the industrial pile fermentation of Qingzhuan tea. *Food Res. Int.* **2024**, *178*, 113979. [CrossRef]
21. Granato, D.; Grevink, R.; Zielinski, A.A.F.; Nunes, D.S.; van Ruth, S.M. Analytical Strategy Coupled with Response Surface Methodology to Maximize the Extraction of Antioxidants from Ternary Mixtures of Green, Yellow, and Red Teas (*Camellia sinensis var. sinensis*). *J. Agric. Food Chem.* **2014**, *62*, 10283–10296. [CrossRef]

22. Rudge, R.E.D.; Fuhrmann, P.L.; Scheermeijer, R.; van der Zanden, E.M.; Dijksman, J.A.; Scholten, E. A tribological approach to astringency perception and astringency prevention. *Food Hydrocoll.* **2021**, *121*, 106951. [CrossRef]
23. Yuan, H.; Luo, J.; Lyu, M.; Jiang, S.; Qiu, Y.; Tian, X.; Liu, L.; Liu, S.; Ouyang, Y.; Wang, W. An integrated approach to Q-marker discovery and quality assessment of edible *Chrysanthemum* flowers based on chromatogram–effect relationship and bioinformatics analyses. *Ind. Crop. Prod.* **2022**, *188*, 115745. [CrossRef]
24. Gibbins, H.L.; Carpenter, G.H. Alternative Mechanisms of Astringency—What is the Role of Saliva. *J. Texture Stud.* **2013**, *44*, 364–375. [CrossRef]
25. Ma, S.; Lee, H.; Liang, Y.; Zhou, F. Astringent Mouthfeel as a Consequence of Lubrication Failure. *Angew. Chem. (Int. Ed. Engl.)* **2016**, *55*, 5793–5797. [CrossRef] [PubMed]
26. Luo, D.; Deng, T.; Yuan, W.; Deng, H.; Jin, M. Plasma metabolomic study in Chinese patients with wet age-related macular degeneration. *BMC Ophthalmol.* **2017**, *17*, 165. [CrossRef] [PubMed]
27. Fraser, K.; Lane, G.A.; Otter, D.E.; Hemar, Y.; Quek, S.; Harrison, S.J.; Rasmussen, S. Analysis of metabolic markers of tea origin by UHPLC and high resolution mass spectrometry. Tea—From bushes to mugs: Composition, stability and health aspects. *Food Res. Int.* **2013**, *53*, 827–835. [CrossRef]
28. Yang, C.; Hu, Z.; Lu, M.; Li, P.; Tan, J.; Chen, M.; Lv, H.; Zhu, Y.; Zhang, Y.; Guo, L.; et al. Application of metabolomics profiling in the analysis of metabolites and taste quality in different subtypes of white tea. *Food Res. Int.* **2018**, *106*, 909–919. [CrossRef] [PubMed]
29. Lin, N.; Liu, X.; Zhu, W.; Cheng, X.; Wang, X.; Wan, X.; Liu, L. Ambient Ultraviolet B Signal Modulates Tea Flavor Characteristics via Shifting a Metabolic Flux in Flavonoid Biosynthesis. *J. Agric. Food Chem.* **2021**, *69*, 3401–3414. [CrossRef] [PubMed]
30. Roland, W.S.U.; van Buren, L.; Gruppen, H.; Driesse, M.; Gouka, R.J.; Smit, G.; Vincken, J. Bitter Taste Receptor Activation by Flavonoids and Isoflavonoids: Modeled Structural Requirements for Activation of hTAS2R14 and hTAS2R39. *J. Agric. Food Chem.* **2013**, *61*, 10454–10466. [CrossRef]
31. Nakaya, A.; Katayama, T.; Itoh, M.; Hiranuka, K.; Kawashima, S.; Moriya, Y.; Okuda, S.; Tanaka, M.; Tokimatsu, T.; Yamanishi, Y.; et al. KEGG OC: A large-scale automatic construction of taxonomy-based ortholog clusters. *Nucleic Acids Res.* **2013**, *41*, D353–D357. [CrossRef]
32. Hodaei, M.; Rahimmalek, M.; Arzani, A.; Talebi, M. The effect of water stress on phytochemical accumulation, bioactive compounds and expression of key genes involved in flavonoid biosynthesis in *Chrysanthemum morifolium* L. *Ind. Crop Prod.* **2018**, *120*, 295–304. [CrossRef]
33. Li, Q.; Jin, Y.; Jiang, R.; Xu, Y.; Zhang, Y.; Luo, Y.; Huang, J.; Wang, K.; Liu, Z. Dynamic changes in the metabolite profile and taste characteristics of Fu brick tea during the manufacturing process. *Food Chem.* **2021**, *344*, 128576. [CrossRef]
34. Falcone Ferreyra, M.L.; Rius, S.P.; Casati, P. Flavonoids: Biosynthesis, biological functions, and biotechnological applications. *Front. Plant Sci.* **2012**, *3*, 222. [CrossRef] [PubMed]
35. Cao, Q.Q.; Zou, C.; Zhang, Y.H.; Du, Q.Z.; Yin, J.F.; Shi, J.; Xue, S.; Xu, Y.Q. Improving the taste of autumn green tea with tannase. *Food Chem.* **2019**, *277*, 432–437. [CrossRef] [PubMed]
36. Liu, W.; Feng, Y.; Yu, S.; Fan, Z.; Li, X.; Li, J.; Yin, H. The Flavonoid Biosynthesis Network in Plants. *Int. J. Mol. Sci.* **2021**, *22*, 12824. [CrossRef] [PubMed]
37. Malgorzata, R.; Magdalena, B. Decomposition of Flavonols in the Presence of Saliva. *Appl. Sci.* **2020**, *10*, 7511. [CrossRef]
38. Yuan, J.; Huang, J.; Wu, G.; Tong, J.; Xie, G.; Duan, J.; Qin, M. Multiple responses optimization of ultrasonic-assisted extraction by response surface methodology (RSM) for rapid analysis of bioactive compounds in the flower head of *Chrysanthemum morifolium* Ramat. *Industrial Crops and Products.* **2015**, *74*, 192–199. [CrossRef]
39. Kim, M.; Son, H.; Kim, Y.; Misaka, T.; Rhyu, M. Umami–bitter interactions: The suppression of bitterness by umami peptides via human bitter taste receptor. *Biochem. Biophys. Res. Commun.* **2015**, *456*, 586–590. [CrossRef]

Disclaimer/Publisher's Note: The statements, opinions and data contained in all publications are solely those of the individual author(s) and contributor(s) and not of MDPI and/or the editor(s). MDPI and/or the editor(s) disclaim responsibility for any injury to people or property resulting from any ideas, methods, instructions or products referred to in the content.

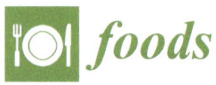

Article

GC–MS Combined with Fast GC E-Nose for the Analysis of Volatile Components of Chamomile (*Matricaria chamomilla* L.)

Jiayu Lu [1,2], Zheng Jiang [1,2], Jingjie Dang [1,2], Dishuai Li [1,2], Daixin Yu [1,2], Cheng Qu [3,*] and Qinan Wu [1,2,*]

[1] Jiangsu Collaborative Innovation Center of Chinese Medicinal Resources Industrialization, Nanjing University of Chinese Medicine, Nanjing 210023, China; lujiayu5210@163.com (J.L.); jyjiangzheng@163.com (Z.J.); 20223110@njucm.edu.cn (J.D.); 20210651@njucm.edu.cn (D.L.); yudaixin0616@163.com (D.Y.)
[2] State Key Laboratory on Technologies for Chinese Medicine Pharmaceutical Process Control and Intelligent Manufacture, Nanjing University of Chinese Medicine, Nanjing 210023, China
[3] School of Pharmacy, Nanjing University of Chinese Medicine, Nanjing 210023, China
* Correspondence: qucheng@njucm.edu.cn (C.Q.); wuqn@njucm.edu.cn (Q.W.)

Abstract: Chamomile has become one of the world's most popular herbal teas due to its unique properties. Chamomile is widely used in dietary supplements, cosmetics, and herbal products. This study aimed to investigate the volatile aromatic components in chamomile. Two analytical techniques, gas chromatography–mass spectrometry (GC-MS) and an ultra-fast gas chromatography electronic nose, were employed to examine samples from Xinjiang (XJ), Shandong (SD), and Hebei (HB) in China, and imported samples from Germany (GER). The results revealed that all chamomile samples contained specific sesquiterpene compounds, including α-bisabolol, bisabolol oxide, bisabolone oxide, and chamazulene. Additionally, forty potential aroma components were identified by the electronic nose. The primary odor components of chamomile were characterized by fruity and spicy notes. The primary differences in the components of chamomile oil were identified as (E)-β-farnesene, chamazulene, α-bisabolol oxide B, spathulenol and α-bisabolone oxide A. Significant differences in aroma compounds included geosmin, butanoic acid, 2-butene, norfuraneol, γ-terpinene. This study demonstrates that GC–MS and the ultra-fast gas chromatography electronic nose can preliminarily distinguish chamomile from different areas, providing a method and guidance for the selection of origin and sensory evaluation of chamomile. The current study is limited by the sample size and it provides preliminary conclusions. Future studies with a larger sample size are warranted to further improve these findings.

Keywords: *Matricaria chamomilla*; HERACLES Neo; GC-MS; flavor; volatile components

Citation: Lu, J.; Jiang, Z.; Dang, J.; Li, D.; Yu, D.; Qu, C.; Wu, Q. GC–MS Combined with Fast GC E-Nose for the Analysis of Volatile Components of Chamomile (*Matricaria chamomilla* L.). *Foods* **2024**, *13*, 1865. https://doi.org/10.3390/foods13121865

Academic Editors: Salvador Maestre Pérez and Shahab A. Shamsi

Received: 6 May 2024
Revised: 9 June 2024
Accepted: 11 June 2024
Published: 13 June 2024

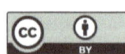

Copyright: © 2024 by the authors. Licensee MDPI, Basel, Switzerland. This article is an open access article distributed under the terms and conditions of the Creative Commons Attribution (CC BY) license (https://creativecommons.org/licenses/by/4.0/).

1. Introduction

Chamomile (*Matricaria chamomilla* L.) is one of the most important, widely used aromatic and medicinal plants, belonging to the Asteraceae family. It has been used both as food and medicine for its aroma, anti-inflammatory, analgesic, and antibacterial properties [1,2]. Its extracts, oils, and teas are utilized worldwide to treat various ailments, including stomach issues, spasms, dermatitis, chronic headaches, constipation, anhidrosis, joint swelling, and urinary system diseases [3,4]. Chamomile is also used in skincare and cosmetic products, such as face creams, shampoos, and conditioners. Additionally, it is employed in traditional medicines of Asian countries including India, China, and Japan. In Chinese traditional medicine, it is incorporated into proprietary medicines [5]. Chamomile is widely cultivated, primarily in Eastern Europe, North America, South America, and parts of Asia. Market assessments forecast that global demand for chamomile will exceed USD 400 billion by 2025 [6].

The most commonly used components of chamomile are its essential oils, which promote relaxation and provide calming effects on the nervous system. Additionally, its aromatic components are extracted for flavoring beverages and as additives in perfumes [7,8]. Chamomile's volatile organic compounds (VOCs), mainly consisting of monoterpenes and sesquiterpenes, include bisabolol and its oxides, chamazulene, farnesene, and cineole. These components are primarily found in the volatile oil and have calming, antidepressant, and antimicrobial effects, underscoring their substantial market value and research significance [9]. Research on chamomile's volatile components typically utilizes gas chromatography–mass spectrometry (GC-MS), requiring extraction of volatile oils and involving tedious sample preparation and time-consuming analysis [10]. However, this method lacks the capability to accurately gauge or describe the aroma [11]. Volatile components influence the quality of floral teas, with aromatic teas generally scoring higher in sensory evaluations [12,13]. In addition to traditional olfactory sensory evaluations, ultra-fast gas chromatography electronic noses (E-noses) have been used in the sensory evaluation of food and pharmaceuticals [14]. These devices can identify unknown odor types and qualitatively analyze volatile components within 1–3 min. Research on dry ginger's odor components revealed that its overall aroma is spicy and fragrant, aligning with its sensory evaluation [15]. Additionally, the high-temperature extraction of volatile oils often degrades thermosensitive metabolites through carbocation formation or concerted cyclic rearrangements into their structural analogs, altering the composition [16,17]. Therefore, developing a rapid, non-destructive method for analyzing and describing the aroma of chamomile is essential for assessing its overall aroma information and quality.

This study employed gas chromatography–mass spectrometry (GC-MS) and ultra-fast gas chromatography electronic nose technology to analyze the volatile oil components and aroma profiles of chamomile. This is the first study to use an electronic nose to analyze the aroma of chamomile. These results provide a comprehensive analysis of chamomile's volatile components, contributing to a better understanding of its aroma compounds and sensory evaluations.

2. Materials and Methods

2.1. Instruments and Reagents

The HERACLES Neo ultra-fast gas chromatography electronic nose (Alpha Mos, Toulouse, France), equipped with a PAL RSI automatic headspace sampler, MXT-5 non-polar capillary column, and MXT-1701 medium-polarity capillary column, was used for the aroma analysis of chamomile. Additionally, the GA-380N low-noise air pump and the GH-380 high-purity hydrogen generator (Beijing Zhong Xing Hui Li Technology Development Co., Ltd., Beijing, China) were utilized for the analysis. The Agilent 7890B gas chromatograph and Agilent 7000C triple quadrupole mass spectrometer (Agilent Technologies, Santa Clara, CA, USA) were used for gas phase and mass spectrometric analysis of chamomile volatile oils.

An electronic analytical balance (AUX220, Shimadzu Corporation, Kyoto, Japan) was used for weighing. Sample drying was performed using an electric hot air oven (9140A DHG, Shanghai Jinghong Experimental Equipment Co., Ltd., Shanghai, China). A temperature-regulated electric heating mantle (PTHW3000 mL, Gong Yi Yu Hua Instruments Co., Ltd., Gongyi, China) was employed for the heating process. The SAGA-10TY laboratory ultrapure water system (Nanjing EasyPure Development Co., Ltd., Nanjing, China) provided ultrapure water for the experiments.

Mixed reference substances used in the experiment included n-alkanes (lot A0168401, containing 0.02–53.27 g of normal alkanes (C6–C16) per 100 g, Restek Corporation, Bellefonte, PA, USA), and a C7-C40 mixed standard (lot number S08HB193959, Shanghai Yuan Ye Co., Ltd., Shanghai, China). The n-hexane (lot K2212140) and n-hexadecane (lot J1217041) were sourced from Aladdin Chemical Reagents Co., Ltd., Nanjing, China, and the anhydrous sodium sulfate (lot 1503023670) was obtained from Nanjing Chemical Reagents Co., Ltd., Nanjing, China.

2.2. Chamomile Samples

A total of 15 chamomile samples were collected in 2023 from major chamomile-producing areas in China. The samples originated from Xinjiang (XJ), Shandong (SD), and Hebei (HB), with geographical coordinates ranging from 80°09′ to 121°00′ East and 35°35′ to 49°10′ North (Figure 1). The German samples consisted of three different brands of chamomile collected in Germany. Each chamomile sample was ground into a fine powder using a high-speed grinder, and passed through a No. 1 sieve (850 μm ± 29 μm) as specified in the Chinese Pharmacopoeia for experimental use.

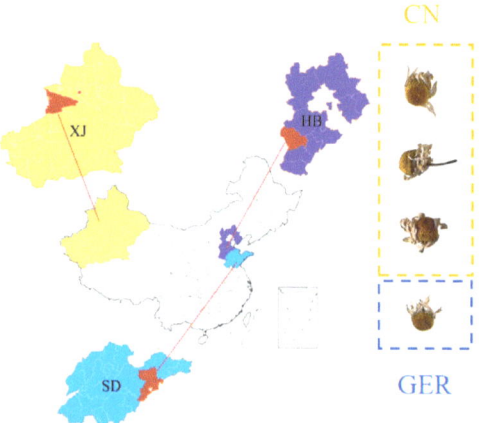

Figure 1. Regional information of chamomile from China (SD: Shandong; XJ: Xinjiang; HB: Hebei); CN: Samples from China; GER: Samples from Germany.

2.3. Determination of Volatile Oil Content

The method is based on the determination of volatile oil content as described in the Chinese Pharmacopoeia, with modifications [18]. Approximately 75 g of the sample (equivalent to 0.5 to 1.0 mL of volatile oil) were weighed and placed in a round-bottom flask. Then, 1500 mL of ultrapure water (or an appropriate amount) and a few zeolites were added. After shaking and mixing, the flask was connected to a volatile oil determiner and a reflux condenser. Water was added from the top of the condenser until it filled the scale part of the volatile oil determiner and overflowed into the flask. The mixture was then slowly heated to boiling with a temperature-regulated electric heating mantle and maintained at a consistent boil for 4 h [19]. The piston at the bottom of the determiner was opened after a short pause, and water was slowly released until the top of the oil layer reached 5 mm above the zero mark on the scale. The piston was opened again to lower the oil layer until its upper end was level with the zero mark, after the solution had been left to stand for 1 h. The volume of volatile oil was then read, and the content (%) of volatile oil in the test sample was calculated.

2.4. Volatile Oil GC–MS Analysis

55 μL of hexadecane was diluted to 50 mL with n-hexane to serve as the internal standard solution. Chamomile essential oil was dried over anhydrous sodium sulfate for the test sample solution. An amount of 10 μL of the essential oil was then extracted and diluted to 1 mL with the internal standard solution, serving as the sample solution for analysis.

The gas chromatographic conditions were based on the method described by Elahe Piri et al., with some modifications [20]: split mode injection with an injection volume of 1 μL, carrier gas helium (purity 99.999%) at a flow rate of 1.0 mL/min, injector temperature 250 °C, and split ratio 30:1. The oven temperature program started at 50 °C, held for 3 min, then increased at 5 °C/min to 250 °C, and held for 5 min. The total GC runtime was 48 min. The chromatographic column used was an Agilent 19091S-433I HP-5ms Inert, with temperature limits of 0 °C to 325 °C (maximum 340 °C): 30 m × 250 μm × 0.25 μm.

The mass spectrometry conditions were as follows: the ionization method was electron ionization (EI) with a quadrupole temperature of 150 °C, ion source temperature of 230 °C, mass scan range m/z 30.0 to 500.0 amu, interface temperature 280 °C, and full scan mode at an electron energy of 70 eV.

2.5. Ultra-Fast Gas Chromatography Electronic Nose Analysis

2.5.1. Single-Factor Investigation

Sample Quantity: The injection volume was set at 3000 μL, with an incubation temperature of 60 °C and an incubation time of 20 min. The impact of different quantities (0.2 g, 0.3 g, 0.4 g, 0.5 g, 1.0 g) of the same chamomile sample (ID S-7) on the chromatographic peak area was investigated. Results indicated that the peak area increased with the sample quantity. No noticeable increase in peak area was observed for sample quantities of 0.5 g or 1 g. Therefore, a sample weight of 0.5 g was selected based on the relationship between sample weight and peak area.

Injection Volume: A 0.5 g sample of chamomile was analyzed, with the incubation temperature set at 60 °C and the incubation time at 20 min. The effect of different injection volumes (1000 μL, 2000 μL, 3000 μL, 4000 μL, 5000 μL) on the odor chromatographic peak area was examined. Results showed that peak area increased with the injection volume, thus the chosen injection volume was 5000 μL.

Incubation Temperature: A 0.5 g sample of chamomile was analyzed, with an incubation time of 20 min and an injection volume of 5000 μL. The impact of various incubation temperatures (40 °C, 50 °C, 60 °C, 70 °C) on the odor chromatographic peak area was explored. As the temperature increased, the chromatographic peak response gradually increased. Chamomile contains aromatic volatile oils, and lower temperatures are closer to real environmental conditions. According to the instrument's instructions, temperatures below 50 °C are considered low. The maximum chromatographic peak response was observed at 50 °C, so the incubation temperature was set at 50 °C.

Incubation Time: A 0.5 g sample of chamomile was analyzed, with an incubation temperature of 50 °C and an injection volume of 5000 μL. The influence of different incubation times (10 min, 15 min, 20 min, 25 min, 30 min) on the odor chromatographic peak area was assessed. The results demonstrated that the peak area became saturated and stable at an incubation time of 20 min. Therefore, the chosen incubation time was 20 min

2.5.2. Sample Analysis

A 0.5 g sample of chamomile was placed in a 20 mL headspace vial specifically designed for electronic nose analysis and sealed with a PTFE gasket. The HERACLES Neo Analyzer is an advanced, fast gas-phase electronic nose with a built-in pre-concentration trap [21], unlike the standard metal oxide semiconductor (MOS) electronic noses, which rely on metal oxide sensors. Initially, each sample is placed in an incubator to concentrate the volatile components in the gas phase of the headspace vial until equilibrium is reached. The gaseous sample is then transferred to the pre-concentration trap, where the captured components are quickly released and separated in the MXT-5 and MXT-1701 columns, allowing for rapid separation. The concentrated odors are detected using two hydrogen flame ionization detectors (FIDs). Alpha Soft-17.0 software is used to record the signals, and each sample is tested three times in parallel.

The instrument conditions were modified based on preliminary research conducted in our laboratory. The chromatographic columns used are a low polarity MXT-5 (5% diphenyl/95% dimethyl polysiloxane, 10 m × 0.18 mm, 0.4 μm) and a medium polarity MXT-1701 (14% cyanopropylphenyl/86% dimethyl polysiloxane, 10 m × 0.18 mm, 0.4 μm) metal capillary columns. The headspace vial volume is 20 mL; sample quantity is 0.5 g; injection volume is 5000 μL; shaking temperature is 50 °C; shaking time is 20 min; injection speed is 125 µL/s; injection duration is 45 s; injection port temperature is 200 °C; initial temperature of the capture trap is 40 °C; hydrogen is used as the carrier gas at a flow rate of 1.0 mL/min, with a capture trap diversion rate of 10 mL/min; the capture duration is 50 s; final temperature of the capture trap is 240 °C; initial column temperature is 50 °C. The temperature program ramps from 1 °C/s to 80 °C, then 3 °C/s to 250 °C, holding for 21 s. Acquisition time is 110 s; FID gain is 12 [15].

2.5.3. Methodological Investigation

Precision: Six chamomile samples (ID S-7) were precisely weighed, each at 0.5 g, and analyzed under the detection conditions described in Section 2.5.2. Ten common peaks were identified, with their chromatographic peak areas and retention times recorded. Results showed that the RSD values for the peak areas of the ten common peaks ranged from 2.60% to 7.12%, and were all below 10.00%; RSD values for their retention times ranged from 0.03% to 0.14%, and were all below 3.0%, indicating good instrument precision.

Reproducibility: Six parallel preparations of chamomile samples (ID S-7) were precisely weighed. The analysis was conducted according to the method described in Section 2.5.2. Ten common peaks were recorded, along with their chromatographic peak areas and retention times. Results showed that the RSD values for the peak areas of the ten common peaks ranged from 1.15% to 6.94%, and were all below 10.00%; RSD values for their retention times ranged from 0.02% to 0.06%, and were all below 3.0%, indicating good reproducibility of the experiment.

Stability: The same chamomile sample (ID S-7) was precisely weighed at 0.5 g at 0, 2, 4, 8, 12, 24 h and analyzed under the detection conditions described in Section 2.5.2. Ten common peaks were recorded, along with their chromatographic peak areas and retention times. Results showed that the RSD values for the peak areas of the ten common peaks ranged from 1.34% to 8.63%, and were all below 10.00%. RSD values for their retention times ranged from 0.03% to 0.15%, and were all below 3.0%, indicating good stability within 24 h.

2.6. Qualitative and Quantitative Analysis

GC–MS analysis was employed to analyze a solution of n-alkanes (C7-C40) under identical conditions to calculate the retention index (RI) values of various volatile compounds in chamomile essential oil. The NIST 14 library was used to identify unknown compounds by comparing the mass spectral information with published RI values. Typically, higher R-matching values in the NIST library are considered the first indicator for identifying unknown compounds. Additionally, a difference of no more than 30 between experimental RI values and reported RI values is regarded as an important criterion for identification [22]. To quantitatively analyze different components, n-hexadecane was added as an internal standard in each sample. The relative content of each component in the essential oil was determined by the ratio of the analyzed peak area to the internal standard.

The flavor components analyzed by the fast gas chromatography electronic nose (e-nose) were calibrated using mixed n-alkanes (C6 to C16 standards [23]) for calculating RI values, and potential compounds were identified through comparison with the AroChemBase database.

2.7. Chemometric Analysis

Chemometric analyses were conducted using SIMCA–P software (Version 14.1, Umetrics, Sweden) for principal component analysis (PCA), partial least squares discriminant analysis (PLS–DA), and orthogonal partial least squares discriminant analysis (OPLS–DA). Discriminant factor analysis (DFA) was carried out using the HERACLES fast gas chromatography electronic nose software Alpha Soft (version 17.0, Toulouse, France).

3. Results
3.1. Chamomile Volatile Oil

The yield of essential oil from chamomile has always been a concern in agricultural science and the commodity economy, as higher content of volatile oils in chamomile is generally considered indicative of better quality [24].The essential oil content of 18 batches of chamomile herbs ranged from 0.43% to 1.38%, with an average of 0.80%. The average essential oil contents of chamomile samples from different areas were 0.87% for Xinjiang, 1.02% for Shandong, 0.52% for Hebei, and 0.87% for Germany.

3.2. GC–MS Identification of Chamomile Volatile Oil Components

In this experiment, 16 volatile components were identified from chamomile samples from different areas, including 13 terpenoids, one aliphatic hydrocarbon, one ester, and one ketone. The relative content of each substance was determined by comparing the peak area of each batch's chromatographic peaks with that of the internal standard, as shown in Table S2. All the essential oils were blue, due to the formation of chamazulene under high-temperature conditions. During distillation, high temperatures can lead to the formation of chamazulene, which imparts a blue color to the oil. However, supercritical CO_2 extraction avoids this type of thermal degradation. As a result, oils extracted using this method do not exhibit the blue coloration associated with chamazulene formation [25]. Among the volatile oil components of chamomile, besides chamazulene, the oxygenated sesquiterpenes are the most characteristic, with bisabolol oxide B, α-bisabolol, bisabolone oxide, and bisabolol oxide A being the most notable compounds [18]. Chamazulene offers photoprotective effects on the human keratinocyte cell line (HaCaT) and provides ultraviolet blocking capabilities [26]; α-Bisabolol inhibited glioblastoma cell migration and invasion by downregulating central mucoepidermoid tumor (c-Met); α-Bisabolol oxide A from chamomile flowers is reported to inhibit the migration of Caco-2 colon cancer cells and deactivate the vascular epidermal growth factor receptor-2 (VEGFR2) angiogenic enzymes [27].

This experiment determined the average relative content of chamazulene from the three sources to be: XJ 0.71 µg/mL, SD 2.14 µg/mL, HB 0.45 µg/mL, and GER 0.22 µg/mL. The combined average relative content of bisabolol and its oxides (β-bisabolol, α-bisabolol oxide B, bisabolol oxide B, α-bisabolone oxide A, α-bisabolol, α-bisabolol oxide A) was: XJ 3.41 µg/mL, SD 4.68 µg/mL, HB 2.84 µg/mL, and GER 1.83 µg/mL. The results indicate that samples from Shandong (CN) have the highest oil content and levels of characteristic components, although these differences could be attributed to climate, soil, cultivation methods, etc. [28]. This can to some extent assess the quality of chamomile [29]. We generated a histogram to show intuitive representation of the differences in volatile oil components from different sources (Figure 2).

3.3. Discrimination of Chamomile by GC–MS
3.3.1. PCA (Principal Component Analysis)

Principal component analysis (PCA) was conducted to investigate the differences in volatile oils of different chamomile samples. The common peak areas of chamomile volatile oils were used as variables, and PCA was performed using SIMCA 14.1 software, as shown in Figure 3A. The results revealed that the first two principal components accounted for 82.30% of the total variance (PC1 62.80%, PC2 19.50%), with R2X = 0.995 and a model predictive ability Q2(cum) = 0.746 (>0.5), indicating that the model can adequately reflect the sample information and explain and predict the total variance well.

The PCA was conducted using the first two principal components, t [1] and t [2], which together explain a significant portion of the variance in the dataset (R2X [1] = 0.628 and R2X [2] = 0.195). XJ samples are represented by green dots, forming a distinct cluster. This indicates a unique volatile oil profile that separates XJ samples from others. SD samples are represented by blue dots, forming a distinct cluster in the upper right quadrant. The separation from XJ samples suggests significant differences in the volatile oil components.

HB samples are represented by red dots, and these samples form a separate cluster in the lower left quadrant. This indicates that HB samples also have a unique volatile oil profile. GER samples are represented by yellow dots, clustering tightly in the lower left region, suggesting that German chamomile samples have a distinct volatile profile that is closer to that of HB samples but still unique.

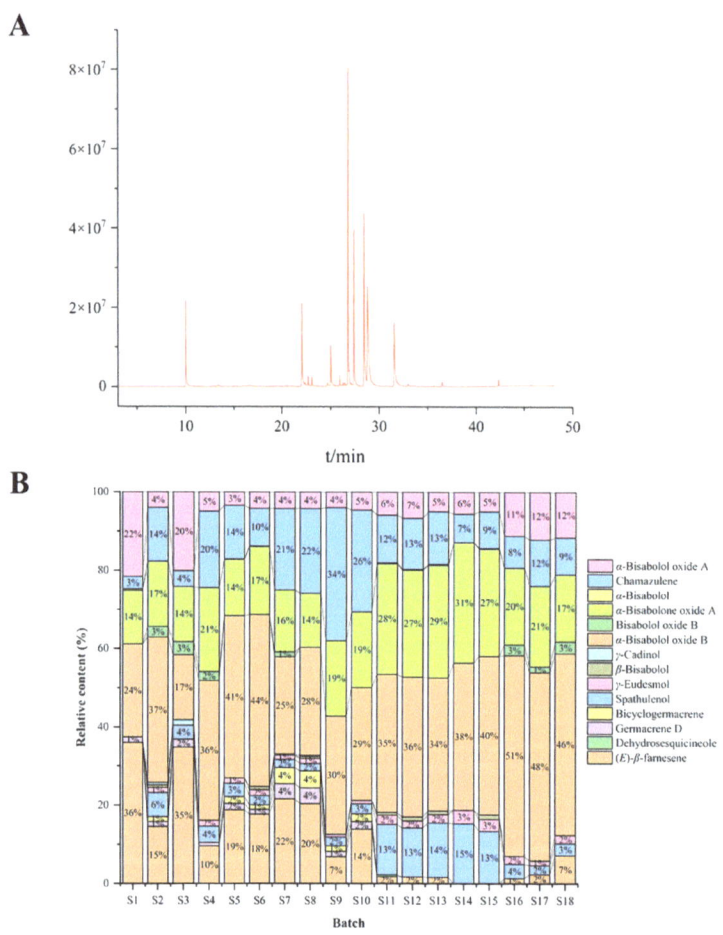

Figure 2. (**A**) Chromatogram example; (**B**) Histogram of volatile oil component distribution; S1–S18: Corresponding sample name from Table 1.

Table 1. Sample information.

No.	Sources	No.	Sources	No.	Sources
S1	XJ	S7	SD	S13	HB
S2	XJ	S8	SD	S14	HB
S3	XJ	S9	SD	S15	HB
S4	XJ	S10	SD	S16	GER
S5	XJ	S11	HB	S17	GER
S6	SD	S12	HB	S18	GER

No.: The number of each sample; Sources: Source information of the sample; XJ: Xinjiang Province, China; SD: Shandong Province, China; HB: Hebei Province, China; GER: Samples collected in Germany.

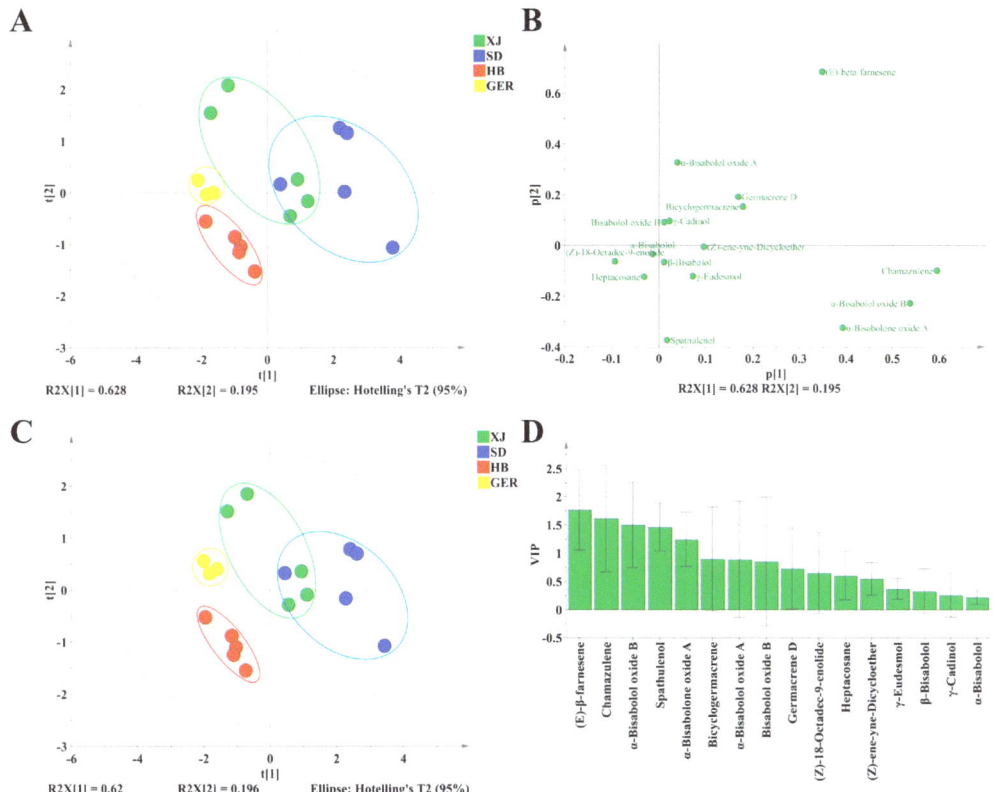

Figure 3. (**A**) Score plots of PCA Model; (**B**) Loading scatter plots of PCA Model; (**C**) Score plots of PLS–DA Model; (**D**) Variable importance factor (VIP) plots.

There is clear separation between the samples from different areas, indicating that the volatile oil profiles may be region-specific. Some overlap between XJ and SD samples suggests that, while they have distinct profiles, there might be some similarities in certain components. This differentiation can be attributed to various factors such as climate, soil, and cultivation practices. The clustering pattern highlights the potential for using PCA and volatile oil profiles to distinguish and authenticate chamomile samples from different geographical origins.

The scatter plot illustrates the loadings of volatile oil components from chamomile samples on the first two principal components (Figure 3). This analysis helps identify which specific volatile compounds are most influential in differentiating the chamomile samples. (E)-β-farnesene is positioned with high positive loadings on both p [1] and p [2], indicating it is a major contributor to the variance and differentiation of samples. Chamazulene and α-bisabol oxide B are positioned with high positive loadings on p [1], suggesting these compounds significantly influence the first principal component. α-bisabolol oxide A is positioned with high positive loadings on p [2], indicating its significant influence on the second principal component.

The loading scatter plots of the PCA effectively highlight the volatile compounds that may play vital roles in differentiating chamomile samples. The identified key compounds, such as (E)-β-farnesene, chamazulene, and α-bisabol oxide B, can be further investigated for their potential as markers for geographic origin.

3.3.2. PLS–DA (Partial Least Squares Discriminant Analysis)

PCA is an unsupervised analysis method that cannot ignore intra-group differences and random errors when determining differential components. This study employed a supervised PLS–DA analysis model to explore the differences in volatile oils of chamomile from different areas and to identify potential differential compounds, as shown in Figure 3.

The results demonstrate that the 18 batches of chamomile were categorized into four groups, with samples from the same area clustering together. The model exhibited good explanatory and predictive capabilities, with R2X = 0.914, R2Y = 0.802, and Q2 = 0.566. The PLS–DA results provided preliminary validation of the PCA model. The 200 permutation tests yielded R^2X = 0.192 and Q2Y = -0.548, both of which are below the thresholds of 0.3 and 0.05. This indicates that the model is reliable and not overfitted, as shown in Figure S1.

The VIP value is used to assess the relative importance of each variable in the PLS–DA model. A higher VIP value indicates a greater contribution of that variable to the model's explanation. Variables with VIP values greater than 1 are not only statistically significant but also practically important. They may represent key biomarkers, environmental factors, or other important explanatory variables [21]. The analysis of the variable importance in projection (VIP) scores revealed that five components had VIP values greater than 1: (E)-β-farnesene, chamazulene, α-bisabolol oxide B, spathulenol, and α-bisabolone oxide A. These compounds are the most characteristic oxygenated sesquiterpenes and bicyclic terpenes in chamomile volatile oils, typically extracted from natural chamomile sources [18,28]. Therefore, these five components are considered potential differentiating substances for the volatile oils from the three distinct areas of chamomile (Figure 3).

3.4. Identification of Chamomile Using the Rapid Gas Chromatography Electronic Nose Method

3.4.1. Rapid Gas Chromatography Electronic Nose Determination Results

The retention index (RI) of the compounds obtained by GC–MS primarily range between 1500 and 2200, failing to capture data for compounds with retention indices below 1500. The ultra-fast gas chromatography electronic nose acts as a rapid olfactory analyzer that can enrich volatile components at low temperatures (50 °C) and collect information for compounds with RIs less than 1500. This system simulates human olfaction to provide sensory information about volatile components. Two sets of electronic nose chromatogram data were obtained and imported into Origin software (Version 2024), resulting in the generation of a chamomile medicinal material odor fingerprint map, as seen in Figure 4. It is observable that the main peak levels of the SD samples are higher than those from the other sources, indicating a more intense odor and greater aromaticity, suggesting a relatively higher quality. The chromatogram results indicate that chamomile odor components were well separated in the MXT-5 chromatographic column, which displayed a rich variety of components. Consequently, the MXT-5 column was selected as the primary identification column, with the MXT-1701 column as a secondary identification column.

Peaks with an area greater than 1000 and good separation were chosen for further analysis [15]. Forty odor compounds were identified within 110 s by Alpha Soft electronic nose software (Version 17.0) and the AroChemBase database (17.0), and their sensory characteristics were acquired. Figure 4 presents relevant information on these odor components, including nine terpenes, five esters, five aldehydes, three ketones, two alcohols, two alkanes, and three carboxylic acids. The results indicate that the aroma of chamomile is categorized into several major groups, with the primary aromas being fruity and spicy. Fifteen components were identified with a fruity odor, including methyl crotonate, ethyl butyrate, (Z)-3-hexenal, butanoic acid, myrcene, octanal, γ-terpinene, 3-nonanone, p-cymenene, n-nonanal, cymen-8-ol, (Z)-3-hexenyl hexanoate, n-hexyl-hexanoate, β-caryophyllene, and methyl dodecanoate. Six components were identified with a spicy flavor, including ethanol, 1-propanol, pentanoic acid, 5-methylfurfural, α-phellandrene, and 2 pentadecanone, which aligns with the apple-like fragrance of chamomile [2,30].

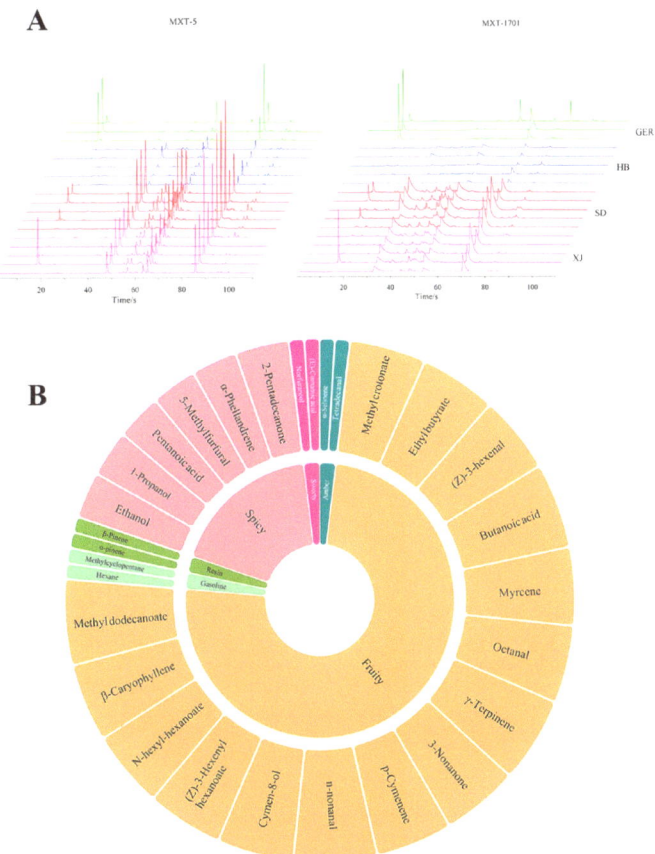

Figure 4. (**A**) Chamomile electronic nose fingerprint diagram; (**B**) Flavor wheel diagram of chamomile odor; inner circle: odor descriptors, outer circle: the identified compounds.

The aroma components identified in this experiment, including β-caryophyllene, α-pinene, β-pinene, and α-phellandrene, are consistent with those reported in the literature for chamomile [31], further enhancing the credibility of the electronic nose in characterizing odors. The relative abundance of compounds such as butanoic acid, ethyl ester, 3-nonanone, and geosmin was highest among the odor components and was classified as fruity and spicy odors, likely representing key factors influencing the aroma of chamomile. Since high temperatures can lead to the degradation of volatile components in chamomile, the electronic nose, to a certain extent, accurately reflects the information on volatile components of chamomile, providing a reference for the analysis of chamomile's odor components [32,33].

3.4.2. PCA

The ultra-fast gas chromatography electronic nose can detect distinctive aromas quickly, making it suitable for the rapid identification of the areas of medicinal materials. Based on the aroma information obtained from the ultra-fast gas chromatography electronic nose, the common odor peak areas of chamomile (with an integrated peak area greater than 1000) were used as variables for PCA analysis using SIMCA 14.1 software, as shown in Figure 5. The results show that the two principal components from the PCA score plot account for a cumulative contribution rate of 89.60% (PC1 63.60%, PC2 16.40%), with a model predictive Q2 value of 0.896 (>0.5), indicating that the model effectively reflects the odor information present in the samples.

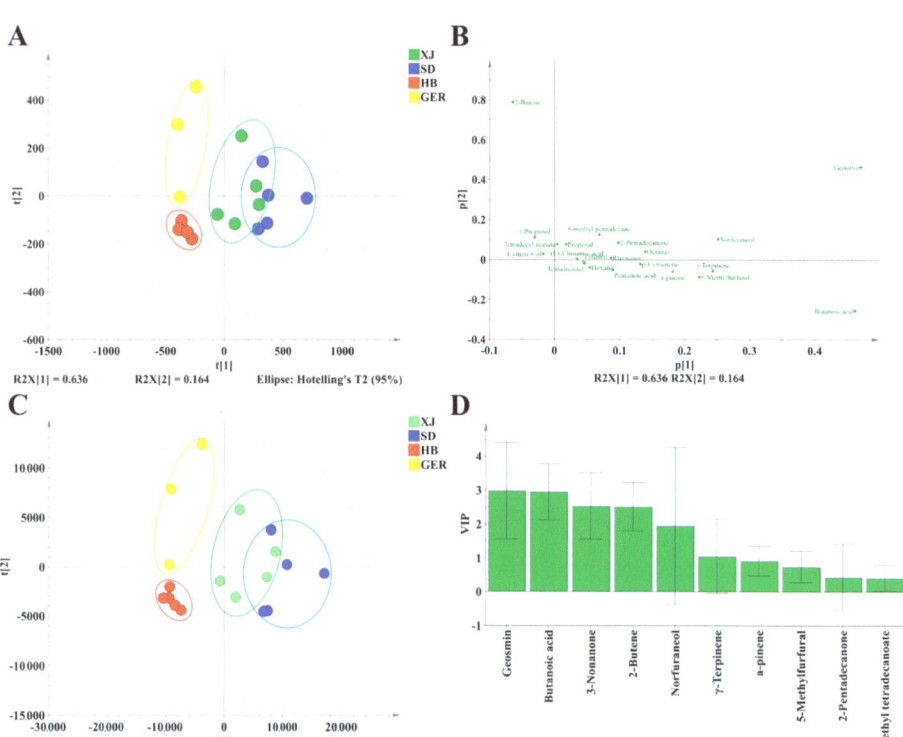

Figure 5. (**A**) Score plots of PCA model; (**B**) Loading scatter plots of PCA model; (**C**) Score plots of PLS–DA model; (**D**) Variable importance factor (VIP) plots.

There is clear separation between the samples from different areas, suggesting that the aroma components may be area-specific. PCA results show that XJ and SD samples can be distinguished; however, they are closer in distance compared to the HB and GER samples. This indicates that while geographical location and climate differences between XJ and SD contribute to their odor differences, they do not fully account for them. This suggests that other factors, such as germplasm or cultivation methods, may influence the aroma of chamomile. It also indicates that while they have distinct profiles, there might be some similarities in certain components. The inter-group variation among Shandong samples is larger, which may be related to coastal climate conditions. High temperatures and heavy rainfall could affect the harvesting and drying of chamomile, ultimately impacting quality.

The figure illustrates that samples from Hebei showed smaller inter-group differences, which may be related to geographical location, agricultural production methods, similar climatic conditions, and farming practices. These results indicate that the ultra-fast gas chromatography electronic nose can effectively analyze the aroma components of chamomile. The detected aroma characteristics have the potential to serve as discriminative indicators for identifying different chamomile samples.

3.4.3. Establishment of the DFA Discrimination Model

Discriminant factor analysis (DFA) is a model that extends differentiation among groups while compressing variations within the same group based on PCA [34]. This method facilitates a more intuitive discrimination of odor differences in chamomile from various sources and validates the PCA results.

In this study, DFA analysis of odor data from different chamomile samples was performed by Alpha Soft 17.0 software, which is a unique software package included with the electronic nose (Figure 6). The results show that the two-dimensional DFA score plot distinctly categorizes chamomile samples from different origins into four areas. The discriminant factors DF1 and DF2 contribute 46.791% and 40.935% respectively, with a cumulative contribution of 87.726%. This indicates that the DFA model effectively differentiates the geographical areas of chamomile and further verifies that the ultra-fast gas chromatography electronic nose can be used for rapid and accurate identification of chamomile from different sources [35]. The two-dimensional DFA plot clearly divides chamomile from different sources into four distinct areas, with the largest model distance between the samples from Germany and others, indicating significant odor differences between chamomile from China and Germany. The odor characteristics of chamomile are influenced by various factors such as geographical location, climatic conditions, and production methods.

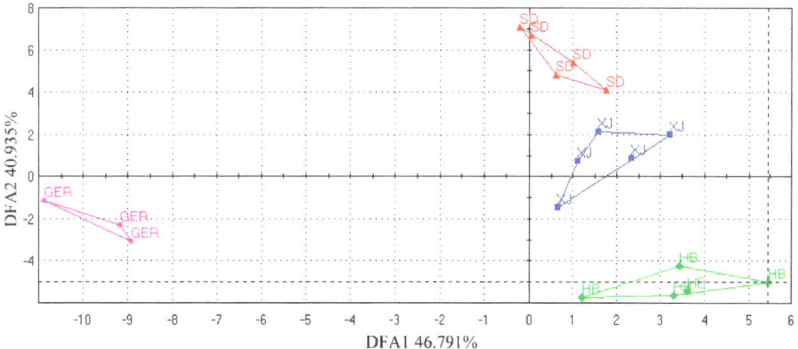

Figure 6. Discriminant function analysis.

3.4.4. Study on Odor Biomarkers of Chamomile from Different Areas

PCA cannot overlook intra-group differences and random errors when identifying differential components. A PLS–DA model was employed to further explore the odor differences of chamomile samples (Figure 5). The results divided 18 batches of chamomile into four categories, with samples from the same area clustering together. The model's R2X = 0.996, R2Y = 0.727, and Q2 = 0.509, indicate good explanatory and predictive capabilities. A 200 permutation test yielded R2X = 0.293 and Q2Y = −0.416, which are both below 0.3 and 0.05, respectively, demonstrating the model's reliability and the absence of overfitting (Figure S1).

The VIP scores were plotted (Figure 5) to identify the characteristic aroma components affecting classification. Components with VIP values greater than 1 were selected as key aroma indicators influencing different chamomile samples. The analysis identified six components with VIP values greater than 1: geosmin, butanoic acid, 3-noanone, 2-butene, norfuraneol, and γ-terpinene. These components serve as important variables in the model analysis and may represent the substances responsible for the aroma differences among chamomile samples. The aroma characteristics identified by the electronic nose suggest that these six components predominantly exhibit fruity and spicy odors.

PCA and PLS–DA score plots showed that the GER samples were considerably distant from the CN samples, indicating a completely diverse aroma profile. Therefore, an OPLS–DA model was used to further explain the flavor differentials between GER and CN samples, and the scatter plots and flavor variables (VIP > 1.0) are shown in Figure 7. Comparing GER to XJ samples, n-nonanal, 5-methyfurfural, butanoic acid, and ethyl butyrate had a greater effect in discrimination, exhibiting the main flavors of spicy and fruity. The main flavor differentials between GER and SD samples were 3-nonanone, α-phellandrene, 5-methyfurfural and p-cymenene, also exhibiting spicy and fruity flavors. GER samples showed differences from HB samples in flavor compounds such as 2-pentadecanone, octanal, γ-terpinene, and α-pinene. Overall, the primary odor components distinguishing GER from CN samples were characterized by spicy and fruity notes.

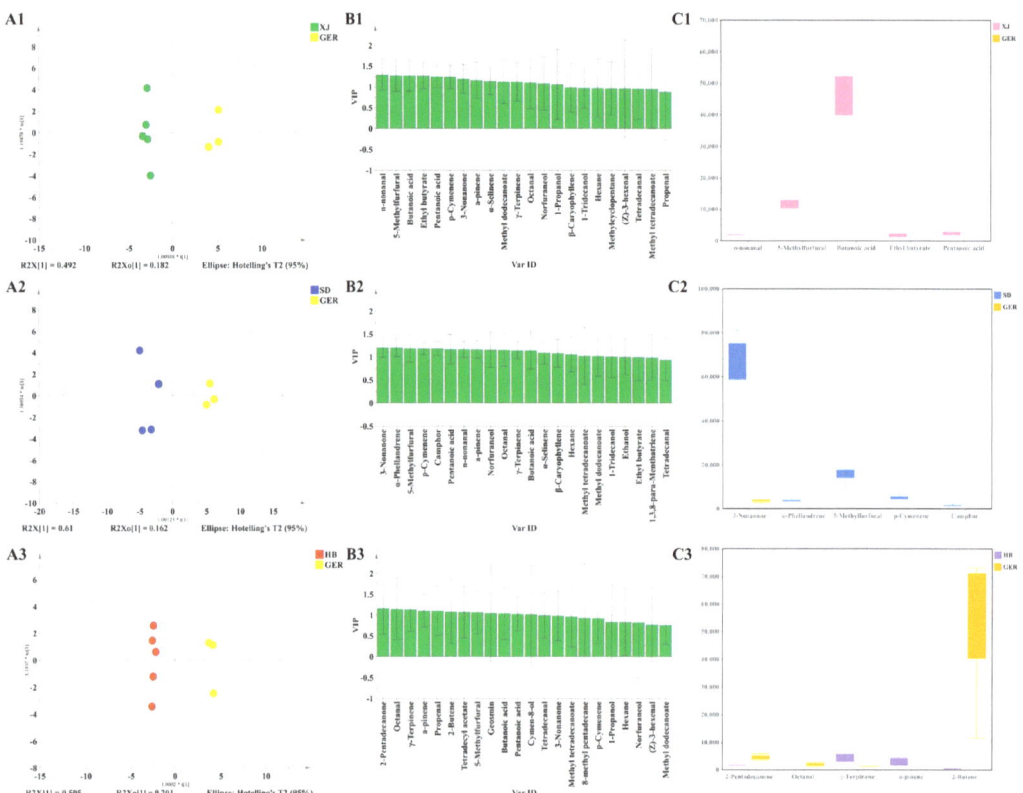

Figure 7. Score scatter plots (**A1–A3**); VIP plots (**B1–B3**); Comparison of the main difference compounds (**C1–C3**).

Generally, chamomile is known for its apple-like fragrance and is extensively used in various fragrances and flavorings. Although highly responsive irritant components can be characterized by the electronic nose system, the influence of other odors, such as minty or woody, should not be underestimated. Only by integrating all aspects of the odor profiles can the authenticity of the quality assessment for chamomile be ensured.

4. Discussion

Previous studies have focused on the volatile oil components of chamomile and their effects. The characteristic components of the oil are mainly chamazulene and oxygenated sesquiterpenes, including bisabolol oxide B, α-bisabolol, bisabolone oxide, and bisabolol oxide A [18]. Our research confirmed the existence of these components in different chamomile samples, suggesting that these compounds can serve as identification markers for chamomile. Additionally, differences in the volatile oil content of chamomile were discovered; the SD samples exhibited the highest concentrations of chamazulene and bisabolol, indicating superior quality [24]. PCA analysis based on GC–MS indicated that volatile oil components could be used to distinguish chamomile samples. Furthermore, PLS–DA analysis initially explored the key volatile oil components distinguishing the different groups of chamomile, identifying (E)-β-farnesene, chamazulene, α-bisabolol oxide B, spathulenol, and α-bisabolone oxide A.

The ultra-fast gas chromatography electronic nose technology can extract major aroma components from chamomile and provide corresponding sensory information within 110 s [36]. Sensory evaluation results indicate that the primary aromas of chamomile are concentrated on sweet and spicy odors, consistent with the general records of chamomile scent [2,30]. The electronic nose results indicate that the SD samples have the most intense odor, possess higher aromaticity, and are of better quality. This is the first attempt to distinguish different chamomile samples using the electronic nose, with the finding that the electronic nose results could preliminarily discriminate chamomile samples from four areas. Subsequently, DFA was used to perform group discrimination from different dimensions, validating the PCA results. Finally, PLS-DA was employed to identify potential differentiators between GER and CN samples: geosmin, butanoic acid, 3-nonanone, 2-butene, norfuraneol, and γ-terpinene. Additionally, we conducted OPLS–DA to analyze the differentiating compounds between GER and each specific CN sample. The combination of the two techniques not only provides the relative content of volatile oil components from chamomile originating in different areas but also analyzes the comprehensive aroma characteristics, offering a rapid, accurate, and feasible strategy for analyzing the volatile components of chamomile. This provides new insights for the quality evaluation of chamomile and technological support for the future development of chamomile tea and the traditional Chinese medicine industry.

Compared to traditional methods relying on human olfactory experience to judge the authenticity and quality of aromatic products, the ultra-fast gas chromatography electronic nose offers unique advantages of speed, non-destructiveness, objective evaluation results, and effective avoidance of human-related errors. This technology enables the swift identification of odor profiles and precise differentiation based on the region and authenticity of samples [37]. Although electronic nose technology is widely used in odor recognition and related fields, its application in aromatic product research may encounter challenges in specificity and exclusivity of identification results. This is primarily because electronic nose technology often targets specific natural substances, such as hydrocarbons and alcohols, when developing odor component databases.

The multivariate analysis results showed some distinction between different groups. However, the representativeness of these results is limited by the small number of chamomile samples analyzed in this study. Future research will increase the sample size to better capture the differences between various types of chamomile.

5. Conclusions

This study is the first to explore the application of GC–MS and ultra-fast gas chromatography electronic nose technology for distinguishing the components of chamomile samples. A comprehensive comparison of the volatile components of chamomile at different boiling points was conducted, and a rapid analysis technique based on the ultra-fast gas chromatography electronic nose was developed specifically for chamomile. Using GC–MS and the ultra-fast gas chromatography electronic nose, 16 volatile oil components and forty aroma components were identified. This study provided a comprehensive analysis of the volatile oils and aromatic components of chamomile, examining both the identified volatile oil components and those volatiles present at low temperatures. The analysis of high-temperature (GC–MS) and low-temperature (e-nose) products revealed that this chamomile contains characteristic components, such as bisabolol derivatives and chamazulene. The aroma profile of chamomile was attributed to fruity and spicy notes, aligning with the "apple-like" meaning of its name. This analysis offers viable strategies for quality assessment and differentiation of chamomile from various sources, potentially reducing adulteration in high-value agricultural and herbal products and enhancing consumer satisfaction. The findings are constrained by the limited sample size. Future research should include a larger number of samples to enhance these findings.

Supplementary Materials: The following are available online at https://www.mdpi.com/article/10.3390/foods13121865/s1, Table S1: The formula, and sensory description of flavor components in chamomile by fast GC e-nose. Table S2: Volatile oil composition of chamomile. Table S3: Electronic nose raw data. Figure S1: Results of Permutation. Figure S2: Results of Single-Factor Investigations.

Author Contributions: Conceptualization, J.L.; methodology, J.L. and Z.J.; software, D.Y.; validation, D.Y. and J.D.; formal analysis, D.L. and J.D.; investigation, J.L.; resources, Q.W.; and C.Q.; data curation, J.L.; writing—original draft preparation, J.L.; writing—review and editing, J.L. and C.Q.; supervision, C.Q. and Q.W.; project administration, Q.W.; funding acquisition, Q.W. and C.Q. All authors have read and agreed to the published version of the manuscript.

Funding: This research was funded by the Research of Assurance Ability Improvement of Chinese Medicinal Resources (2023).

Institutional Review Board Statement: Not applicable.

Informed Consent Statement: Not applicable.

Data Availability Statement: The original contributions presented in the study are included in the article/supplementary material, further inquiries can be directed to the corresponding authors.

Acknowledgments: This study would like to acknowledge the help with sample collection by Tang Hai-tao from Jiangsu Suzhong Pharmaceutical Group Medicine Co., Ltd.

Conflicts of Interest: The authors declare no conflicts of interest.

References

1. El, M.; Borjac, M. Matricaria chamomilla: A valuable insight into recent advances in medicinal uses and pharmacological activities. *Phytochem. Rev.* **2022**, *21*, 1913–1940.
2. Sah, A.; Naseef, P. A Comprehensive Study of Therapeutic Applications of Chamomile. *Pharmaceuticals* **2022**, *15*, 1284. [CrossRef] [PubMed]
3. Srivastava, K.; Shankar, E. Chamomile: A herbal medicine of the past with bright future. *Mol. Med. Rep.* **2010**, *3*, 895–901. [PubMed]
4. Rafieiolhossaini, M.; Adams, A. Fast quality assessment of German chamomile (*Matricaria chamomilla* L.) by headspace solid-phase microextraction: Influence of flower development stage. *Nat. Prod. Commun.* **2012**, *7*, 97–100. [CrossRef]
5. Dai, L.; Li, Y. Chamomile: A Review of Its Traditional Uses, Chemical Constituents, Pharmacological Activities and Quality Control Studies. *Molecules* **2022**, *28*, 133. [CrossRef] [PubMed]
6. Shakya, P.; Thakur, R. GGE biplot and regression based multi-environment investigations for higher yield and essential oil content in German chamomile (*Matricaria chamomilla* L.). *Ind. Crops Prod.* **2023**, *193*, 116145. [CrossRef]
7. Fernandes, J.; Reboredo, H. Elemental Composition of Commercial Herbal Tea Plants and Respective Infusions. *Plants* **2022**, *11*, 1412. [CrossRef] [PubMed]
8. Raal, A.; Orav, A. Content of essential oil, terpenoids and polyphenols in commercial chamomile (*Chamomilla recutita* L. Rauschert) teas from different countries. *Food Chem.* **2012**, *131*, 632–638. [CrossRef]
9. De, P.; Ercolano, G. Chamomile essential oils exert anti-inflammatory effects involving human and murine macrophages: Evidence to support a therapeutic action. *J. Ethnopharmacol.* **2023**, *311*, 116391.
10. Can, D.; Demir, U. Psychopharmacological profile of Chamomile (*Matricaria recutita* L.) essential oil in mice. *Phytomedicine* **2012**, *19*, 306–310. [CrossRef]
11. Liu, J.; Yuan, Q. Phyllotaxis development: A lesson from the Asteraceae family. *Trends Plant Sci.* **2021**, *26*, 873–875. [CrossRef] [PubMed]
12. An, H.; Ou, X. Study on the key volatile compounds and aroma quality of jasmine tea with different scenting technology. *Food Chem.* **2022**, *385*, 132718. [CrossRef] [PubMed]
13. Baranauskiene, R.; Venskutonis, R. Valorisation of Roman chamomile (*Chamaemelum nobile* L.) herb by comprehensive evaluation of hydrodistilled aroma and residual non-volatile fractions. *Food Res. Int.* **2022**, *160*, 111715. [CrossRef] [PubMed]
14. Melucci, D.; Bendini, A. Rapid direct analysis to discriminate geographic origin of extra virgin olive oils by flash gas chromatography electronic nose and chemometrics. *Food Chem.* **2016**, *204*, 263–273. [CrossRef] [PubMed]
15. Yu, D.X.; Zhang, X.; Guo, S.; Yan, H.; Wang, J.M.; Zhou, J.Q.; Yang, J.; Duan, J.A. Headspace GC/MS and fast GC e-nose combined with chemometric analysis to identify the varieties and geographical origins of ginger (*Zingiber officinale* Roscoe). *Food Chem.* **2022**, *396*, 133672. [CrossRef] [PubMed]
16. Orav, A.; Raal, A. Content and composition of the essential oil of *Chamomilla recutita* (L.) Rauschert from some European countries. *Nat. Prod. Res.* **2010**, *24*, 48–55. [CrossRef] [PubMed]
17. Mahanta, P.; Bora, K. Thermolabile essential oils, aromas and flavours: Degradation pathways, effect of thermal processing and alteration of sensory quality. *Food Res. Int.* **2021**, *145*, 110404. [CrossRef]

18. Formisano, C.; Delfine, S. Correlation among environmental factors, chemical composition and antioxidative properties of essential oil and extracts of chamomile (*Matricaria chamomilla* L.) collected in Molise (South-central Italy). *Ind. Crops Prod.* **2015**, *63*, 256–263. [CrossRef]
19. Satyal, P.; Shrestha, S.; Setzer, W.N. Composition and Bioactivities of an (*E*)-beta-Farnesene Chemotype of Chamomile (*Matricaria chamomilla*) Essential Oil from Nepal. *Nat. Prod. Commun.* **2015**, *10*, 1453–1457.
20. Piri, E.; Mahmoodi Sourestani, M.; Khaleghi, E.; Mottaghipisheh, J.; Zomborszki, Z.P.; Hohmann, J.; Csupor, D. Chemo-Diversity and Antiradical Potential of Twelve *Matricaria chamomilla* L. Populations from Iran: Proof of Ecological Effects. *Molecules* **2019**, *24*, 1315. [CrossRef]
21. Dai, Y.; Yu, R. Flavorand taste change rules of Sophora Flavescentis Radix processed using ancient classical method:an exploration based on intelligent sensory analysis. *Zhongguo Zhong Yao Za Zhi* **2021**, *46*, 6410–6416. [PubMed]
22. Biancolillo, A.; Aloia, R. Organosulfur volatile profiles in Italian red garlic (*Allium sativum* L.) varieties investigated by HS-SPME/GC-MS and chemometrics. *Food Control* **2022**, *131*, 108477. [CrossRef]
23. Li, M.X.; Qin, Y.W.; Li, Y.; Zhang, J.B.; De, J.; Qu, L.Y.; Gong, J.W.; Jia, A.M.; Mao, C.Q.; Lu, T.L. Rapid identification and differential markers of Curcumae Radix decoction pieces of different sources based on Heracles Neo ultra-fast gas phase electronic nose. *China J. Chin. Mater. Medica* **2023**, *48*, 1518–1525.
24. Alhasan, S.; Khadim, A. Effect of Applying Different Levels of Nitrogen Fertilizer on Growth and Essential Oil of Chamomile (*Matricaria chamomilla* L.). *IOP Conf. Ser. Earth Environ. Sci.* **2022**, *1060*, 012102. [CrossRef]
25. Zengin, G.; Mollica, A. A Comparative Study of Chamomile Essential Oils and Lipophilic Extracts Obtained by Conventional and Greener Extraction Techniques: Chemometric Approach to Chemical Composition and Biological Activity. *Separations* **2023**, *10*, 18. [CrossRef]
26. Zhou, Y.; He, L.; Wang, W.; Wei, G.; Ma, L.; Liu, H.; Yao, L. Artemisia sieversiana Ehrhart ex Willd. Essential Oil and Its Main Component, Chamazulene: Their Photoprotective Effect against UVB-Induced Cellular Damage and Potential as Novel Natural Sunscreen Additives. *ACS Sustain. Chem. Eng.* **2023**, *11*, 17675–17686. [CrossRef]
27. Shaaban, M.; El-Hagrassi, A.M.; Osman, A.F.; Soltan, M.M. Bioactive compounds from Matricaria chamomilla: Structure identification, in vitro antiproliferative, antimigratory, antiangiogenic, and antiadenoviral activities. *Z. Naturforschung C J. Biosci.* **2022**, *77*, 85–94. [CrossRef] [PubMed]
28. Singh, O.; Khanam, Z. Chamomile (*Matricaria chamomilla* L.): An overview. *Pharmacogn. Rev.* **2011**, *5*, 82–95. [CrossRef] [PubMed]
29. Mckay, J.; Blumberg, B. A review of the bioactivity and potential health benefits of chamomile tea (*Matricaria recutita* L.). *Phytother. Res.* **2006**, *20*, 519–530. [CrossRef]
30. Chauhan, R.; Singh, S. A Comprehensive Review on Biology, Genetic Improvement, Agro and Process Technology of German Chamomile (*Matricaria chamomilla* L.). *Plants* **2021**, *11*, 29. [CrossRef]
31. Zhao, Y. Study on the Chemical Composition and Quality Standards of Uighur Medicine Chamomile. Ph.D. Thesis, China Academy of Chinese Medical Sciences, Beijing, China, 2018; p. 72.
32. Flemming, M.; Kraus, B. Revisited anti-inflammatory activity of matricine in vitro: Comparison with chamazulene. *Fitoterapia* **2015**, *106*, 122–128. [CrossRef] [PubMed]
33. Ramadan, M.; Goeters, S. Chamazulene carboxylic acid and matricin: A natural profen and its natural prodrug, identified through similarity to synthetic drug substances. *J. Nat. Prod.* **2006**, *69*, 1041–1045. [CrossRef] [PubMed]
34. Qiu, H.; Qu, K. Analysis of thermal oxidation of different multi-element oleogels based on carnauba wax, sitosterol/lecithin, and ethyl cellulose by classical oxidation determination method combined with the electronic nose. *Food Chem.* **2023**, *405*, 134970. [CrossRef] [PubMed]
35. Flambeau, J.; Lee, W. Discrimination and geographical origin prediction of washed specialty Bourbon coffee from different coffee growing areas in Rwanda by using electronic nose and electronic tongue. *Food Sci. Biotechnol.* **2017**, *26*, 1245–1254. [CrossRef] [PubMed]
36. Zhang, K.; Wang, J.; Fan, X.; Zhu, G.; Lu, T.; Xue, R. Discrimination between raw and ginger juice processed Magnoliae officinalis cortex based on HPLC and Heracles NEO ultra-fast gas phase electronic nose. *Phytochem. Anal.* **2022**, *33*, 722–734. [CrossRef]
37. Zhang, M.; Wang, X. Species discrimination among three kinds of puffer fish using an electronic nose combined with olfactory sensory evaluation. *Sensors* **2012**, *12*, 12562–12571. [CrossRef]

Disclaimer/Publisher's Note: The statements, opinions and data contained in all publications are solely those of the individual author(s) and contributor(s) and not of MDPI and/or the editor(s). MDPI and/or the editor(s) disclaim responsibility for any injury to people or property resulting from any ideas, methods, instructions or products referred to in the content.

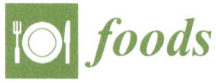

Article

Functional Tea Extract Inhibits Cell Growth, Induces Apoptosis, and Causes G0/G1 Arrest in Human Hepatocellular Carcinoma Cell Line Possibly through Reduction in Telomerase Activity

Yuan Chen [1,2,3], Changsong Chen [1,2,*], Jiaxing Xiang [1,4,†], Ruizhen Gao [1,4,†], Guojun Wang [5] and Wenquan Yu [1,2,*]

1. Tea Research Institute, Fujian Academy of Agricultural Sciences, Fuzhou 350003, China; chenyuan@faas.cn (Y.C.); 19949533447@163.com (J.X.); 18639424217@163.com (R.G.)
2. Fujian Academy of Agricultural Sciences, Fuzhou 350003, China
3. Agricultural Product Processing Research Institute, Fujian Academy of Agricultural Sciences, Fuzhou 350003, China
4. Horticulture College, Fujian Agriculture and Forestry University, Fuzhou 350003, China
5. Harbor Branch Oceanographic Institute, Florida Atlantic University, 5600 U.S. 1, Fort Pierce, FL 34946, USA; guojunwang@fau.edu
* Correspondence: ccs6536597@163.com (C.C.); wenquan_yu@yeah.net (W.Y.)
† These authors contributed equally to this work.

Abstract: The functional tea CFT-1 has been introduced into China as a nutraceutical beverage according to the "Healthy China" national project. The effects on human hepatocellular carcinoma (HCC) cells remain unclear and were investigated with the functional tea extract (purity > 98%). The morphological changes in the cells were observed with microscopes. Cell proliferation, migration, cycle distribution, and apoptotic effects were assessed by MTT, Transwell assays, and flow cytometry, respectively, while telomerase inhibition was evaluated with telomerase PCR ELISA assay kits. The CFT-1 treatment resulted in cell shrinkage, nuclear pyknosis, and chromatin condensation. CFT-1 suppressed the growth of Hep3B cells with IC50 of 143 μg/mL by inducing apoptosis and G0/G1 arrest in Hep3B cells. As for the molecular mechanism, CFT-1 treatment can effectively reduce the telomerase activity. The functional tea extract inhibits cell growth in human HCC by inducing apoptosis and G0/G1 arrest, possibly through a reduction in telomerase activity. These results indicate that CFT-1 extract exhibited in vitro anticancer activities and provided insights into the future development and utilization of CFT-1 as functional foods to inhibit the proliferation of HCC cells.

Keywords: hepatocellular carcinoma; Hep3B; growth inhibition; apoptosis; cell cycle arrest; telomerase

1. Introduction

Liver cancer is a frequently occurring malignancy with a poor prognosis and a high mortality rate, and is the second leading cause of cancer-related deaths [1]. Hepatocellular carcinoma (HCC), as an aggressive tumor, accounts for 90% of primary liver cancers and constitutes the third leading cause of cancer mortality worldwide [2–4]. The main therapeutic methods, including surgery, radiotherapy, and chemotherapy, often have limited effects on the tumors, but huge side effects on the human body. HCC is notoriously characterized by a poor prognosis and high mortality rate owing to the high rates of metastasis and recurrence [5–7]. There are a variety of risk factors, such as infection with viral hepatitis, hepatic cirrhosis, obesity, and consumption of dietary hepatocarcinogens [8,9]. According to epidemiologic studies, it has been shown that regular tea consumption is associated with a decreased risk of various carcinomas, including breast cancer [10], bladder or kidney cancer [11,12], liver cancer [13,14], lung cancer [15], upper aerodigestive tract cancer [16], and others. Therefore, cancer prevention is of great significance. One potential way to fight cancers is to develop a functional food that has a highly inhibitive effect on cancer cells but low toxicity on healthy cells.

As the most abundant and active ingredient in tea, (−)-epigallocatechin-3-gallate (EGCG) has raised considerable interest in the development of anti-cancer drugs [17–19]. Mechanism studies suggested that in a variety of cancer cells, EGCG inhibits telomerase activity by down-regulating the protein expression, which eventually leads to the suppression of cell viability and induction of apoptosis [20]. Telomerase, a ribonucleoprotein acting to elongate telomeres, has been directly implicated in tumorigenesis and shown to be expressed in approximately 90% of all cancers [21]. Accumulating literature has demonstrated the ability of EGCG to inhibit the growth and proliferation of hepatocellular tumors through the induction of apoptosis and modulation of autophagic and anti-angiogenetic activities [22]. Recently, a new tea plant strain, Camellia sinensis CV, was developed.CFT-1 extract (CFT-1) was introduced into China as a nutraceutical beverage according to the "Healthy China" national project, which aims at exploring the resources of crops that are rich in nutrients and functional ingredients. CFT-1 is rich in EGCG, which is almost twice as abundant as in the nationwide popular tea Fuyun No. 6 [23]. Furthermore, CFT-1 has larger amounts of antioxidants, which are believed to have benefits in terms of preventing cancer. However, to the best of our knowledge, there is no study exploring the health benefits or pharmacological activity of CFT-1, especially in the prevention and treatment of human HCC.

The aim of this study was to conduct a preliminary study on the antitumor activity and mechanism of CFT-1 extracts to support the development and synthesis of new, efficient, and low-toxicity anti-tumor lead compounds. We hypothesized that possible molecular mechanisms would be related to the effect of CFT-1 on telomerase activity.

2. Materials and Methods

2.1. Reagents

The experimental samples were extracted from the functional tea CFT-1 with purity >98%. Human Hep3B hepatoma cells were provided by the Fujian Medical University biochemistry and molecular biology laboratory. MTT (3-[4,5-dimethylthiazol-2-yl]-2,5-diphenyltetrazolium bromide) and all other chemicals employed in this study were of analytical grade and purchased from Sigma-Aldrich Co. Fetal bovine serum, Dulbecco's Modified Eagle's medium (DMEM), and penicillin–streptomycin were obtained from Thermo Fisher Scientific, Inc. Telomerase PCR ELISA kit was purchased from Boehringer Mannheim.

Gallic acid (GA), (−)-gallocatechin (GC), caffeine (CAF), theophylline (THEO), (−)-epigallocatechin (EGC), (+)-catechin (C), chlorogenic acid (CHL), theobromine (TB), caffeic acid (CAA), (−)-epicatechin (EC), (−)-epigallocatechin gallate (EGCG), p-coumaric acid (COU), (−)-gallocatechin gallate (GCG), ferulic acid (FER), sinapic acid (SIN), epicatechin gallate (ECG), rutin (RUT), myricetin (MYR), quercetin (QUE), and kaempferol (KAE) were purchased from Sigma (St. Louis, MO, USA), and the purity of the reagents was above 95%. The acetonitrile (HPLC grade) was purchased from Merck KgaA (Darmstadt, Germany), and all other reagents, including methanol and formic acid, were purchased from Sinopharm Chemical Reagent Co., Ltd. (Shanghai, China). Ultrapure water was obtained from a Milli-Q water system (Millipore, Bedford, MA, USA).

2.2. Preparation of CFT-1 Extract

Tea samples underwent initial drying at 35 °C for 2 h, followed by crushing into powders and passage through a 40-mesh screen (304 stainless steel sieve, Yongkang Jielong Industrial and Trade Co., Ltd., Jinhua, China). The selection of this specific mesh screen aimed to optimize the extraction procedure, achieving elevated dissolution rates while minimizing material loss. An aliquot of 3 g of sample powder was weighed into an Erlenmeyer flask, and 150 mL of water was added. The mixture was shaken for 15 min at room temperature and centrifuged at 8000 rpm for 15 min at 4 °C. This extraction process was repeated once. The supernatants from the two extracts were combined, diluted to 50 mL with water, and analyzed.

2.3. HPLC-DAD Analysis

In this study, a HPLC-DAD system was employed for the analysis. The instrument used for this analysis was the Ultimate 3000 HPLC (Thermo Fisher Scientific, Milan, Italy). Prior to HPLC analysis, the extract was filtered through a 0.22 μm microporous membrane, and 1 μL of the filtered extract was injected into the HPLC system. Chromatographic separation was performed using a reverse-phase column (Merck Lichrospher RP-18, 250 mm × 4.6 mm, Darmstadt, Germany). Mobile phases A and B were 0.1% formic acid and acetonitrile, respectively. The gradient elution procedure was: 0 min, 94% A; 11 min, 93% A; 12 min, 92% A; 18 min, 90% A; 48 min, 82% A; 56.8 min, 82% A; 58 min, 69% A; 68 min, 52% A; 70 min, 6% A. The analysis duration for each specimen was 20 min, inclusive of a 4 min column equilibration period. The column temperature and flow rate were maintained at 30 °C and 0.8 mL·min^{-1}, respectively. For detection, two wavelengths, 280 and 340 nm, were compared in this study using the DAD integrated into the HPLC system. The developed HPLC method was validated according to ICH guidelines to ensure fulfillment of current regulatory standards.

2.4. Cell Culture and Treatment

Human HCC Hep3B cells were purchased from Shanghai Cell Bank, Chinese Academy of Sciences (Shanghai, China). Hep3B cells were cultured with DMEM supplemented with 10% heat-inactivated FBS and 1% penicillin–streptomycin solution in 5% CO_2 at 37 °C. Human HCC cell line Hep3B was selected as our study model. To evaluate the effect of CFT-1 exact in HCC cell line Hep3B, the extract of functional tea CFT-1 (brown powder) was weighted and dissolved in a variety of volumes of Milli Q water to produce the desired drug concentrations (containing approximately 143 mg/g of EGCG). These samples were then ultrafiltered for the following use. For the CFT-1 treatment, the solution of CFT-1 extract was added to the Hep3B cells and incubated for 48 h followed by examinations. Cell morphology was examined and photographed using a Nikon TS2 inverted microscope at a magnification of ×100.

2.5. Cell Viability Assay

Hep3B cell viability was measured with an MTT assay according to previous publications. Briefly, Hep3B cells were seeded in 96-well culture plates at a density of 1×10^4 cells per well. After incubation for 24 h, cells were treated with different concentrations of CFT-1 extract for 48 h. Then, 20 μL MTT solution (5 mg/mL) was added to each well, and the cells were incubated at 37 °C for an additional 4 h. After removing the supernatants, 200 μL dimethyl sulfoxide (DMSO) was added to each well. The optical density (OD) was measured at 450 nm using a microplate reader. Cell viability was calculated using the following formula:

$$\text{Cell viability (\%)} = (OD_{\text{experimental group}} - OD_{\text{blank control}}) / (OD_{\text{control group}} - OD_{\text{blank control}}) \times 100\%$$

2.6. Colony Formation Assay

A colony formation assay was carried out according to a previous publication with minor modifications [24]. Specifically, 200 cells/10 mL of Hep3B were plated onto a 10 cm dish and incubated for 24 h prior to drug treatment. Then, the cells were exposed to CFT-1 extract followed by incubation for an additional 20 days. The colony formation ability was observed after fixing with 4% paraformaldehyde and staining with 0.1% crystal violet.

2.7. Transwell Migration Assay

The effect of CFT-1 extract on Hep3B cells was evaluated using a modified Boyden chamber model as previously reported [25]. The Transwell insert was placed back onto the 24-well plate, and the lower chamber was filled with 0.6 mL of DMEM containing 20% FBS with or without 143 µg/mL (IC50) of CFT-1. Human Hep3B cells (5×10^4 cells/well) in 200 µL medium were plated to the upper chamber. After 5 h of incubation at 37 °C, all non-migrated cells were removed from the upper face of the Transwell membrane, and migrated cells were fixed with methanol, stained with 0.1% crystal violet, and counted under an Olympus light microscope at a magnification of ×100. The formula was calculated as: relative cell counts per field = number of migrated cells in sample/number of migrated cells in control × 100%.

2.8. Cell Cycle Analysis

The effect of CFT-1 extract on the cell cycle distribution was measured with PI staining according to a previous publication. Hep3B cells were treated with 143 µg/mL CFT-1 or vehicle control in 6-well culture plates for 48 h. Approximately 1×10^6 cells were collected, washed with PBS, and fixed with 70% ethanol at −20 °C overnight. After centrifugation, cells were then resuspended in 1 mL staining solution (50 µg/mL PI, 20 µg/mL RNAase). After incubation for 30 min at room temperature in the dark, samples were analyzed with a flow cytometer. The percentage of cells in various phases of the cell cycle was determined using FlowJo software.

2.9. Apoptosis Analysis

Cell apoptosis was determined using an annexin V-FITC kit according to the manual. Briefly, Hep3B cells were treated with or without 143 µg/mL CFT-1 extract for 48 h prior to analysis. Cells were then collected and washed twice with cold PBS. Then, they were stained with Annexin V and PI in binding buffer at room temperature for 15 min. Cells were then analyzed using flow cytometry.

2.10. Telomerase Activity Assay

Telomerase activity in Hep3B cells was measured using a telomerase PCR ELISA assay kit according to the manual. Briefly, after treatment with CFT-1 extract or vehicle control for 48 h, the cells were collected, lysed, and homogenized in 200 µL of lysis buffer. After 30 min of incubation on ice, the lysates were centrifuged and the supernatants were collected. Protein concentration was measured using a BCA reagent. Then, 5 µg of cell extract was used in the following PCR amplification step, and aliquots (5 µL) of PCR product were analyzed using ELISA assay.

2.11. Statistical Analysis

All experiments were performed in triplicate, and the results are expressed as the mean ± SD. Data were analyzed using SPSS software. Comparisons between groups were performed using t-test. Differences were considered statistically significant at p-values < 0.05.

3. Results

3.1. Characterization of CFT-1 Tea Extract

Figure S1 shows the quantitative results of the identification of the compounds contained in CFT-1 extracts using HPLC. The concentrations of various compounds in the extract were measured and reported as follows (Table 1).

Table 1. The concentrations of various compounds in CFT-1 tea extract.

Compound	Concentration (mg/g)
GA	0.39 ± 0.04
GC	1.78 ± 0.18
CAF	43.89 ± 4.4
EGC	79.73 ± 10.03
C	4.00 ± 0.29
CHL	0.14 ± 0.00
TB	0.65 ± 0.05
EC	3.25 ± 0.29
EGCG	143.83 ± 11.63
COU	0.20 ± 0.02
GCG	2.86 ± 0.22
FER	15.05 ± 1.2
SIN	0.10 ± 0.01
ECG	41.84 ± 3.20
RUT	2.07 ± 0.08
MYR	0.49 ± 0.03
QUE	0.02 ± 0.00
KAE	0.03 ± 0.00

3.2. CFT-1 Treatment Induced Morphologic Alterations in Hep3B Cells

Morphology and structure are the material basis of function, and malignant tumor cells have typical cytological characteristics: a large nucleocytoplasmic ratio and multiple large nucleoli with nucleolar edge aggregation phenomenon, all of which are signs of rapid growth of tumor cells. The cell surface has dense and slender microvilli, which facilitate the exchange of substances between the tumor and the outside world for malignant proliferation, as well as facilitating metastasis and attachment to other tissues. Morphological differentiation and maturation are markers of malignant tumor cell differentiation.

We firstly investigated the effect of CFT-1 extract on Hep3B cells by examining the morphological changes in cells which were exposed to different concentrations of CFT-1. As shown in Figure 1, in comparison with the untreated cells (control group), Hep3B cells treated with CFT-1 extract (100 μg/mL) clearly showed enhanced amounts of shrinkage of the cell body, compaction of the nucleus, and condensation of chromatin, which together are regarded as typical apoptotic features [26]. On this basis, we were interested in investigating the anti-cancer activity of CFT-1 on Hep3B cells.

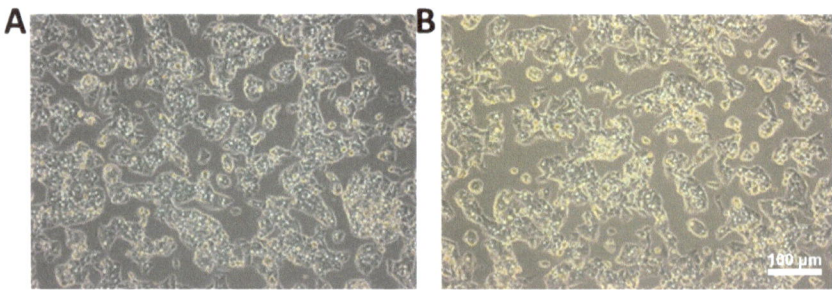

Figure 1. Morphology of cells treated with CFT-1 extract. (A) Hep3B cells treated with vehicle control. (B) Hep3B cells treated with CFT-1 extract (100 μg/mL). Scale bar = 100 μm.

3.3. CFT-1 Treatment Suppressed the Cell Growth, Colony Formation, and Migration of Hep3B Cells

Suppression of cell growth, colony formation, and migration in Hep3B cells is a common goal in cancer research, aiming to develop strategies to inhibit the aggressive behavior of HCC, which is often associated with high proliferation and metastatic potential.

Research on the effects of natural compounds on Hep3B cells often focuses on identifying substances with anti-cancer properties that can suppress cell growth, colony formation, and migration. EGCG has been investigated for its potential anticancer properties, including its ability to suppress cell growth and induce apoptosis in Hep3B cells.

Liver cancer cells grow actively, and the magnitude of absorbance values in MTT experiments can reflect the number of live cells. Therefore, the MTT colorimetric method can be used to quantitatively determine the effect of anticancer drugs on human cancer cells based on their quantity and metabolic activity [27]. We incubated Hep3B cells with CFT-1 at different concentrations (10, 30, 50, 70, 90, 100 µg/mL) for 48 h, and then examined the cell viability with MTT assay. It was seen that CFT-1 treatment obviously reduced the cell viability in a dose-dependent manner (Table 2). The half-maximal inhibitory concentration (IC50) of CFT-1 against Hep3B cells was about 143 µg/mL after 48 h incubation. It was noted that this potency is comparable to the reported activity of chemical EGCG on HCC cell lines (e.g., HepG2: IC50 = 74.7 µg/mL, SMMC7721: IC50 = 59.6 µg/mL; SK-hep1: IC50 = 61.3 µg/mL). As referenced above, EGCG is the major component of green tea, with great promise as a cancer preventive. Our results suggest that CFT-1 has great anti-cancer potential.

Table 2. Inhibition of cell growth of Hep3B by CFT-1 extract.

Concentration of CFT-1 (µg/mL)	Growth Inhibition (%)
10	2.9 ± 0.3
30	14.6 ± 1.2
50	20.7 ± 1.1
70	28.7 ± 1.6
90	35.4 ± 2.1
100	40.3 ± 2.8
143	50.1 ± 3.1

We also assessed the effect of CFT-1 on the colony formation of Hep3B cells. As shown in Figure 2, it can be seen the CFT-1 treatment (143 µg/mL, 48 h) dramatically limited the colony formation by reducing both the number and size of the colonies. In other words, CFT-1 treatment resulted in much fewer and smaller colonies compared to the untreated Hep3B cells (Figure 2A,B). Quantitative analysis indicated that the colony formation of Hep3B cells was reduced to 32.01% by CFT-1 (Figure 2C). Furthermore, CFT-1-treated cells appeared to be less densely packed as compared with untreated cells.

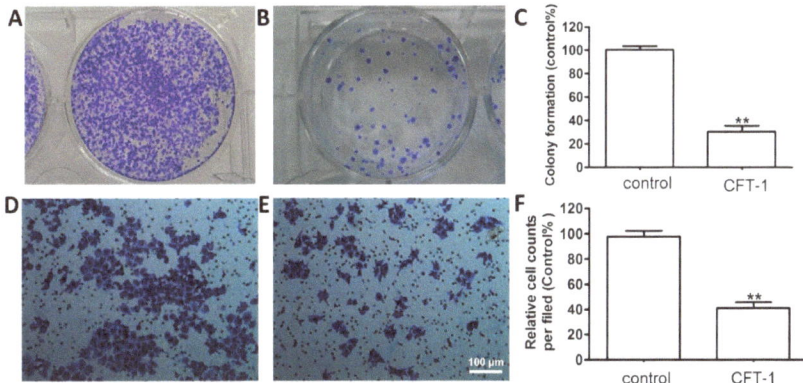

Figure 2. Effect of CFT-1 treatment on colony formation ability and mobility of Hep3B cells. (**A–C**) Colony formation of Hep3B cells treated with 143 µg/mL CFT-1. (**D–F**) Transwell assays demonstrating the migration ability of Hep3B cells treated by 143 µg/mL CFT-1. ** $p < 0.01$. Scale bar = 100 µm.

We further determined the influence of CFT-1 on the cell mobility with the Transwell migration assay. As shown in Figure 2D,E, the migration of Hep3B cells was significantly suppressed by CFT-1 treatment. Specifically, the number of migrated Hep3B cells in the treated group was reduced by more than 41.7% as compared to the vehicle control cells (Figure 2F).

3.4. CFT-1 Treatment-Induced Apoptosis and G0/G1 Arrest in Hep3B Cells

Apoptosis and G0/G1 arrest are two important cellular processes that researchers often study in the context of cancer, including in Hep3B cells, which are a commonly used HCC (liver cancer) cell line. These processes are relevant because they play key roles in controlling cell growth, preventing uncontrolled proliferation, and influencing the response to various treatments. Apoptosis, or programmed cell death, is a regulated process that eliminates damaged or unwanted cells. Inducing apoptosis in cancer cells is a common goal in cancer research and therapy. Researchers often explore different compounds or treatments that can trigger apoptosis in Hep3B cells. These may include chemotherapy drugs, targeted therapies, or experimental agents designed to promote apoptotic pathways. The cell cycle consists of different phases, and G0/G1 arrest refers to a halt in the G0 and G1 phases. This arrest prevents cells from progressing into the S phase, where DNA replication occurs.

The above results confirm that CFT-1 exerts anti-cancer potential against the human Hep3B cell line by suppressing cell growth, colony formation, and cell migration. To investigate the mechanism of action, we assessed the cell death in CFT-1-treated Hep3B cells with flow cytometry. This was based on the observation of morphologic alterations caused by CFT-1, e.g., cell body shrinkage, nucleus compaction, and chromatin condensation, which together suggest an apoptotic process. We treated Hep3B cells with 143 μg/mL CFT-1 for 48 h. As shown in Figure 3, CFT-1 treatment significantly promoted apoptosis in Hep3B cells. The total apoptotic rate of Hep3B cells in the untreated control group was only 5.7%, indicating that the natural apoptotic rate of Hep3B cells was very low. Quantitative analysis indicated that the percentage of apoptotic cells increased from 5.7% to 14.8% after CFT-1 treatment.

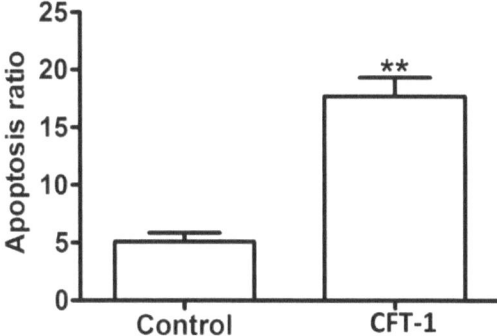

Figure 3. Effect of CFT-1 treatment on apoptosis of Hep3B cells. ** $p < 0.01$.

Apoptosis and cell proliferation inhibition could be mediated by the dysregulation of cell cycle progression [28]. On this basis, we examined the cell cycle distribution with flow cytometry. After 48 h of incubation, it was shown that CFT-1 treatment resulted in a significant increase in the percentage of cells in the G0/G1 phase (73.07%) compared to the untreated cells (59.66%), while it decreased the percentage of cells in the S phase from 30.98% to 19.69% (Figure 4A–C). This is in agreement with the suppressed cell proliferation in CFT-1-treated cells. On this basis, it can be concluded that CFT-1 induces G0/G1 phase arrest in the Hep3B cell line. Notably, this conclusion coincides with previous studies on EGCG [29].

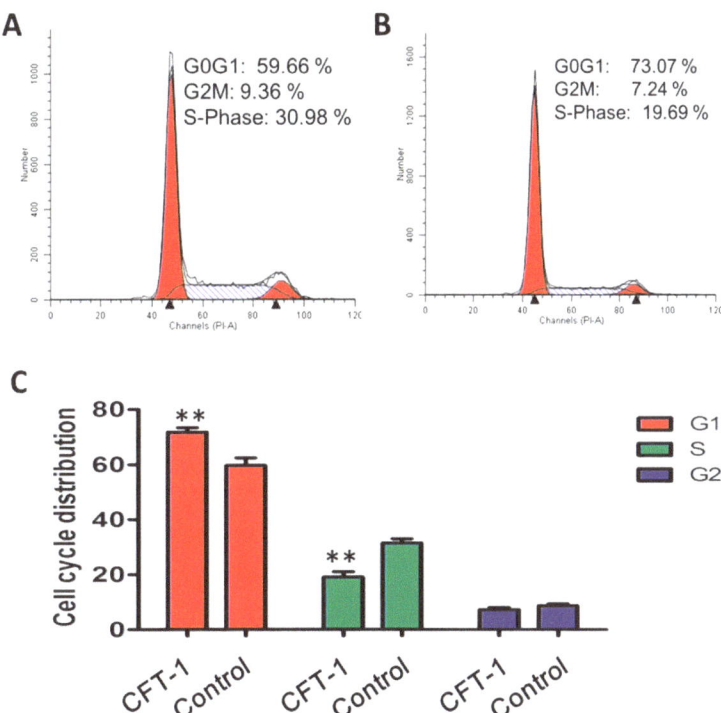

Figure 4. Effect of CFT-1 treatment on the Hep3B cell cycle. (**A**) The cell cycle distribution of untreated Hep3B cells. (**B**) The cell cycle distribution of Hep3B cells treated with 143 µg/mL CFT-1 for 48 h. (**C**) Quantification of cell cycle distribution results. ** $p < 0.01$.

3.5. CFT-1 Treatment Reduces the Telomerase Activity in Hep3B Cells

Telomerase activity in liver cancer cells, such as HCC, is an area of interest in cancer research. Hep3B cell is the most common type of liver cancer, and understanding the role of telomerase in its development and progression is crucial. In many cases of liver cancer, increased telomerase activity is observed. The upregulation of telomerase allows cancer cells to maintain the lengths of their telomeres, promoting continuous cell division and contributing to the unchecked growth characteristic of cancer. Researchers study the mechanisms regulating telomerase activity in liver cancer cells to identify potential therapeutic targets. Inhibiting telomerase activity could be a strategy to limit the proliferation of liver cancer cells.

It is obvious that there is an agreement between our results for CFT-1 and previous studies on EGCG. EGCG, as the most abundant active ingredient in green tea, plays an essential role in preventing the occurrence and development of carcinomas [30–32]. To gain insight into the possible molecular basis behind the anti-proliferative ability of CFT-1, we referred to the available knowledge about the molecular target(s) of EGCG. According to previous studies, EGCG has been shown to inhibit telomerase activity considerably in several different cancer cell lines by repressing the target mRNA expression [33,34]. Telomerase seems to play a primary role in the cancer-fighting virtues of EGCG.

On this basis, we hypothesized that CFT-1 exerts its pharmacological activity possibly through turning down the activity of telomerase. To validate this hypothesis, we examined the influence of CFT-1 extract on the telomerase activity with a telomerase–PCR–ELISA assay kit. As shown in Figure 5, CFT-1 treatment (143 µg/mL, 48 h) resulted in a significant decrease of 205.65% in the telomerase activity in Hep3B cells, suggesting a possible basis for the performance of CFT-1 on human HCC.

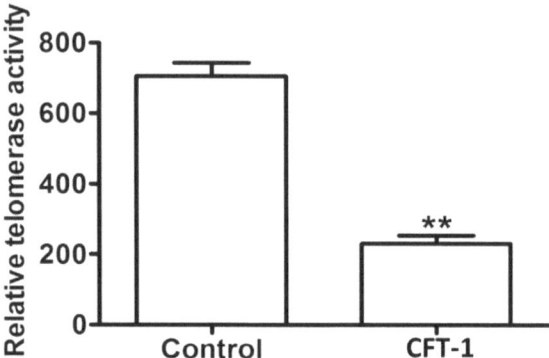

Figure 5. Effect of CFT-1 treatment (143 µg/mL, 48 h) on telomerase activity in Hep3B cells. ** $p < 0.01$.

4. Discussion

Tea-based chemoprevention has gained increasing attention in recent years for the prevention of cancer. EGCG has been widely studied for its role in the chemoprevention of various tumors. Research has shown that EGCG can affect signaling pathways, induce cell apoptosis, promote cell growth arrest, and prevent cancer. As the primary active ingredient, EGCG has already shown great potential in cancer treatment. EGCG, accounting for 59% of the total catechin content, has been confirmed to have chemopreventive and chemotherapeutic effects against cancer [35]. For instance, Mayr et al. reported that EGCG also has a synergistic cytotoxic effect with conventional chemotherapy, e.g., cisplatin, in biliary tract cancer cell lines [36]. Recently, the EGCG-rich functional tea (CFT-1) has been introduced in China as a nutraceutical beverage. It is highly popular for its possible functions against cancer and other diseases. However, its health benefits and pharmacological activity remain unclear.

In the present study, we aimed to assess the anti-cancer effect of CFT-1 on the selected human Hep3B cell line. As a result, we observed dramatic alterations in cell morphology caused by CFT-1, including large amounts of cell body shrinkage, nucleus compaction, and chromatin condensation. We also found significant inhibition of proliferation, colony formation, and migration in CFT-1 treated Hep3B cells, which, together, definitely indicated the great potential of CFT-1 against human HCC. Specifically, we determined the IC50 value (143 µg/mL) of CFT-1 on Hep3B cells after 48 h of incubation. This is very close to the previously reported activity of EGCG on HCC cell lines, suggesting the strong potency of CFT-1. To gain insight into the mechanism of action, we assessed the cell death and cell cycle distribution associated with the CFT-1 treatment. Our results showed that CFT-1 significantly induced apoptosis and cell cycle arrest at the G0/G1 phase in human HCC Hep3B cells. Consistently, it was reported that EGCG inhibits cell growth, induces apoptosis, and causes G0/G1 arrest in different carcinomas [37], suggesting the similarity of action modes between CFT-1 and EGCG.

Currently available reports focus specifically on the molecular target telomerase, which is responsible for elongating telomeres [38]. Telomerase is directly implicated in tumorigenesis and is regarded as a promising anti-cancer target. To explore the possible molecular basis of the mechanism for CFT-1 tea, we assessed its influence on the telomerase activity. The CFT-1 tea has a significant inhibitory effect on tumor cell growth in vitro, and its inhibitory effect gradually increases with the increase in tea concentration. Our results showed that CFT-1 can strongly affect the enzyme in Hep3B cells by reducing the activity by more than half. On this basis, it could be suggested that CFT-1 suppresses the growth of Hep3B cells by inducing apoptosis and G0/G1 cell cycle arrest, possibly through a reduction in telomerase activity.

5. Conclusions

Overall, CFT-1 can inhibit the proliferation of HCC cells in vitro. Our work clearly shows the promise of CFT-1 as effective chemopreventatives and chemotherapy against human HCC. And CFT 1 tea is better than common tea in terms of protecting the liver effectively and preventing the development of cancer. These results provide a basis for the development of a functional food based on tea.

Supplementary Materials: The following supporting information can be downloaded at: https://www.mdpi.com/article/10.3390/foods13121867/s1, Figure S1: HPLC chromatograms of (A) CFT-1 extract and (B) standards. 1. Gallic acid (GA), 2. (−)-gallocatechin (GC), 3. caffeine (CAF), 4. theophylline (THEO), 5. (−)- epigallocatechin (EGC), 6. (+)-catechin (C), 7. chlorogenic acid (CHL), 8. theobromine (TB), 9. caffeic acid (CAA), 10. (−)-epicatechin (EC), 11. (−)-epigallocatechin gallate (EGCG), 12. p-coumaric acid (COU), 13. (−)-gallocatechin gallate (GCG), 14. ferulic acid (FER), 15. sinapic acid (SIN), 16. epicatechin gallate (ECG), 17. rutin (RUT), 18. myricetin (MYR), 19. quercetin (QUE), 20. kaempferol (KAE).

Author Contributions: Writing—original draft preparation, Y.C.; methodology, Y.C. and C.C.; writing—review and editing, R.G., J.X., and W.Y.; guiding paper writing skills and planning experimental designs, G.W. and W.Y. All authors have read and agreed to the published version of the manuscript.

Funding: This work was supported by Fujian Academy of Agricultural Science Projects (Grant No. ZYTS2019019), the Fujian Province Foreign Cooperation Projects China (No 2021I0034) and the Foreign Cooperation Projects of Fujian Academy of Agricultural Sciences (No. DWHZ-2022-21).

Institutional Review Board Statement: Not applicable.

Informed Consent Statement: Not applicable.

Data Availability Statement: The original contributions presented in the study are included in the article/supplementary material, further inquiries can be directed to the corresponding authors.

Conflicts of Interest: The authors declare that there are no conflicts of interest.

References

1. Sung, H.; Ferlay, J.; Siegel, R.L.; Laversanne, M.; Soerjomataram, I.; Jemal, A.; Bray, F. Global Cancer Statistics 2020: GLOBOCAN Estimates of Incidence and Mortality Worldwide for 36 Cancers in 185 Countries. *CA Cancer J. Clin.* **2021**, *71*, 209–249. [CrossRef] [PubMed]
2. Zhang, C.H.; Cheng, Y.; Zhang, S.; Fan, J.; Gao, Q. Changing epidemiology of hepatocellular carcinoma in Asia. *Liver Int.* **2022**, *42*, 2029–2041. [CrossRef] [PubMed]
3. Singal, A.G.; Kanwal, F.; Llovet, J.M. Global trends in hepatocellular carcinoma epidemiology: Implications for screening, prevention and therapy. *Nat. Rev. Clin. Oncol.* **2023**, *20*, 864–884. [CrossRef] [PubMed]
4. Donne, R.; Lujambio, A. The liver cancer immune microenvironment: Therapeutic implications for hepatocellular carcinoma. *Hepatology* **2023**, *77*, 1773–1796. [CrossRef] [PubMed]
5. Zhou, J.; Sun, H.; Wang, Z.; Cong, W.; Wang, J.; Zeng, M.; Zhou, W.; Bie, P.; Liu, L.; Wen, T.; et al. Guidelines for the Diagnosis and Treatment of Hepatocellular Carcinoma (2019 Edition). *Liver Cancer* **2020**, *9*, 682–720. [CrossRef]
6. Xia, Y.; Li, J.; Liu, G.; Wang, K.; Qian, G.; Lu, Z.; Yang, T.; Yan, Z.; Lei, Z.; Si, A.; et al. Long-term Effects of Repeat Hepatectomy vs. Percutaneous Radiofrequency Ablation Among Patients with Recurrent Hepatocellular Carcinoma: A Randomized Clinical Trial. *JAMA Oncol.* **2020**, *6*, 255–263. [CrossRef] [PubMed]
7. Torimura, T.; Iwamoto, H. Treatment and the prognosis of hepatocellular carcinoma in Asia. *Liver Int.* **2022**, *42*, 2042–2054. [CrossRef]
8. McGlynn, K.A.; Petrick, J.L.; El-Serag, H.B. Epidemiology of Hepatocellular Carcinoma. *Hepatology* **2021**, *73* (Suppl. 1), 4–13. [CrossRef]
9. Sagnelli, E.; Macera, M.; Russo, A.; Coppola, N.; Sagnelli, C. Epidemiological and etiological variations in hepatocellular carcinoma. *Infection* **2020**, *48*, 7–17. [CrossRef]
10. Zhang, D.; Nichols, H.B.; Troester, M.; Cai, J.; Bensen, J.T.; Sandler, D.P. Tea consumption and breast cancer risk in a cohort of women with family history of breast cancer. *Int. J. Cancer* **2020**, *147*, 876–886. [CrossRef]
11. Al-Zalabani, A.H.; Wesselius, A.; Yi-Wen Yu, E.; van den Brandt, P.; Grant, E.J.; White, E.; Skeie, G.; Liedberg, F.; Weiderpass, E.; Zeegers, M.P. Tea consumption and risk of bladder cancer in the Bladder Cancer Epidemiology and Nutritional Determinants (BLEND) Study: Pooled analysis of 12 international cohort studies. *Clin. Nutr.* **2022**, *41*, 1122–1130. [CrossRef] [PubMed]

12. Chen, Y.; Abe, S.K.; Inoue, M.; Yamaji, T.; Iwasaki, M.; Nomura, S.; Hashizume, M.; Tsugane, S.; Sawada, N.; Group, J.S. Green tea and coffee consumption and risk of kidney cancer in Japanese adults. *Sci. Rep.* **2022**, *12*, 20274. [CrossRef] [PubMed]
13. Kim, T.L.; Jeong, G.H.; Yang, J.W.; Lee, K.H.; Kronbichler, A.; van der Vliet, H.J.; Grosso, G.; Galvano, F.; Aune, D.; Kim, J.Y.; et al. Tea Consumption and Risk of Cancer: An Umbrella Review and Meta-Analysis of Observational Studies. *Adv. Nutr.* **2020**, *11*, 1437–1452. [CrossRef] [PubMed]
14. Xu, X.Y.; Zhao, C.N.; Cao, S.Y.; Tang, G.Y.; Gan, R.Y.; Li, H.B. Effects and mechanisms of tea for the prevention and management of cancers: An updated review. *Crit. Rev. Food Sci. Nutr.* **2020**, *60*, 1693–1705. [CrossRef] [PubMed]
15. Seow, W.J.; Koh, W.P.; Jin, A.; Wang, R.; Yuan, J.M. Associations between tea and coffee beverage consumption and the risk of lung cancer in the Singaporean Chinese population. *Eur. J. Nutr.* **2020**, *59*, 3083–3091. [CrossRef] [PubMed]
16. Rodríguez-Molinero, J.; Migueláñez-Medrán, B.d.C.; Puente-Gutiérrez, C.; Delgado-Somolinos, E.; Martín Carreras-Presas, C.; Fernández-Farhall, J.; López-Sánchez, A.F. Association between Oral Cancer and Diet: An Update. *Nutrients* **2021**, *13*, 1299. [CrossRef] [PubMed]
17. Alam, M.; Ali, S.; Ashraf, G.M.; Bilgrami, A.L.; Yadav, D.K.; Hassan, M.I. Epigallocatechin 3-gallate: From green tea to cancer therapeutics. *Food Chem.* **2022**, *379*, 132135. [CrossRef] [PubMed]
18. Almatroodi, S.A.; Almatroudi, A.; Khan, A.A.; Alhumaydhi, F.A.; Alsahli, M.A.; Rahmani, A.H. Potential Therapeutic Targets of Epigallocatechin Gallate (EGCG), the Most Abundant Catechin in Green Tea, and Its Role in the Therapy of Various Types of Cancer. *Molecules* **2020**, *25*, 3146. [CrossRef] [PubMed]
19. Kazi, J.; Sen, R.; Ganguly, S.; Jha, T.; Ganguly, S.; Chatterjee Debnath, M. Folate decorated epigallocatechin-3-gallate (EGCG) loaded PLGA nanoparticles; in-vitro and in-vivo targeting efficacy against MDA-MB-231 tumor xenograft. *Int. J. Pharm.* **2020**, *585*, 119449. [CrossRef]
20. Parekh, N.; Garg, A.; Choudhary, R.; Gupta, M.; Kaur, G.; Ramniwas, S.; Shahwan, M.; Tuli, H.S.; Sethi, G. The Role of Natural Flavonoids as Telomerase Inhibitors in Suppressing Cancer Growth. *Pharmaceuticals* **2023**, *16*, 605. [CrossRef]
21. Tsatsakis, A.; Oikonomopoulou, T.; Nikolouzakis, T.K.; Vakonaki, E.; Tzatzarakis, M.; Flamourakis, M.; Renieri, E.; Fragkiadaki, P.; Iliaki, E.; Bachlitzanaki, M.; et al. Role of telomere length in human carcinogenesis (Review). *Int. J. Oncol.* **2023**, *63*, 78. [CrossRef] [PubMed]
22. Kang, Q.; Tong, Y.; Gowd, V.; Wang, M.; Chen, F.; Cheng, K.W. Oral administration of EGCG solution equivalent to daily achievable dosages of regular tea drinkers effectively suppresses miR483-3p induced metastasis of hepatocellular carcinoma cells in mice. *Food Funct.* **2021**, *12*, 3381–3392. [CrossRef] [PubMed]
23. Liao, S.; Lin, J.; Liu, J.; Chen, T.; Xu, M.; Zheng, J. Chemoprevention of elite tea variety CFT-1 rich in EGCG against chemically induced liver cancer in rats. *Food Sci. Nutr.* **2019**, *7*, 2647–2665. [CrossRef] [PubMed]
24. Liao, R.; Chen, X.; Cao, Q.; Bai, L.; Ma, C.; Dai, Z.; Dong, C. AMD1 promotes breast cancer aggressiveness via a spermidine-eIF5A hypusination-TCF4 axis. *Breast Cancer Res.* **2024**, *26*, 70. [CrossRef] [PubMed]
25. Merckens, A.; Sieler, M.; Keil, S.; Dittmar, T. Altered Phenotypes of Breast Epithelial × Breast Cancer Hybrids after ZEB1 Knock-Out. *Int. J. Mol. Sci.* **2023**, *24*, 17310. [CrossRef] [PubMed]
26. Monier, B.; Suzanne, M. Orchestration of Force Generation and Nuclear Collapse in Apoptotic Cells. *Int. J. Mol. Sci.* **2021**, *22*, 10257. [CrossRef] [PubMed]
27. Bala, R.; Pareek, B.; Umar, A.; Arora, S.; Singh, D.; Chaudhary, A.; Alkhanjaf, A.A.M.; Almadiy, A.A.; Algadi, H.; Kumar, R.; et al. In-vitro cytotoxicity of nickel oxide nanoparticles against L-6 cell-lines: MMP, MTT and ROS studies. *Environ. Res.* **2022**, *215*, 114257. [CrossRef] [PubMed]
28. Liu, J.; Peng, Y.; Wei, W. Cell cycle on the crossroad of tumorigenesis and cancer therapy. *Trends Cell Biol.* **2022**, *32*, 30–44. [CrossRef] [PubMed]
29. Niu, X.; Liu, Z.; Wang, J.; Wu, D. Green tea EGCG inhibits naive CD4(+) T cell division and progression in mice: An integration of network pharmacology, molecular docking and experimental validation. *Curr. Res. Food Sci.* **2023**, *7*, 100537. [CrossRef]
30. Bimonte, S.; Cascella, M.; Barbieri, A.; Arra, C.; Cuomo, A. Current shreds of evidence on the anticancer role of EGCG in triple negative breast cancer: An update of the current state of knowledge. *Infect. Agent. Cancer* **2020**, *15*, 2. [CrossRef]
31. Ferrari, E.; Bettuzzi, S.; Naponelli, V. The Potential of Epigallocatechin Gallate (EGCG) in Targeting Autophagy for Cancer Treatment: A Narrative Review. *Int. J. Mol. Sci.* **2022**, *23*, 6075. [CrossRef] [PubMed]
32. Aggarwal, V.; Tuli, H.S.; Tania, M.; Srivastava, S.; Ritzer, E.E.; Pandey, A.; Aggarwal, D.; Barwal, T.S.; Jain, A.; Kaur, G.; et al. Molecular mechanisms of action of epigallocatechin gallate in cancer: Recent trends and advancement. *Semin. Cancer Biol.* **2022**, *80*, 256–275. [CrossRef] [PubMed]
33. Talib, W.H.; Awajan, D.; Alqudah, A.; Alsawwaf, R.; Althunibat, R.; Abu AlRoos, M.; Al Safadi, A.; Abu Asab, S.; Hadi, R.W.; Al Kury, L.T. Targeting Cancer Hallmarks with Epigallocatechin Gallate (EGCG): Mechanistic Basis and Therapeutic Targets. *Molecules* **2024**, *29*, 1373. [CrossRef] [PubMed]
34. Huang, Y.-J.; Wang, K.-L.; Chen, H.-Y.; Chiang, Y.-F.; Hsia, S.-M. Protective Effects of Epigallocatechin Gallate (EGCG) on Endometrial, Breast, and Ovarian Cancers. *Biomolecules* **2020**, *10*, 1481. [CrossRef]
35. Rady, I.; Mohamed, H.; Rady, M.; Siddiqui, I.A.; Mukhtar, H. Cancer preventive and therapeutic effects of EGCG, the major polyphenol in green tea. *Egypt. J. Basic. Appl. Sci.* **2018**, *5*, 1–23. [CrossRef]

36. Mayr, C.; Wagner, A.; Neureiter, D.; Pichler, M.; Jakab, M.; Illig, R.; Berr, F.; Kiesslich, T. The green tea catechin epigallocatechin gallate induces cell cycle arrest and shows potential synergism with cisplatin in biliary tract cancer cells. *BMC Complement. Altern. Med.* **2015**, *15*, 194. [CrossRef] [PubMed]
37. Peng, H.; Lin, X.; Wang, Y.; Chen, J.; Zhao, Q.; Chen, S.; Cheng, Q.; Chen, C.; Sang, T.; Zhou, H.; et al. Epigallocatechin gallate suppresses mitotic clonal expansion and adipogenic differentiation of preadipocytes through impeding JAK2/STAT3-mediated transcriptional cascades. *Phytomedicine* **2024**, *129*, 155563. [CrossRef]
38. Guterres, A.N.; Villanueva, J. Targeting telomerase for cancer therapy. *Oncogene* **2020**, *39*, 5811–5824. [CrossRef]

Disclaimer/Publisher's Note: The statements, opinions and data contained in all publications are solely those of the individual author(s) and contributor(s) and not of MDPI and/or the editor(s). MDPI and/or the editor(s) disclaim responsibility for any injury to people or property resulting from any ideas, methods, instructions or products referred to in the content.

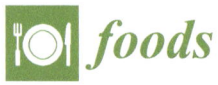

Article

The Potential Mechanisms of Catechins in Tea for Anti-Hypertension: An Integration of Network Pharmacology, Molecular Docking, and Molecular Dynamics Simulation

Yanming Tuo [1], Xiaofeng Lu [1], Fang Tao [1], Marat Tukhvatshin [1], Fumin Xiang [1], Xi Wang [1], Yutao Shi [1,2], Jinke Lin [1,*] and Yunfei Hu [3,*]

1. College of Horticulture, Fujian Agriculture and Forestry University, Fuzhou 350002, China; tuo3152022@163.com (Y.T.); lxfitea21@163.com (X.L.); whitehydrangea@163.com (F.T.); marattukhvatshin@mail.ru (M.T.); fuminrz@163.com (F.X.); wx553829422@163.com (X.W.); ytshi@wuyiu.edu.cn (Y.S.)
2. College of Tea and Food Sciences, Wuyi University, Wuyishan 354300, China
3. Anxi College of Tea Science, Fujian Agriculture and Forestry University, Fuzhou 350002, China
* Correspondence: 000q020008@fafu.edu.cn (J.L.); huyunfei@fafu.edu.cn (Y.H.)

Abstract: Catechins, a class of polyphenolic compounds found in tea, have attracted significant attention due to their numerous health benefits, particularly for the treatment and protection of hypertension. However, the potential targets and mechanisms of action of catechins in combating hypertension remain unclear. This study systematically investigates the anti-hypertensive mechanisms of tea catechins using network pharmacology, molecular docking, and molecular dynamics simulation techniques. The results indicate that 23 potential anti-hypertensive targets for eight catechin components were predicted through public databases. The analysis of protein–protein interaction (PPI) identified three key targets (MMP9, BCL2, and HIF1A). KEGG pathway and GO enrichment analyses revealed that these key targets play significant roles in regulating vascular smooth muscle contraction, promoting angiogenesis, and mediating vascular endothelial growth factor receptor signaling. The molecular docking results demonstrate that the key targets (MMP9, BCL2, and HIF1A) effectively bind with catechin components (CG, GCG, ECG, and EGCG) through hydrogen bonds and hydrophobic interactions. Molecular dynamics simulations further confirmed the stability of the binding between catechins and the targets. This study systematically elucidates the potential mechanisms by which tea catechins treat anti-hypertension and provides a theoretical basis for the development and application of tea catechins as functional additives for the prevention of hypertension.

Keywords: tea; catechins; hypertension; network pharmacology; molecular docking; molecular dynamics simulation

Citation: Tuo, Y.; Lu, X.; Tao, F.; Tukhvatshin, M.; Xiang, F.; Wang, X.; Shi, Y.; Lin, J.; Hu, Y. The Potential Mechanisms of Catechins in Tea for Anti-Hypertension: An Integration of Network Pharmacology, Molecular Docking, and Molecular Dynamics Simulation. *Foods* **2024**, *13*, 2685. https://doi.org/10.3390/foods13172685

Academic Editor: Ivana Generalic Mekinic

Received: 6 August 2024
Revised: 22 August 2024
Accepted: 23 August 2024
Published: 26 August 2024

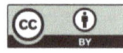

Copyright: © 2024 by the authors. Licensee MDPI, Basel, Switzerland. This article is an open access article distributed under the terms and conditions of the Creative Commons Attribution (CC BY) license (https://creativecommons.org/licenses/by/4.0/).

1. Introduction

Tea is one of the three major non-alcoholic beverages consumed worldwide. Tea polyphenols, important natural components found within tea, possess various health benefits [1,2]. Among these, catechins constitute the primary portion of tea polyphenols, accounting for approximately 80% of the total. The main catechins include catechin gallate (CG), epicatechin gallate (ECG), gallocatechin gallate (GCG), epigallocatechin gallate (EGCG), catechin (C), epicatechin (EC), gallocatechin (GC), and epigallocatechin (EGC) [3,4]. Catechins are crucial components responsible for the numerous health benefits conferred by tea. Research has shown that catechins possess potential health benefits in antioxidation, anti-hypertension, and hypoglycemia, thus offering new possibilities for hypertension (HTN) treatment and prevention [5–8].

The long-term condition of hypertension has emerged as a critical global healthcare issue, presenting a significant challenge in the field of public health [9]. According to the World Health Organization (WHO), the number of individuals with hypertension is expected to reach approximately 1.56 billion by 2025 [10]. Hypertension, while not the primary cause of mortality, can lead to complications such as cardiovascular disease, heart failure, and renal failure [11,12]. Hypertensive patients, who experience prolonged elevated blood pressure, endure increased pressure on the vascular walls, leading to conditions such as atherosclerosis and vascular sclerosis, which in turn result in vascular narrowing, blockage, or rupture [13]. Thus, there is an urgent need to develop effective treatment and prevention strategies to address this global health problem.

In recent years, natural products have become a focus of hypertension treatment research due to their lower side effects and higher safety profiles. Tea catechins, as significant natural products, have shown potential anti-hypertensive effects. Studies have indicated that improving arterial elasticity is another mechanism for preventing hypertension. An epidemiological study with a cross-sectional design, which included 6589 adults aged 40–75 years in Wuyishan, Fujian Province, China, suggested that habitual tea drinking may protect against arterial stiffness [14]. Additionally, the consumption of green and black tea has been associated with reduced risks of cardiovascular disease and certain cancers [15]. These health benefits are typically attributed to the polyphenolic compounds in tea [16]. Garcia et al. [17] investigated the effects of green tea on blood pressure and sympathetic nerve excitation in an L-NAME-induced hypertensive rat model. The results showed that L-NAME-treated rats exhibited elevated blood pressure (165 mmHg) compared to control rats (103 mmHg), while green tea treatment reduced hypertension (119 mmHg). In vivo experiments have demonstrated the anti-hypertensive effects of a catechin-rich diet in rats [18]. Catechins may alleviate vascular dysfunction in hypertensive mice by regulating oxidative stress and endothelial nitric oxide synthase (eNOS) [19].

Despite the potential anti-hypertensive effects of tea catechins, further research is needed to explore their active components, mechanisms of action, and targets in hypertension treatment. To gain a deeper understanding of the pharmacological mechanisms by which drugs treat diseases, researchers have increasingly employed various computational methods, including network pharmacology, molecular docking, and molecular dynamics simulation [20]. Network pharmacology, an emerging research approach, integrates systems biology, network analysis, and pharmacology and is frequently employed to investigate the multi-target effects of complex natural compounds [21]. Molecular docking is a computational simulation method used to predict the binding modes and affinities between small molecules (drugs) and protein receptors (targets) [22]. Molecular dynamics simulation further verifies and optimizes the binding modes between these small molecules and protein receptors, providing a more precise molecular level understanding [23].

In this study, we aim to comprehensively elucidate the anti-hypertensive potential of tea catechin components, identify their targets, and explore their mechanisms of action using a combined approach of network pharmacology, molecular docking, and molecular dynamics simulation. This research will provide a theoretical basis for the further application of tea catechins in the biomedical field. The complete research process is illustrated in Figure 1.

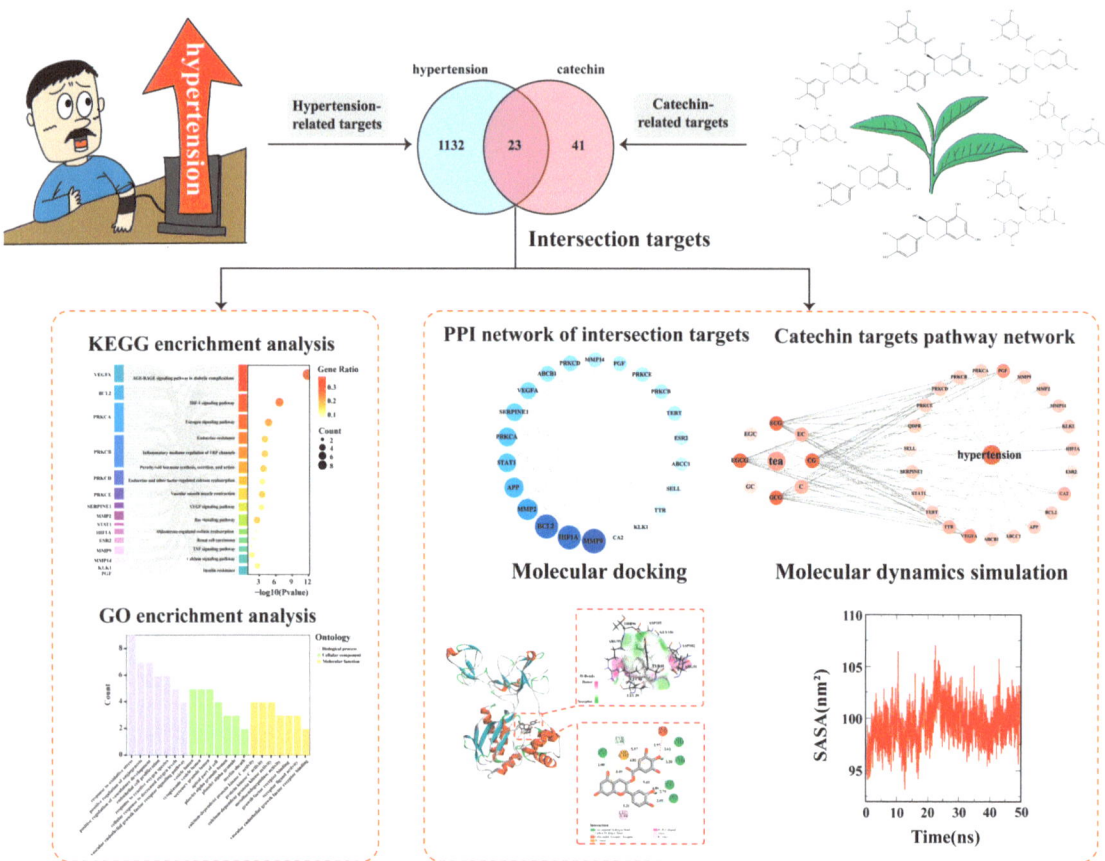

Figure 1. Network pharmacology regulatory mechanisms of catechins in anti-hypertension.

2. Materials and Methods

2.1. Collection of Catechin Targets

The isomeric SMILES numbers for the eight catechin components—catechin (C), epicatechin (EC), gallocatechin (GC), epigallocatechin (EGC), catechin gallate (CG), epicatechin gallate (ECG), gallocatechin gallate (GCG), and epigallocatechin gallate (EGCG)—were obtained from the PubChem database (https://pubchem.ncbi.nlm.nih.gov/, accessed on 14 July 2024), with their structures illustrated in Figure 2. Subsequently, the predicted targets of catechins were identified using the isomeric SMILES numbers through the SEA Search Server (https://sea.bkslab.org/, accessed on 14 July 2024) and the SwissTargetPrediction (http://www.swisstargetprediction.ch/, accessed on 14 July 2024) databases. The predicted targets from the two databases were then merged, and duplicates were removed, resulting in the collection of potential targets for the eight catechin components. Furthermore, the catechin–targets network was constructed and visualized using Cytoscape 3.9.1.

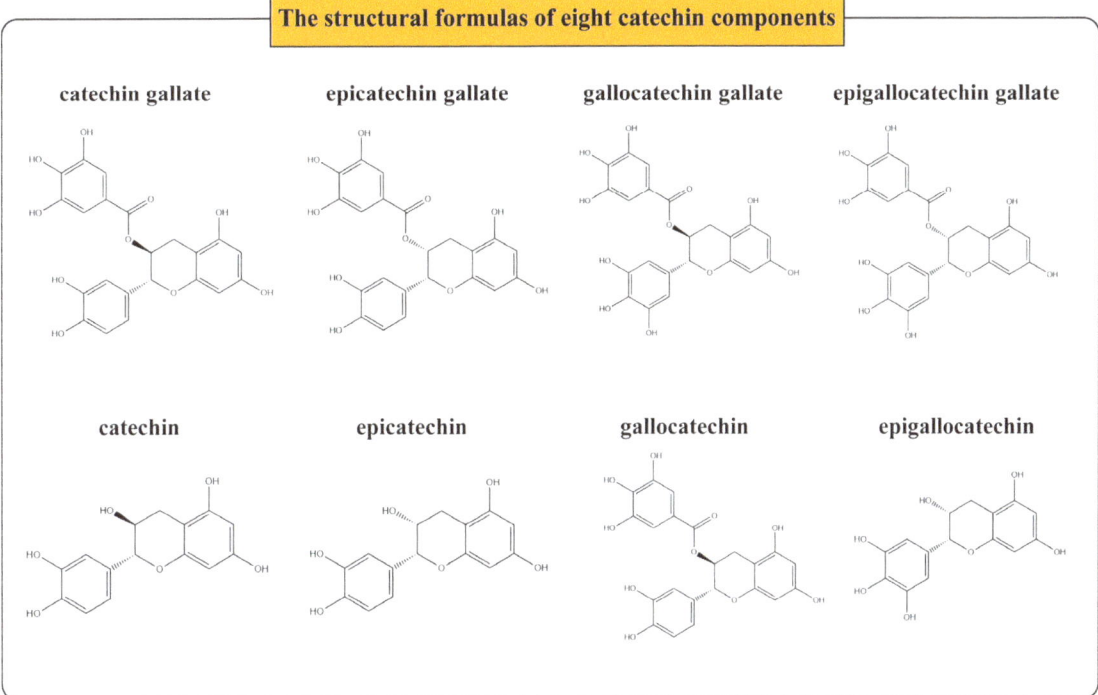

Figure 2. Structural formulas of eight catechin components.

2.2. Screening of Hypertension-Related Targets

Hypertension-related targets were retrieved from three disease databases: DisGeNET (https://www.disgenet.org/, accessed on 15 July 2024), OMIM (https://omim.org/, accessed on 15 July 2024), and GeneCards (https://www.genecards.org/, accessed on 15 July 2024), using the keyword "hypertension". The screening criteria were set as a score of gda ≥ 0.1 in the DisGeNET database and a relevance score ≥ 5 in the GeneCards database. The hypertension-related targets from the three databases were then merged, and duplicate targets were removed.

2.3. Screening of Key Targets and Construction and Analysis of the Protein–Protein Interaction (PPI) Network

To explore the potential targets of catechins in treating hypertension, an intersection analysis was performed between the catechin targets and hypertension targets, and a Venn diagram was generated using the online platform (https://cloud.metware.cn/, accessed on 21 July 2024). The intersecting targets were imported into the STRING database (http://string-db.org/, accessed on 21 July 2024) to construct the PPI network of the target proteins [24]. "Homo sapiens" was selected as the species, and the minimum interaction score threshold was set to 0.4, with other parameters set to default. The network was visualized using Cytoscape 3.9.1 software, and the Network Analysis plugin was employed to calculate the degree value of each target. Key targets were identified based on their degree values, and molecular docking studies were subsequently conducted on the top three key proteins with the highest degree values.

2.4. GO and KEGG Pathway Enrichment Analyses

To further investigate the biological functions of the key target genes, GO and KEGG enrichment analyses were performed using the "clusterProfiler" package, with a p-value threshold set at $p < 0.05$. GO functional analysis predicted gene functions across three categories: biological process (BP), cellular component (CC), and molecular function (MF), while KEGG pathway enrichment analysis identified key pathways associated with the anti-hypertensive targets of catechins. Both GO and KEGG analysis results were visualized using an online tool (https://cloud.metware.cn/, accessed on 21 July 2024).

2.5. Molecular Docking

The SDF format ligand files for the eight catechin components were obtained from the PubChem database (https://pubchem.ncbi.nlm.nih.gov/, accessed on 23 July 2024), and the three-dimensional structure models of the proteins MMP9 (PDB ID: 1L6J), HIF1A (PDB ID: 4H6J), and BCL2 (PDB ID: 5FCG) were obtained from the UniProt database (https://www.uniprot.org/, accessed on 23 July 2024) [25]. Molecular docking was conducted using AutoDock Vina 1.2.5 [26], and the docking results were further analyzed and visualized using Discovery Studio 2019 software.

2.6. Molecular Dynamics Simulation

To explore the stability of the protein–ligand interactions in greater depth, molecular dynamics (MD) simulations were performed on four complexes: CG-MMP9, GCG-MMP9, ECG-HIF1A, and EGCG-BCL2, using GROMACS 2020.6 software. The AMBER99SB force field and SPC water model were utilized, with the system temperature set at 300 K and the simulation time at 50 ns. The energy minimization phase employed the steepest descent method, followed by energy equilibration to stabilize the system before completing the MD simulation. The binding free energies were calculated using the MM/GBSA method, and the resulting MD simulation data were visualized using Xmgrace software 5.1.25 [27].

3. Results

3.1. Screening of Potential Targets for the Anti-Hypertensive Effects of Catechin Components

For the eight catechin components, 51 and 48 targets were predicted from the SEA Search Server and Swiss Target Prediction databases, respectively. After removing duplicate targets, 64 unique targets for the catechin components were identified, and a tea–catechin–targets network was constructed using Cytoscape 3.9.1 (Figure 3A, Supplementary Table S1). Among these, ECG had the most associated potential targets (61), followed by EGCG (60), GCG (60), CG (59), C (24), EC (24), GC (13), and EGC (13). Additionally, hypertension-related targets were gathered from multiple databases, resulting in 784 targets from DisGeNET, 683 from GeneCards, and 75 from OMIM. After removing duplicates, 1155 hypertension-related targets were obtained (Supplementary Table S2). A Venn diagram was used to identify the intersecting targets between the predicted catechin targets and hypertension targets. The analysis identified 23 targets as potential candidates for the anti-hypertensive action of catechins (Figure 3B).

3.2. Protein–Protein Interaction (PPI) Network Analysis and Key Target Screening

The PPI network for the 23 intersecting targets was constructed using the STRING database and visualized with Cytoscape 3.9.1 software (Figure 3C). The PPI network comprised 22 nodes and 150 edges, with node size and color varying according to their degree value (Supplementary Table S3). The degree value represents the number of edges connected to a node, indicating its importance. Among the targets, MMP9, BCL2, and HIF1A exhibited the highest degree values, with degrees of 15, 14, and 14, respectively, identifying them as potential key targets.

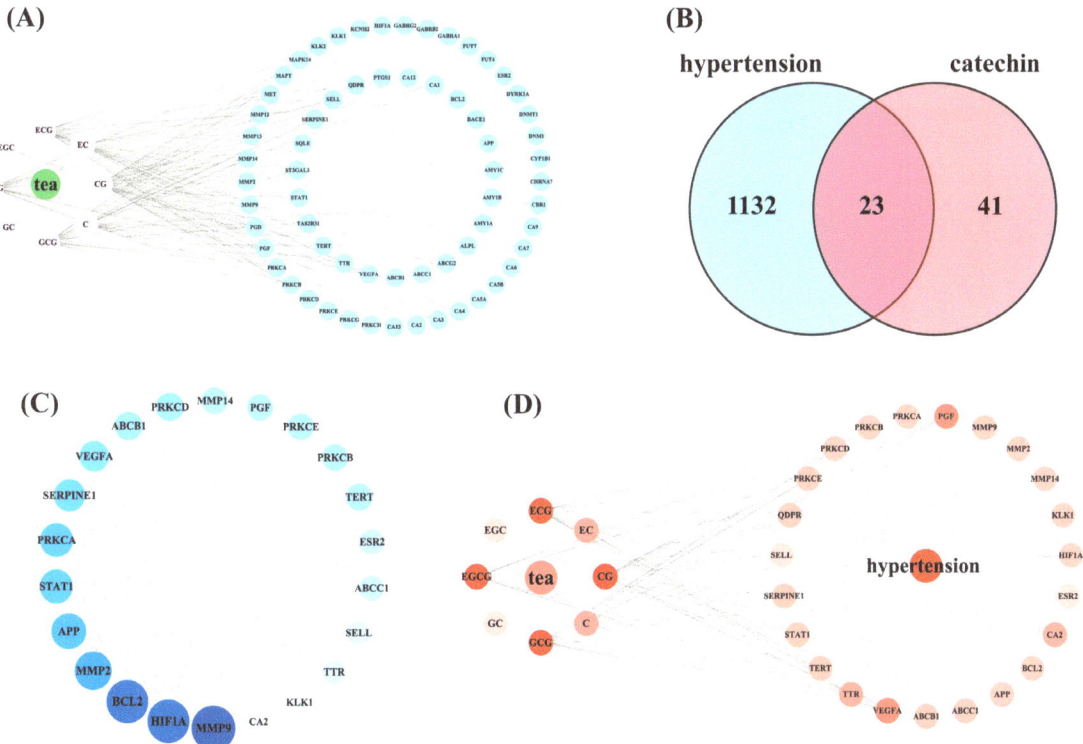

Figure 3. (**A**) Construction of the tea–catechin–targets network. (**B**) Venn diagram of predicted catechin targets and hypertension-related targets. (**C**) PPI network of intersecting targets. (**D**) tea–catechin–targets–hypertension network diagram.

To determine the key catechin components for anti-hypertension, an interaction network between the eight catechin components and the intersecting targets was constructed (Figure 3D). Notably, all these catechin components interacted with multiple targets. Among the eight catechin components, GCG, EGCG, ECG, and CG had the highest degree values (degree = 22), followed by C and EC (degree = 7) and, lastly, CG and EGC (degree = 3) (Supplementary Table S4). In summary, GCG, EGCG, ECG, and CG are likely the essential catechin components for combating hypertension.

3.3. Functional Enrichment Analysis of Key Targets

To comprehensively understand the mechanisms by which catechin components act on hypertension at the system level, KEGG and GO enrichment analyses were performed on the 23 intersecting targets. KEGG enrichment analysis revealed that the 23 intersecting targets were enriched in 90 signaling pathways ($p < 0.05$, Supplementary Table S5), including the vascular smooth muscle contraction (hsa04270), aldosterone-regulated sodium reabsorption (hsa04960), renal cell carcinoma (hsa05211), and TNF signaling pathway (hsa04668), among others (Figure 4A). Additionally, the GO enrichment results show that the targets were enriched in 1063 biological processes (BPs), seven cellular components (CCs), and 89 molecular functions (MFs) (Supplementary Table S6, $p < 0.05$). As illustrated in Figure 4B, in the BP category, the main enrichments were in positive regulation of angiogenesis (GO:0045766), endothelial cell proliferation (GO:0001935), and vascular endothelial growth factor receptor signaling pathway (GO:0048010). In the CC category, the primary enrichments were in platelet alpha granule lumen (GO:0031093), platelet alpha granule (GO:0031091), and apical part of cell (GO:0045177). In the MF category, significant enrichments included calcium-dependent protein kinase C activity (GO:0010857), vascular endothelial growth factor receptor binding (GO:0005172), and metalloendopeptidase activity (GO:0004222). The results of the KEGG pathway and GO enrichment analyses suggest that the key targets play important roles in regulating vascular smooth muscle contraction, promoting angiogenesis, and mediating vascular endothelial growth factor receptor signaling processes.

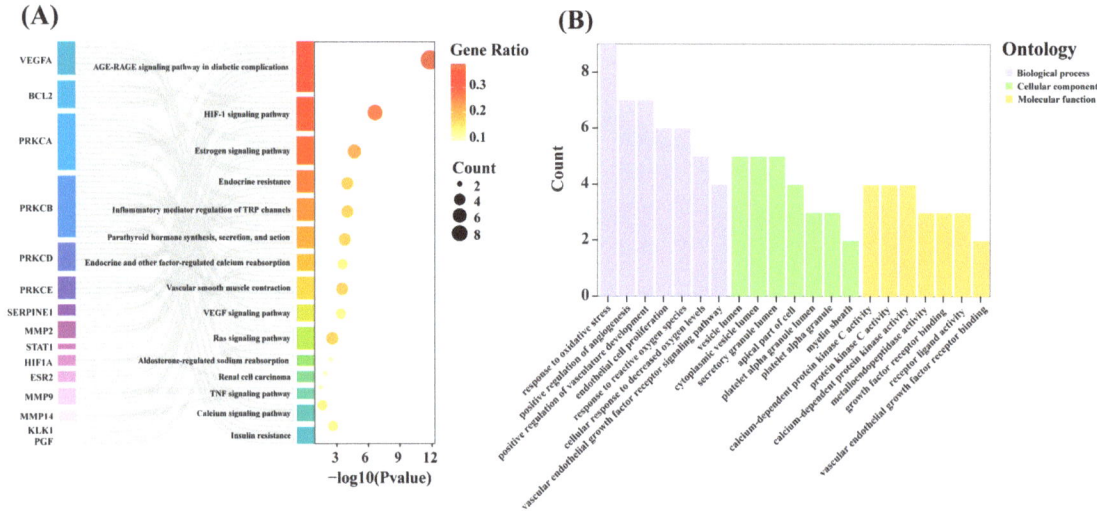

Figure 4. (**A**) KEGG pathway analysis of key targets. (**B**) GO enrichment analysis of key targets.

3.4. Molecular Docking Verification

Molecular docking was employed to evaluate the binding affinities of four catechin components with three key target genes (MMP9, HIF1A, and BCL2). The results show that the docking scores for the four catechin components with the three targets ranged from −6.2 kcal/mol to −8.9 kcal/mol (Table 1). Lower docking scores indicate stronger binding affinities, with scores < −5.0 kcal/mol indicating potential binding and scores < −7.0 kcal/mol denoting strong binding affinities [28]. For MMP9, CG and GCG exhibited the strongest binding affinities, both scoring −8.9 kcal/mol. For HIF1A and BCL2, the strongest binding ligands were ECG and EGCG, with docking scores of −8.8 kcal/mol and −6.7 kcal/mol, respectively. The reference drug enalapril had docking scores of −7.1 kcal/mol, −6.7 kcal/mol, and −6.0 kcal/mol with MMP9, HIF1A, and BCL2, respectively. Compared to the reference drug enalapril, these significant compounds demonstrated stronger binding affinities to the key targets.

The binding mechanisms between the three key targets and their selected catechin ligands are shown in Figure 5. The binding pockets of MMP9, HIF1A, and BCL2 were tightly occupied by CG, GCG, ECG, and EGCG, stabilized by hydrogen bonds and hydrophobic interactions (Supplementary Table S7). In MMP9, CG formed hydrogen bonds with LEU39 (2.75 Å), ASP185 (2.61 Å), GLY186 (2.20 Å), ARG51 (2.00 Å), ARG95 (2.69 Å and 2.67 Å), and TYR48 (3.00 Å) and hydrophobic interactions with TYR48 (5.57 Å), LEU39 (5.43 Å and 4.89 Å), and LEU44 (5.21 Å) (Figure 5A). GCG in MMP9 formed hydrogen bonds with ASP182 (2.98 Å), THR96 (2.74 Å), GLY186 (2.50 Å), TYR52 (2.14 Å), ARG51 (2.05 Å), ARG95 (2.60 Å), and TYR48 (2.98 Å) and hydrophobic interactions with TYR48 (5.55 Å), LEU39 (5.41 Å and 4.92 Å), and LEU44 (5.15 Å) (Figure 5B). In HIF1A, ECG formed hydrogen bonds with TYR325 (2.30 Å), LYS465 (2.28 Å), ARG440 (1.94 Å), and VAL464 (2.51 Å) and hydrophobic interactions with PRO360 (4.95 Å), VAL464 (5.49 Å), PRO360 (4.74 Å), LYS328 (4.47 Å), VAL464 (4.32 Å), and PRO360 (5.18 Å) (Figure 5C). EGCG in BCL2 formed hydrogen bonds with VAL117 (2.70 Å), GLU113 (2.89 Å), LYS24 (2.27 Å), ARG28 (2.22 Å), and SER66 (2.53 Å) and hydrophobic interactions with ARG28 (5.12 Å and 3.82 Å), VAL117 (5.38 Å), and VAL120 (5.13 Å) (Figure 5D). These results indicate that catechin components effectively bind to the core targets through hydrogen bonds and hydrophobic interactions.

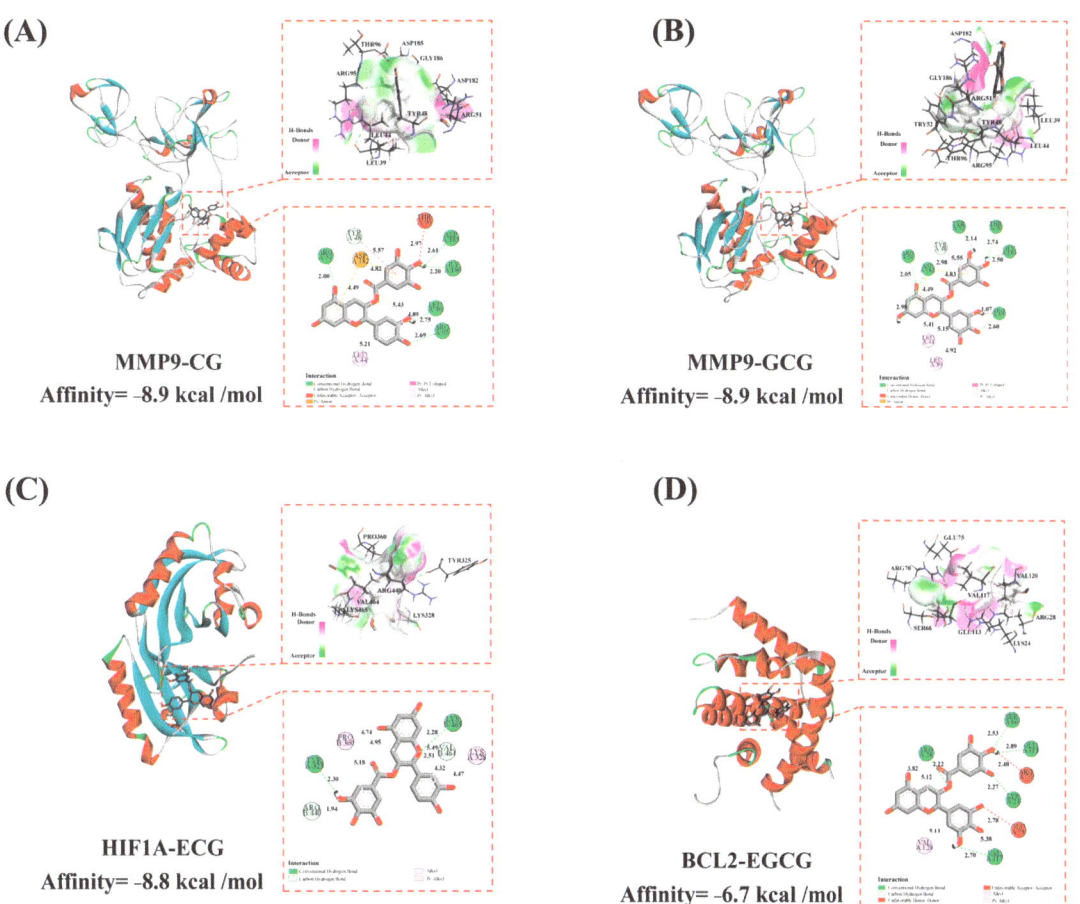

Figure 5. Molecular docking of main catechin components with MMP9, HIF1A, and BCL2. (**A**) Interaction diagram between MMP9 and gallocatechin gallate (GCG). (**B**) Interaction diagram between MMP9 and catechin gallate (CG). (**C**) Interaction diagram between HIF1A and epicatechin gallate (ECG). (**D**) Interaction diagram between BCL2 and epigallocatechin gallate (EGCG).

Table 1. Molecular docking results of catechin components with core targets.

Compound Name	Affinity (kcal/mol)			
	MMP9	HIF1A	BCL2	Mean
CG	−8.9	−8.6	−6.5	−8.0
GCG	−8.9	−8.4	−6.5	−7.9
ECG	−8.0	−8.8	−6.2	−7.7
EGCG	−8.0	−8.5	−6.7	−7.7
Mean	−8.5	−8.6	−6.5	
enalapril	−7.1	−6.7	−6.0	−6.6

3.5. Molecular Dynamics Simulations and Binding Free Energy Calculations

To further explore the stability of protein–ligand interactions, molecular dynamics (MD) simulations were performed on four protein–ligand complexes: MMP9-CG, MMP9-GCG, HIF1A-ECG, and BCL2-EGCG. The root mean square deviation (RMSD) values were used to assess whether the simulation systems reached a stable state, with RMSD values within 1 nm indicating relative stability of protein–ligand interactions in a physiological environment [29]. As shown in Figure 6A, the RMSD values of the four complexes rapidly stabilized at 0.59 ± 0.16 Å, 0.46 ± 0.12 Å, 0.17 ± 0.03 Å, and 0.24 ± 0.05 Å, respectively. The radius of gyration (Rg) was analyzed to evaluate the compactness of receptor–ligand binding. As depicted in Figure 6B, the Rg values of the complexes remained stable throughout the simulation, stabilizing at 2.46 ± 0.03 nm, 2.42 ± 0.03 nm, 1.78 ± 0.01 nm, and 1.61 ± 0.01 nm, respectively. The solvent-accessible surface area (SASA) is an important parameter reflecting protein folding and stability. The SASA values of the four complexes also demonstrated stability, reaching average values of 215.79 ± 2.79 nm^2, 218.87 ± 4.42 nm^2, 115.76 ± 2.49 nm^2, and 99.47 ± 1.90 nm^2, respectively (Figure 6C). The number of hydrogen bonds reflects the strength of protein–ligand binding, with MMP9-GCG showing the highest hydrogen bond density and strength, followed by MMP9-CG, HIF1A-ECG, and BCL2-EGCG (Figure 6D).

The binding free energies (ΔG_{bind}) of the four protein–ligand complexes were further calculated using the MM/GBSA method. Lower ΔG_{bind} values indicate stronger receptor–ligand binding affinity [30]. As shown in Figure 6E, the ΔG_{bind} rankings of the four complexes were MMP9-CG (−29.34 kcal/mol) < MMP9-GCG (−27.7 kcal/mol) < HIF1A-ECG (−24.32 kcal/mol) < BCL2-EGCG (−21.89 kcal/mol), which is consistent with the molecular docking results.

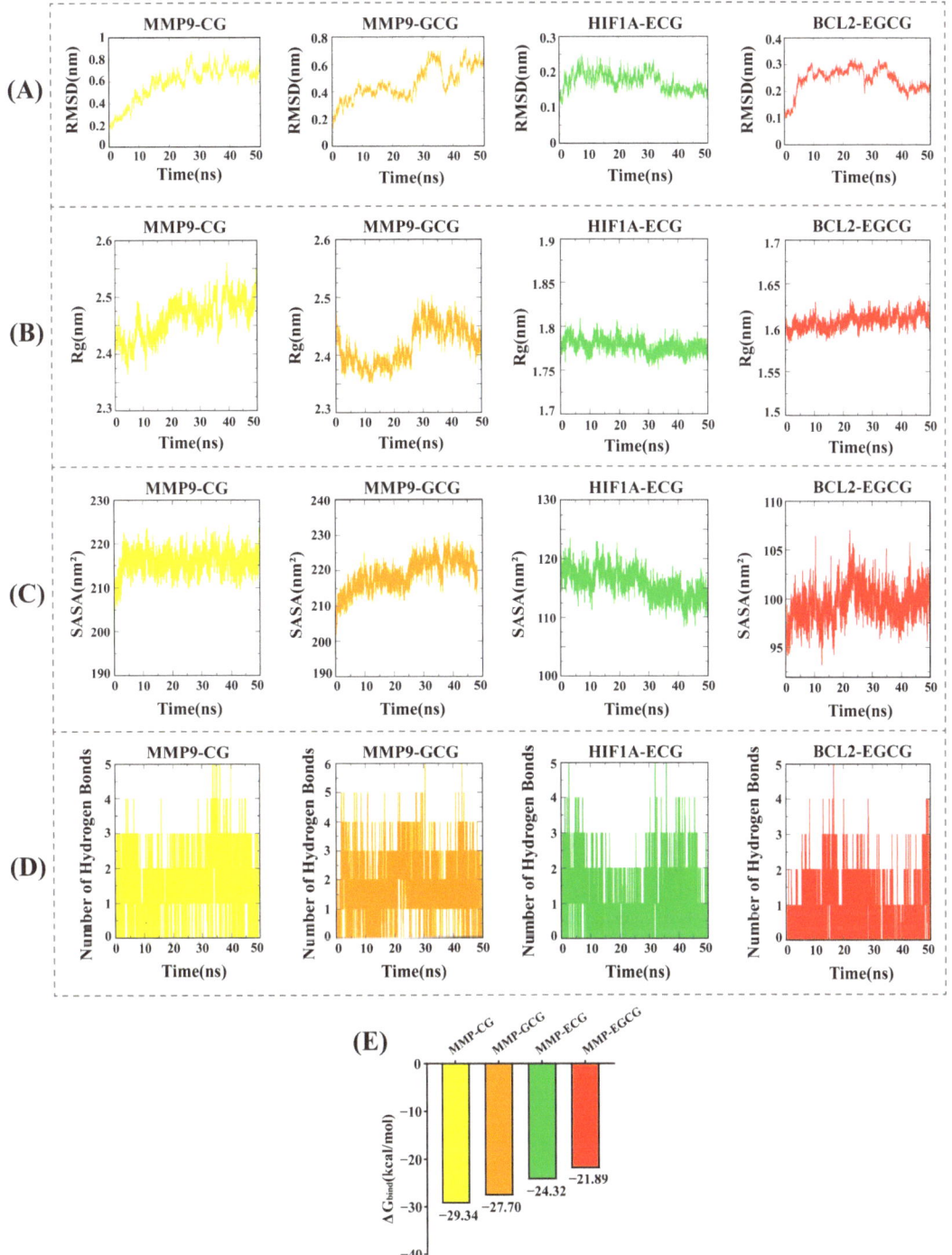

Figure 6. (**A**) RMSD values of the four complexes. (**B**) Radius of gyration (Rg) values of the four complexes. (**C**) Solvent-accessible surface area (SASA) values of the four complexes. (**D**) Number of hydrogen bonds in the four complexes. (**E**) Binding free energies (ΔG_{bind}) of the four complexes.

4. Discussion

Hypertension is increasingly acknowledged as a critical global public health concern due to its chronic nature [9]. Catechins have been confirmed to resist atherosclerosis, regulate intestinal microbiota dysbiosis, improve endothelial cell function, and modulate inflammatory signaling, thereby mitigating the adverse effects of hypertension [18,31]. Network pharmacology, known for its "multi-component, multi-target, and multi-pathway" characteristics, is utilized in this study to investigate the primary targets and potential mechanisms by which catechins exert anti-hypertensive effects, integrating it with computational simulation techniques.

The tea catechin–targets–hypertension network indicates that GCG, EGCG, ECG, and CG have high degree values. Consequently, these key catechin components were further analyzed for their therapeutic effects on hypertension. Chronic inflammation is considered a significant cause of hypertension, and reducing inflammation may aid in the prevention and treatment of hypertension [32]. It has been reported that EGCG, GCG, and CG possess various biological and pharmacological activities, including antioxidant, anti-inflammatory, and anti-angiogenic properties [33–35]. ECG and EGCG in tea play crucial roles in reducing serum cholesterol levels and inhibiting postprandial hyperlipidemia [36]. Redford et al. [37] found through rat experiments that the activation of vascular and neuronal KCNQ5 potassium channels significantly promotes vasodilation in both green and black tea, suggesting that ECG, EGCG, or their optimized derivatives are potential candidates for future anti-hypertensive drug development.

PPI network analysis revealed three potential key targets—MMP9, HIF1A, and BCL2—that are significantly implicated in the treatment of hypertension with catechins. These genes likely play a role in the therapeutic mechanisms by which catechins mitigate hypertension. Studies have shown that the knocking out of matrix metalloproteinase 9 (MMP9) in hypertensive rats can prevent the development of hypertension, proteinuria, glomerular damage, and renal interstitial fibrosis [38]. Cardiovascular diseases significantly impact blood pressure levels, and BCL2, a key anti-apoptotic protein, can serve as a target for modern cardioprotective therapies [39]. HIF1A, a hypoxia-inducible factor, was found to play an essential role in activating the transcriptional cofactor FOG2 in a CMVD mouse model of mild hypertension–diabetes injury, a condition relevant to human disease [40]. Therefore, MMP9, HIF1A, and BCL2 are closely linked to the onset and progression of hypertension, and catechin components may deliver their anti-hypertensive benefits through interactions with these target proteins.

GO and KEGG pathway enrichment analyses revealed key pathways involved in the anti-hypertension effects of catechins. The GO enrichment analysis indicated that the key targets of catechins were primarily enriched in biological processes such as the positive regulation of angiogenesis, the vascular endothelial growth factor receptor signaling pathway, and the vascular endothelial growth factor receptor binding. KEGG pathway enrichment analysis revealed that catechins were involved in several signaling pathways pertinent to hypertension treatment, including vascular smooth muscle contraction, aldosterone-regulated sodium reabsorption, and renal cell carcinoma. Vascular smooth muscle is a crucial component of the blood vessel wall; under hypertensive conditions, its sustained contraction leads to thickening of the vessel wall and increased vascular resistance, thereby elevating blood pressure [41]. Pulmonary arterial hypertension (PAH) is a progressive and complex pulmonary vascular disease, with HIF1A identified as a potential biomarker and therapeutic target for PAH [42]. Aldosterone, a hormone secreted by the adrenal glands, causes sodium and water retention, increasing blood volume and consequently raising blood pressure when at elevated levels, such as in primary aldosteronism [43]. Studies have shown that aldosterone induces MMP9 expression by activating CaMKII through oxidative stress. This exerts direct toxic effects on the myocardium, leading to increased cardiac rupture and mortality post-myocardial infarction in mice [44]. Renal cell carcinoma may contribute to hypertension by activating the renin–angiotensin system and affecting renal structure and function [45]. BCL2 and MMP9 have been found to play significant roles in tumor immunity and may serve as potential novel biomarkers and therapeutic targets for immunotherapy of clear cell renal cell carcinoma (ccRCC) [46,47]. Therefore, catechins achieve their anti-hypertensive effects through the regulation of various biological pathways.

Further, computational simulations were used to explore the binding affinity and mechanisms of catechins with key hypertension-related targets. The molecular docking results show that the docking scores for the four catechin components with the three targets were all less than −5 kcal/mol. The optimal catechin–ligand complexes formed with the three targets were MMP9-CG, MMP9-GCG, HIF1A-ECG, and BCL2-GCG, primarily driven by hydrogen bonding and hydrophobic interactions. Subsequently, molecular dynamics simulations were conducted to analyze the dynamic behavior and stability of the catechin–target complexes over time. The values of RMSD, Rg, and SASA and the number of hydrogen bonds indicated that the four complexes possessed reliable structural stability and compactness. Additionally, the binding free energies (ΔG_{bind}) of the four protein–ligand complexes were analyzed using the MM/PBSA method, showing strong binding affinities, which corroborated the molecular docking results.

This study used network pharmacology to predict three key targets and pathways associated with the anti-hypertensive effects of four catechin components. Futhermore, the binding mechanisms between these catechin components and key targets were investigated using computer simulations. However, this study has certain limitations. Future research should utilize cell experiments and animal models to validate and explore the mechanisms by which catechins regulate hypertension-related pathways in vivo and in vitro, aiming to provide more effective and safer treatment options for patients with hypertension.

5. Conclusions

In this study, network pharmacology and computer simulation were used to explore the potential targets and molecular mechanisms of catechins in anti-hypertension. CG, GCG, ECG, and EGCG were identified as key catechin components for combating hypertension, with MMP9, HIF1A, and BCL2 as potential critical therapeutic targets. Molecular docking and molecular dynamics simulation results illustrate that catechins effectively bind to key targets through hydrogen bonding and hydrophobic interactions. These findings support the potential of catechins as functional additives for treating or preventing hypertension, providing a valuable foundation for further research. However, it is important to note that further pharmacological and clinical studies are required to validate our conclusions.

Supplementary Materials: The following supporting information can be downloaded at: https://www.mdpi.com/article/10.3390/foods13172685/s1, Table S1: Information for 64 potential targets of catechin components; Table S2: Hypertension-related 1155 potential targets in 3 databases; Table S3: PPI network of key targets; Table S4: Catechin-core target degree; Table S5: 90 signaling pathways from KEGG enrichment analysis; Table S6: BP, CC, and MF from GO enrichment analysis; Table S7: Molecular docking data of four key catechin components and core.

Author Contributions: Conceptualization, Y.T. and X.L.; software, F.T.; formal analysis, Y.S.; investigation, F.X. and X.W.; writing—original draft preparation, Y.T.; writing—review and editing, M.T., Y.H., and J.L. All authors have read and agreed to the published version of the manuscript.

Funding: This research was funded by the Ministry of Agriculture and Rural Affairs: The Construction of Anxi Modern Agricultural Industrial Park (KMD18003A), Teaching and Research Team Fund Project of Fujian Agriculture and Forestry University (111418T05). The funders had no role in the design, determination, and interpretation of data or in writing the manuscript.

Institutional Review Board Statement: Not applicable.

Informed Consent Statement: Not applicable.

Data Availability Statement: The original contributions presented in the study are included in the article/supplementary material, further inquiries can be directed to the corresponding authors.

Conflicts of Interest: The authors declare that they have no known competing financial interests or personal relationships that could have appeared to influence the work reported in this paper.

List of Major Abbreviations

Abbreviation	Full name
HTN	hypertension
C	catechin
EC	epicatechin
GC	gallocatechin
EGC	epigallocatechin
CG	catechin gallate
ECG	epicatechin gallate
GCG	gallocatechin gallate
EGCG	epigallocatechin gallate
RMSD	root mean square deviation
Rg	radius of gyration
SASA	solvent-accessible surface area
MD	molecular dynamics
BP	biological process
CC	cellular component
MF	molecular function
PPI	protein–protein interaction
ΔG_{bind}	binding free energies

References

1. Li, H.; Guo, H.; Luo, Q.; Wu, D.-T.; Zou, L.; Liu, Y.; Li, H.-B.; Gan, R.-Y. Current extraction, purification, and identification techniques of tea polyphenols: An updated review. *Crit. Rev. Food Sci. Nutr.* **2021**, *63*, 3912–3930. [CrossRef] [PubMed]
2. Sun, M.-F.; Jiang, C.-L.; Kong, Y.-S.; Luo, J.-L.; Yin, P.; Guo, G.-Y. Recent Advances in Analytical Methods for Determination of Polyphenols in Tea: A Comprehensive Review. *Foods* **2022**, *11*, 1425. [CrossRef] [PubMed]
3. Sabaghi, M.; Hoseyni, S.Z.; Tavasoli, S.; Mozafari, M.; Katouzian, I. Strategies of confining green tea catechin compounds in nano-biopolymeric matrices: A review. *Colloids Surfaces B Biointerfaces* **2021**, *204*, 111781. [CrossRef]
4. Lin, C.; Xia, G.; Liu, S. Modeling and comparison of extraction kinetics of 8 catechins, gallic acid and caffeine from representative white teas. *LWT Food Sci. Technol.* **2017**, *83*, 1–9. [CrossRef]
5. Kim, E.; Hwang, K.; Lee, J.; Han, S.Y.; Kim, E.-M.; Park, J.; Cho, J.Y. Skin Protective Effect of Epigallocatechin Gallate. *Int. J. Mol. Sci.* **2018**, *19*, 173. [CrossRef]
6. Tounekti, T.; Joubert, E.; Hernández, I.; Munné-Bosch, S. Improving the Polyphenol Content of Tea. *Crit. Rev. Plant Sci.* **2012**, *32*, 192–215. [CrossRef]
7. Cao, Y.; Cao, R. Angiogenesis inhibited by drinking tea. *Nature* **1999**, *398*, 381. [CrossRef]
8. Orita, T.; Chogahara, S.; Okuda, M.; Sakao, K.; Miyata, T.; Hou, D.-X. Extraction Efficiency and Alpha-Glucosidase Inhibitory Activities of Green Tea Catechins by Different Infusion Methods. *Foods* **2023**, *12*, 2611. [CrossRef]
9. Qamar, A.; Braunwald, E. Treatment of hypertension addressing a global health problem. *JAMA* **2018**, *320*, 1751–1752. [CrossRef]
10. Khan, M.U.; Aziz, S.; Akram, T.; Amjad, F.; Iqtidar, K.; Nam, Y.; Khan, M.A. Expert Hypertension Detection System Featuring Pulse Plethysmograph Signals and Hybrid Feature Selection and Reduction Scheme. *Sensors* **2021**, *21*, 247. [CrossRef]
11. Grandi, S.M.; Reynier, P.; Platt, R.W.; Basso, O.; Filion, K.B. The timing of onset of hypertensive disorders in pregnancy and the risk of incident hypertension and cardiovascular disease. *Int. J. Cardiol.* **2018**, *270*, 273–275. [CrossRef]
12. On-Nom, N.; Khaengamkham, K.; Kettawan, A.; Rungruang, T.; Suttisansanee, U.; Temviriyanukul, P.; Prangthip, P.; Chupeerach, C. Parboiled Germinated Brown Rice Improves Cardiac Structure and Gene Expression in Hypertensive Rats. *Foods* **2022**, *12*, 9. [CrossRef] [PubMed]
13. Wu, J.; Montaniel, K.R.C.; Saleh, M.A.; Xiao, L.; Chen, W.; Owens, G.K.; Humphrey, J.D.; Majesky, M.W.; Paik, D.T.; Hatzopoulos, A.K.; et al. The Origin of Matrix-Producing Cells That Contribute to Aortic Fibrosis in Hypertension. *Hypertension* **2016**, *67*, 461–468. [CrossRef] [PubMed]
14. Lin, Q.-F.; Qiu, C.-S.; Wang, S.-L.; Huang, L.-F.; Chen, Z.-Y.; Chen, Y.; Chen, G. A Cross-sectional Study of the Relationship Between Habitual Tea Consumption and Arterial Stiffness. *J. Am. Coll. Nutr.* **2015**, *35*, 354–361. [CrossRef]
15. Hodgson, J.M.; Croft, K.D. Tea flavonoids and cardiovascular health. *Mol. Asp. Med.* **2010**, *31*, 495–502. [CrossRef]
16. Hooper, L.; Kroon, P.A.; Rimm, E.B.; Cohn, J.S.; Harvey, I.; Le Cornu, K.A.; Ryder, J.J.; Hall, W.L.; Cassidy, A. Flavonoids, flavonoid-rich foods, and cardiovascular risk: A meta-analysis of randomized controlled trials. *Am. J. Clin. Nutr.* **2008**, *88*, 38–50. [CrossRef] [PubMed]

17. Garcia, M.L.; Pontes, R.B.; Nishi, E.E.; Ibuki, F.K.; Oliveira, V.; Sawaya, A.; Carvalho, P.O.; Nogueira, F.N.; Franco, M.D.; Campos, R.R.; et al. The antioxidant effects of green tea reduces blood pressure and sympathoexcitation in an experimental model of hypertension. *J. Hypertens.* **2017**, *35*, 348–354. [CrossRef]
18. Del Seppia, C.; Federighi, G.; Lapi, D.; Gerosolimo, F.; Scuri, R. Effects of a catechins-enriched diet associated with moderate physical exercise in the prevention of hypertension in spontaneously hypertensive rats. *Sci. Rep.* **2022**, *12*, 17303. [CrossRef]
19. Sabri, N.A.M.; Lee, S.-K.; Murugan, D.D.; Ling, W.C. Epigallocatechin gallate (EGCG) alleviates vascular dysfunction in angiotensin II-infused hypertensive mice by modulating oxidative stress and eNOS. *Sci. Rep.* **2022**, *12*, 17633. [CrossRef]
20. Wang, X.; Wang, Z.-Y.; Zheng, J.-H.; Li, S. TCM network pharmacology: A new trend towards combining computational, experimental and clinical approaches. *Chin. J. Nat. Med.* **2021**, *19*, 1–11. [CrossRef]
21. Zhao, L.; Zhang, H.; Li, N.; Chen, J.; Xu, H.; Wang, Y.; Liang, Q. Network pharmacology, a promising approach to reveal the pharmacology mechanism of Chinese medicine formula. *J. Ethnopharmacol.* **2023**, *309*, 116306. [CrossRef]
22. Yu, Y.; Zhou, M.; Long, X.; Yin, S.; Hu, G.; Yang, X.; Jian, W.; Yu, R. Study on the mechanism of action of colchicine in the treatment of coronary artery disease based on network pharmacology and molecular docking technology. *Front. Pharmacol.* **2023**, *14*, 1147360. [CrossRef] [PubMed]
23. Bai, G.; Pan, Y.; Zhang, Y.; Li, Y.; Wang, J.; Wang, Y.; Teng, W.; Jin, G.; Geng, F.; Cao, J. Research advances of molecular docking and molecular dynamic simulation in recognizing interaction between muscle proteins and exogenous additives. *Food Chem.* **2023**, *429*, 136836. [CrossRef] [PubMed]
24. Szklarczyk, D.; Kirsch, R.; Koutrouli, M.; Nastou, K.; Mehryary, F.; Hachilif, R.; Gable, A.L.; Fang, T.; Doncheva, N.T.; Pyysalo, S.; et al. The STRING database in 2023: Protein-protein association networks and functional enrichment analyses for any sequenced genome of interest. *Nucleic Acids Res.* **2023**, *51*, D638–D646. [CrossRef] [PubMed]
25. Ko, M.; Kim, Y.; Kim, H.H.; Jeong, S.; Ahn, D.; Chung, S.J.; Kim, H. Network pharmacology and molecular docking approaches to elucidate the potential compounds and targets of Saeng-Ji-Hwang-Ko for treatment of type 2 diabetes mellitus. *Comput. Biol. Med.* **2022**, *149*, 106041. [CrossRef]
26. Eberhardt, J.; Santos-Martins, D.; Tillack, A.F.; Forli, S. AutoDock Vina 1.2.0: New Docking Methods, Expanded Force Field, and Python Bindings. *J. Chem. Inf. Model.* **2021**, *61*, 3891–3898. [CrossRef]
27. Dash, S.G.; Kantevari, S.; Guru, S.K.; Naik, P.K. Combination of docetaxel and newly synthesized 9-Br-trimethoxybenzyl-noscapine improve tubulin binding and enhances antitumor activity in breast cancer cells. *Comput. Biol. Med.* **2021**, *139*, 104996. [CrossRef]
28. Li, C.; Wen, R.; Liu, D.; Yan, L.; Gong, Q.; Yu, H. Assessment of the Potential of Sarcandra glabra (Thunb.) Nakai. in Treating Ethanol-Induced Gastric Ulcer in Rats Based on Metabolomics and Network Analysis. *Front. Pharmacol.* **2022**, *13*, 810344. [CrossRef]
29. Sarker, P.; Mitro, A.; Hoque, H.; Hasan, N.; Jewel, G.N.A. Identification of potential novel therapeutic drug target against Elizabethkingia anophelis by integrative pan and subtractive genomic analysis: An in silico approach. *Comput. Biol. Med.* **2023**, *165*, 107436. [CrossRef]
30. Marciniak, A.; Kotynia, A.; Szkatuła, D.; Krzyżak, E. The 2-hydroxy-3-(4-aryl-1-piperazinyl)propyl Phthalimide Derivatives as Prodrugs—Spectroscopic and Theoretical Binding Studies with Plasma Proteins. *Int. J. Mol. Sci.* **2022**, *23*, 7003. [CrossRef]
31. Liu, Y.; Long, Y.; Fang, J.; Liu, G. Advances in the Anti-Atherosclerotic Mechanisms of Epigallocatechin Gallate. *Nutrients* **2024**, *16*, 2074. [CrossRef] [PubMed]
32. Ma, L.-L.; Xiao, H.-B.; Zhang, J.; Liu, Y.-H.; Hu, L.-K.; Chen, N.; Chu, X.; Dong, J.; Yan, Y.-X. Association between systemic immune inflammatory/inflammatory response index and hypertension: A cohort study of functional community. *Nutr. Metab. Cardiovasc. Dis.* **2024**, *34*, 334–342. [CrossRef] [PubMed]
33. Zhang, Y.; Owusu, L.; Duan, W.; Jiang, T.; Zang, S.; Ahmed, A.; Xin, Y. Anti-metastatic and differential effects on protein expression of epigallocatechin-3-gallate in HCCLM6 hepatocellular carcinoma cells. *Int. J. Mol. Med.* **2013**, *32*, 959–964. [CrossRef] [PubMed]
34. Gao, X.; Lin, X.; Li, X.; Zhang, Y.; Chen, Z.; Li, B. Cellular antioxidant, methylglyoxal trapping, and anti-inflammatory activities of cocoa tea (Camellia ptilophylla Chang). *Food Funct.* **2017**, *8*, 2836–2846. [CrossRef]
35. Iijima, T.; Mohri, Y.; Hattori, Y.; Kashima, A.; Kamo, T.; Hirota, M.; Kiyota, H.; Makabe, H. Synthesis of (−)-Epicatechin 3-(3-O-Methylgallate) and (+)-Catechin 3-(3-O-Methylgallate), and Their Anti-Inflammatory Activity. *Chem. Biodivers.* **2009**, *6*, 520–526. [CrossRef]
36. Ikeda, I. Multifunctional effects of green tea catechins on prevention of the metabolic syndrome. *Asia Pac. J. Clin Nutr.* **2008**, *17*, 273–274. [PubMed]
37. Redford, K.E.; Rognant, S.; Jepps, T.A.; Abbott, G.W. KCNQ5 Potassium Channel Activation Underlies Vasodilation by Tea. *Cell. Physiol. Biochem.* **2021**, *55*, 46–64. [CrossRef]
38. Zhang, C.; Mims, P.N.; Zhu, T.; Fan, F.; Roman, R.J. Abstract 097: Knockout of Matrix Metalloproteinase 9 Protects Against Hypertension-induced Renal Disease in Hypertensive Dahl S Rats. *Hypertension* **2017**, *70*, A097. [CrossRef]
39. Korshunova, A.Y.; Blagonravov, M.L.; Neborak, E.V.; Syatkin, S.P.; Sklifasovskaya, A.P.; Semyatov, S.M.; Agostinelli, E. BCL2-regulated apoptotic process in myocardial ischemia-reperfusion injury (Review). *Int. J. Mol. Med.* **2020**, *47*, 23–36. [CrossRef]

40. Guerraty, M.A.; Szapary, H.J.; Berrido, A.; Arany, Z.P.; Rader, D.J. Abstract 219: Role of Transcription Co-Factor Friend of GATA 2 (FOG2) in a Hypertensive-Diabetic Mouse Model of Coronary Microvascular Disease. *Arter. Thromb. Vasc. Biol.* **2018**, *38*, A455. [CrossRef]
41. Touyz, R.M.; Alves-Lopes, R.; Rios, F.J.; Camargo, L.L.; Anagnostopoulou, A.; Arner, A.; Montezano, A.C. Vascular smooth muscle contraction in hypertension. *Cardiovasc. Res.* **2018**, *114*, 529–539. [CrossRef] [PubMed]
42. Wei, R.-Q.; Zhang, W.-M.; Liang, Z.; Piao, C.; Zhu, G. Identification of Signal Pathways and Hub Genes of Pulmonary Arterial Hypertension by Bioinformatic Analysis. *Can. Respir. J.* **2022**, *2022*, 1394088. [CrossRef] [PubMed]
43. Shoemaker, R.; Poglitsch, M.; Davis, D.; Huang, H.; Schadler, A.; Patel, N.; Vignes, K.; Srinivasan, A.; Cockerham, C.; Bauer, J.A.; et al. Association of Elevated Serum Aldosterone Concentrations in Pregnancy with Hypertension. *Biomedicines* **2023**, *11*, 2954. [CrossRef] [PubMed]
44. He, B.J.; Joiner, M.-L.A.; Singh, M.V.; Luczak, E.D.; Swaminathan, P.D.; Koval, O.M.; Kutschke, W.; Allamargot, C.; Yang, J.; Guan, X.; et al. Oxidation of CaMKII determines the cardiotoxic effects of aldosterone. *Nat. Med.* **2011**, *17*, 1610–1618. [CrossRef] [PubMed]
45. Bendtsen, M.A.F.; Grimm, D.; Bauer, J.; Wehland, M.; Wise, P.; Magnusson, N.E.; Infanger, M.; Krüger, M. Hypertension Caused by Lenvatinib and Everolimus in the Treatment of Metastatic Renal Cell Carcinoma. *Int. J. Mol. Sci.* **2017**, *18*, 1736. [CrossRef]
46. Xu, T.; Gao, S.; Liu, J.; Huang, Y.; Chen, K.; Zhang, X. MMP9 and IGFBP1 Regulate Tumor Immune and Drive Tumor Progression in Clear Cell Renal Cell Carcinoma. *J. Cancer* **2021**, *12*, 2243–2257. [CrossRef]
47. Feng, X.; Yan, N.; Sun, W.; Zheng, S.; Jiang, S.; Wang, J.; Guo, C.; Hao, L.; Tian, Y.; Liu, S.; et al. miR-4521-FAM129A axial regulation on ccRCC progression through TIMP-1/MMP2/MMP9 and MDM2/p53/Bcl2/Bax pathways. *Cell Death Discov.* **2019**, *5*, 89. [CrossRef]

Disclaimer/Publisher's Note: The statements, opinions and data contained in all publications are solely those of the individual author(s) and contributor(s) and not of MDPI and/or the editor(s). MDPI and/or the editor(s) disclaim responsibility for any injury to people or property resulting from any ideas, methods, instructions or products referred to in the content.

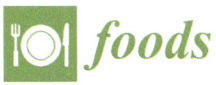

Article

¹H NMR Spectroscopy Combined with Machine-Learning Algorithm for Origin Recognition of Chinese Famous Green Tea Longjing Tea

Zhiwei Hou [1,*,†], Yugu Jin [1,†], Zhe Gu [1], Ran Zhang [1], Zhucheng Su [1] and Sitong Liu [2]

[1] College of Tea Science and Tea Culture, Zhejiang A & F University, 666 Wusu Street, Hangzhou 311300, China; jinyugu0011@163.com (Y.J.); kaaaphapi@163.com (Z.G.); zhangran@163.com (R.Z.); zhuchengsu@zafu.edu.cn (Z.S.)
[2] Hangzhou Tea Research Institute, CHINA COOP, Hangzhou 310016, China; sytoneliu@163.com
* Correspondence: houzhiwei@zafu.edu.cn
† These authors contributed equally to this work.

Abstract: Premium green tea is a high-value agricultural product significantly influenced by its geographical origin, making it susceptible to food fraud. This study utilized nuclear magnetic resonance (NMR) spectroscopy to perform chemical fingerprint analysis on 78 Longjing tea (LJT) samples from both protected designation of origin (PDO) regions (Zhejiang) and non-PDO regions (Sichuan, Guangxi, and Guizhou) in China. Unsupervised algorithms and heatmaps were employed for the visual analysis of the data from PDO and non-PDO teas while exploring the feasibility of linear and nonlinear machine-learning algorithms in discriminating the origin of LJT. The findings revealed that the nonlinear model random forest (92.2%), exhibited superior performance compared to the linear model linear discriminant analysis (85.6%). The random forest model identified 15 key marker metabolites for the geographical origin of LJT, such as kaempferol glycoside, glutamine, and ECG. The results support the conclusion that the integration of NMR with machine-learning classification serves as an effective tool for the quality assessment and origin identification of LJT.

Keywords: NMR; Longjing tea; protected designation of origin; machine learning

Citation: Hou, Z.; Jin, Y.; Gu, Z.; Zhang, R.; Su, Z.; Liu, S. ¹H NMR Spectroscopy Combined with Machine-Learning Algorithm for Origin Recognition of Chinese Famous Green Tea Longjing Tea. *Foods* 2024, *13*, 2702. https://doi.org/10.3390/foods13172702

Academic Editor: Chiara Portesi

Received: 23 July 2024
Revised: 20 August 2024
Accepted: 26 August 2024
Published: 27 August 2024

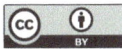

Copyright: © 2024 by the authors. Licensee MDPI, Basel, Switzerland. This article is an open access article distributed under the terms and conditions of the Creative Commons Attribution (CC BY) license (https:// creativecommons.org/licenses/by/ 4.0/).

1. Introduction

Longjing tea is a famous Chinese premium green tea, originating from three regions in Zhejiang Province [1]. According to Chinese national standard (GB/T 18650-2008) [2], flat green tea produced outside the Xihu area and Qiantang area in Hangzhou City, as well as the Yuezhou area in Shaoxing City, Zhejiang Province, cannot be marketed under the label "Longjing Tea" [3]. However, unscrupulous traders often mislabel green tea from other regions as LJT to deceive consumers and gain higher profits [4]. Since consumers are willing to pay a premium for LJT with a protected designation of origin (PDO), this leads to fraudulent behavior in the tea market [5]. Therefore, the development of identification techniques for the origin of LJT is of great significance for the protection of consumers' rights and interests as well as for the quality supervision of the market sector.

Traditional tea origin identification differentiates tea based on attributes such as appearance, aroma, taste, and tea color [6,7]. However, these sensory reviewers require long-term training, are subjective in their conclusions, and are susceptible to environmental factors. Therefore, researchers are keen to develop objective tea quality assessment methods to replace the traditional sensory review. Over the past decade, various methods have been proposed to determine the geographical origin of tea. These methods include analyzing the chemical composition, elemental composition, and spectral fingerprints of tea, as well as by using combinations of these approaches. For instance, Ma et al. employed inductively coupled plasma mass spectrometry (ICP-MS) to differentiate Biluochun green tea samples from three distinct regions [8]. Although the discrimination rate reached 96.4%, the method requires a complex pre-treatment process that consumes significant sample preparation time, making it impractical for constructing the large datasets needed for origin traceability. On the other hand, Yun et al. used head-space gas chromatography-mass spectrometry (HS-GC/MS) to achieve a 100% origin identification rate for several black teas [9]. However, mass spectrometry analyses usually take a long time and depend on the experience of the spectrometry. Many researchers have also tried to differentiate tea origins by analytical methods such as high-performance liquid chromatography (HPLC) [10] and stable isotope ratio mass spectrometry (IRMS) [11]. However, these methods are still inefficient and there is an urgent need to develop faster methods for origin tracing.

NMR spectroscopy is a rapid technique for sample preparation and data acquisition, offering the advantage of minimal sample processing and consistent data generation. This makes it applicable to various purposes in determining the origin of food products [12]. For example, Cui et al. achieved a 95.7% origin discrimination rate for four Huajiao origins using ^{1}H NMR combined with chemometrics [13]. Recently, Cui et al. also achieved a 92.7% discrimination rate for 219 black tea samples from seven origins using ^{1}H NMR combined with a machine-learning algorithm [14]. By combining the fast data acquisition capability of ^{1}H NMR with chemometric analysis methods, it provides a viable solution for tea origin traceability. Widely used analytical and visual chemometrics methods include principal component analysis (PCA) and projection to latent structures discriminant analysis (PLS-DA) [15]. Machinelearning algorithms are increasingly replacing traditional data processing methods due to their potential to improve discriminant performance, minimize the risk of overfitting, and eliminate irrelevant features. These algorithms can be categorized as linear and non-linear. Linear discriminant analysis (LDA) is a commonly used linear approach in machine learning. It assumes that the data in each category is normally distributed and has the same covariance matrix, aiming to find linear combinations of features that best discriminate between multiple categories [16]. However, LDA can only create linear decision boundaries and may not capture the complex relationships in the data. In contrast, random forest (RF) is an ensemble learning method that enhances classification by constructing multiple decision trees during training and outputting the class predictions of each tree [17]. Because RF combines the predictions of multiple trees, it reduces the risk of overfitting and has the ability to handle a wide range of input variables without eliminating any. Moreover, RF can provide feature variables that are more important for discrimination, which helps to understand the key variables that affect the origin of the food. Hence, it is valuable to investigate the efficacy of both linear and nonlinear models in discerning the geographical source of LJT based on metabolite analysis.

This study investigated the application of ^{1}H NMR-based methods combined with machine-learning algorithms in LJT origin identification. By analyzing the metabolic fingerprints of 78 samples from four major LJT-producing regions in China (Zhejiang, Guizhou, Sichuan, and Guangxi), linear (LDA) and non-linear (RF) machine-learning models for origin discrimination were developed. In addition, potential chemical markers for distinguishing LJT origin were revealed. The results of the study can be applied to the origin traceability of LJT and provide a new approach for the quality control of LJT.

2. Materials and Methods

2.1. Longjing Tea Sample Preparation

A total of 78 Longjing tea samples were collected from reliable suppliers (Figure 1a). These samples originated from various regions in China, including Zhejiang (42), Guizhou (12), Sichuan (9), and Guangxi (15). The samples were processed from the raw materials of three varieties of *Camellia sinensis* (Quntizhong, Longjing 43, and Wuniuzao), and their detailed information is shown in Table S1. The authenticity of the samples was confirmed by our collaborators. After the collection of samples, they were transferred to the laboratory in vacuum-sealed packages.

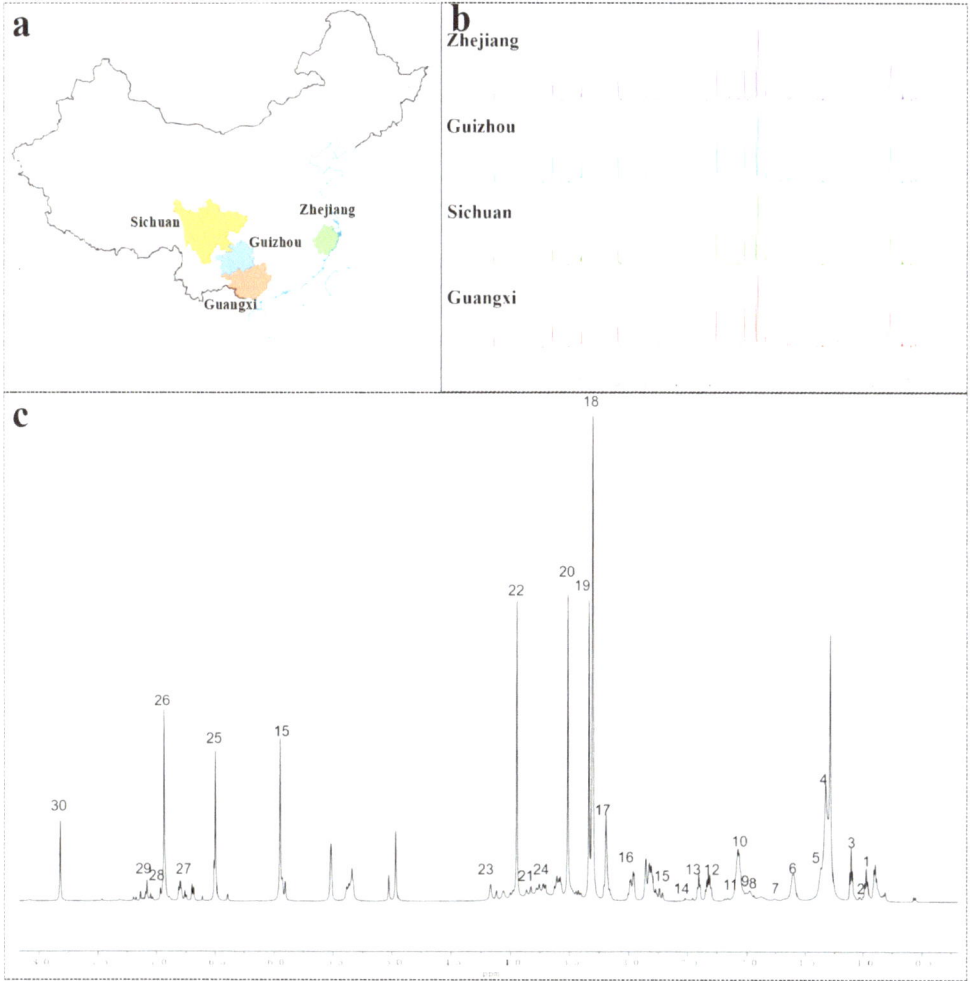

Figure 1. Geographical origin and characteristic ^{1}H NMR profiles of LJT samples. (**a**) Samples of LJT were gathered based on their designated geographical source. (**b**) Comparative ^{1}H NMR spectra of LJT extracts sourced from diverse geographical regions. (**c**) ^{1}H NMR spectrum of LJT depicted in a representative manner.

The extraction procedure follows the methodology outlined by Cui et al. [14]. Initially, all tea samples underwent grinding for a duration of 30 s utilizing an IKA A11basic grinder (manufactured in Germany). Following this, the samples were sifted through a 3 mm mesh sieve. Subsequently, 200 mg of each processed sample was blended with 3 mL of methanol-d4, which contained 0.03% Tetramethylsilane (TMS), and subjected to ultrasonic extraction at 600 W for 10 min. This was followed by centrifugation for 5 min at 15,000× g. Next, 600 µL of the supernatant was carefully collected and transferred into an NMR tube with a diameter of 5 mm. Each tea sample was prepared three times, then measured, and the average was calculated.

2.2. NMR Spectroscopy Detection

NMR detection was conducted in accordance with established methods [14]. All spectra were recorded using a 600 MHz NMR spectrometer (Bruker BioSpin GmbH, Rheinstetten, Germany) equipped with an ultra-low temperature probe. We employed a standard Bruker pulse sequence, with a spectral width spanning from −2 to 14 ppm, a center frequency set at 3600 Hz, and a test temperature maintained at 298 K. The observations were conducted at a frequency of 600 MHz, utilizing a pulse width of 10.25 µs. Each spectrum was acquired over a duration of 4.00 s, with a delay of 1 s between scans, and a total of 31 scans were performed. Corrections for spectral shifts were made based on the TMS signal (δ = 0 ppm) in the ^{1}H NMR spectra. Prior to Fourier transformation, an exponential plus weighting function, corresponding to a linewidth of 0.3 Hz, was implemented.

Regions corresponding to methanol (3.31–3.34 ppm) and TMS (0 ppm) were excluded from the analysis. Signal assignments were verified by comparing with literature sources [13] and cross-referenced using the Human Metabolome Database (HMDB; http://www.hmdb.ca/ (accessed on 5 July 2024)).

2.3. Data Analysis

Phase and baseline corrections were applied to the ^{1}H NMR spectra in the MestReNova software (Version 14.0) using the Whitakker smoothing algorithm, and a displacement calibration was performed based on the TMS internal standard at 0.0 ppm. Data reduction was performed using rectangular bins (0.04 ppm) generated in the MestReNova software, with each bin integrated by summing all intensities within that bin. The bin width of 0.04 ppm represents a compromise between maintaining sufficient data resolution and minimizing the effects of loss of spectral information and peak drift to ensure accurate peak integration. The overall intensity of the spectra was normalized using MestReNova.

PCA and sparse PLS discriminant analysis (sPLS-DA) were performed utilizing the MetaboAnalyst 5.0 online platform (https://www.metaboanalyst.ca (accessed on 5 July 2024)). To mitigate data overfitting and ensure the robustness of supervised analyses, permutation testing (n = 2000) and cross-validation techniques were applied. Additionally, heatmap generation and hierarchical clustering (HC) were conducted using MetaboAnalyst 5.0, with inter-group similarities assessed through Pearson distance metrics. The violin chart was drawn according to the relative value of the peak intensity obtained by the spectral division box.

All machine-learning procedures were executed in MATLAB R2021b (Mathworks, Waltham, MA, USA). The tea samples were divided into a training set (52 samples) and a test set (26 samples) with a 2:1 ratio. To enhance algorithm reliability, a 5-fold cross-validation strategy was employed. Linear Discriminant Analysis (LDA) provided optimal separation by projecting high-dimensional data into a discriminant vector space, thereby extracting classification information and reducing dimensionality. Random forest (RF), an ensemble method, aggregates multiple decision trees through bagging, which involves creating numerous subsets and combining several decision trees. Each subset is randomly sampled with replacement, and certain features are randomly selected as inputs, with the final classification result based on the majority vote. In this study, a random forest with 5000 trees was used to achieve superior classification performance. The efficacy of the machine-learning algorithms was evaluated using a confusion matrix.

3. Results and Discussion

3.1. Metabolomic Analysis of Longjing Tea

In this study, the metabolite composition of 78 LJT samples from four regions was assessed using ^{1}H NMR. The ^{1}H NMR spectra of LJT samples from Zhejiang, Guizhou, Sichuan, and Guangxi are depicted in Figure 1b. Preliminary comparative analysis revealed that LJT from Zhejiang and Guizhou exhibited heightened peaks in the high-field region (0.8–3.5 ppm, corresponding to amino acids) compared to those originating from Sichuan and Guangxi. In the mid-to-low field region (3.5–5.5 ppm, corresponding to carbohydrates), Zhejiang and Sichuan samples displayed similar peaks. In the low-field region above 6 ppm (aromatic compounds), Guizhou and Guangxi samples had higher peaks than those from Zhejiang and Sichuan. These findings suggest that the compound composition of LJT samples varied in different regions.

A representative ^{1}H NMR spectrum of LJT samples can be observed in Figure 1c. Based on previously reported chemical shifts and combined with public metabolomics databases [14,18–20], 30 metabolites were identified (Table 1). LJT extracts contain a diverse array of compounds, including tea polyphenols such as epigallocatechin gallate (EGCG), epicatechin (EC), epigallocatechin (EGC), and epicatechin gallate (ECG). Moreover, they also encompass caffeine and amino acids like theanine, isoleucine, and leucine, as well as organic acids including quinic acid, malic acid, and succinic acid. Additionally, these extracts are characterized by the presence of carbohydrates such as α-glucose, β-glucose, and sucrose. In prior research, it has been observed that the bitter taste and astringency of green tea can be attributed to the existence of EGCG and ECG, which may be influenced by factors like the type and quality of tea leaves. The umami flavor of green tea is primarily attributed to the presence of theanine, which exhibits a strong correlation with the timing of raw material harvest. This suggests that using ^{1}H NMR for metabolite fingerprinting analysis can reflect differences in the quality of the raw materials used in LJT from different regions.

Table 1. Thirty major metabolites were identified through the detection of ^{1}H NMR signals in methanol extracts obtained from LJT samples originating from four distinct geographical locations.

No.	Metabolite	Chemical Shift, in ppm (Multiplicity)
1	Leucine	0.97(d)
2	Isoleucine	1.03, 1.98
3	Theanine	1.10, 2.13, 2.37, 3.19, 3.72
4	Threonine	1.36, 4.23
5	Alanine	1.46 (d), 3.84
6	Arginine	1.68 (m), 1.90 (m)
7	Lysine	1.71 (m), 1.87 (m)
8	Glutamine	2.01
9	Quinic acid	2.05 (m), 3.54 (dd), 4.04 (dd)
10	Acetic acid	2.07
11	Glutamic acid	2.12 (m)
12	Chlorogenic acid	2.17 (m), 5.33 (m)
13	Malic acid	2.37 (dd), 2.63 (dd)
14	Succinic acid	2.52 (s)
15	EGC	2.62, 4.27, 6.06, 6.55, 6.80
16	EGCG	2.72, 3.08, 5.56, 6.59, 6.92
17	ECG	3.08, 4.81, 6.50, 6.95
18	Caffeine	3.22 (s), 3.38 (s), 3.77 (s)
19	Sucrose	3.43, 3.65, 3.70, 4.08, 4.23
20	α-glucose	3.50, 5.16 (d)
21	Theogallin	2.20, 3.84, 4.20
22	Serine	3.83, 3.97 (m)
23	Fructose	3.56, 4.13
24	β-glucose	3.58, 4.58
25	Rutin	4.52 (d), 5.11 (d), 6.39 (d)
26	EC	6.04, 6.11, 6.50, 6.87, 6.99
27	Quercetin glycoside	6.88, 7.63
28	Kaempferol glycoside	6.96
29	Gallic acid	7.07 (s)
30	Theobromine	7.81

3.2. PCA and sPLS-DA Analysis of Longjing Tea Origin

To evaluate the classification accuracy of LJT, PCA was employed using ^{1}H NMR chemical fingerprints. Additionally, it helped in visualizing the distinction between different groups and the variability within each group (Figure 2a). Given that principal components (PCs) are formed by linearly combining the original variables, the visualization of PCA is limited in its ability to capture the entirety of variance [21]. The PCA results indicated an overlap among samples in the PCA score plot, with notable similarities between samples from Guangxi and Guizhou, likely due to their geographical proximity. Interestingly, similarities were also observed between samples from Zhejiang and Sichuan, suggesting that geographical factors significantly influence tea quality [22].

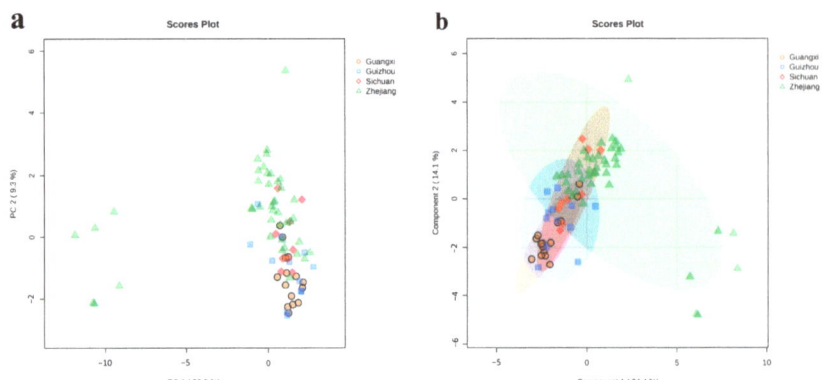

Figure 2. Principal component analysis (PCA) (**a**) and sparse PLS discriminant analysis (sPLS-DA) (**b**) of all 78 LJT samples.

To conduct a more in-depth analysis of the variations in metabolites among the four regions where LJT is produced, we utilized a supervised model known as sPLS-DA to compare and contrast the distinct groups. The sPLS-DA results indicated that distinguishing the four production areas remained challenging (Figure 2b). This difficulty was primarily manifested in the high similarity between samples from Sichuan and Zhejiang, with some samples from Guangxi and Guizhou also overlapping with those from Zhejiang. Previous studies have demonstrated that using supervised models for origin identification can be challenging when samples exhibit highly overlapping or similar metabolite characteristics, posing challenges for the model in recognizing an adequate number of sufficient distinguishing features [23]. LJT from different production areas contains similar primary metabolites; although the concentrations of these metabolites may vary, these differences remain insufficient for the sPLS-DA model to accurately distinguish between the production areas.

3.3. Hierarchical Clustering of Longjing Tea Origins

Heatmap and hierarchical clustering analyses were employed to visualize the metabolites of LJT sourced from various geographical origins (Figure 3). Hierarchical clustering was performed based on the mean values of 25 metabolites selected by ANOVA across samples from four origins. The grouping of LJT samples by origin revealed three hierarchical branches. The first branch includes samples from Guangxi and Guizhou; the second branch comprises samples from Guangxi, Guizhou, and Sichuan; and the third branch indicates that Zhejiang differs from the other three origins. The hierarchical clustering roughly corresponds to the geographical proximity of the origins. LJT from Zhejiang exhibits comparatively elevated levels of polyphenols, amino acids, and alkaloids in comparison to other regions. Conversely, Zhejiang demonstrates relatively diminished concentrations of certain organic acids (such as acetic acid, succinic acid, and chlorogenic acid) and sucrose when compared to the aforementioned regions. The main flavor components of tea are amino acids (umami), flavonoids (bitter and astringent), and alkaloids (bitter) [24]. Therefore, the differences in these substances in the LJT provide clues for origin discrimination and quality assessment.

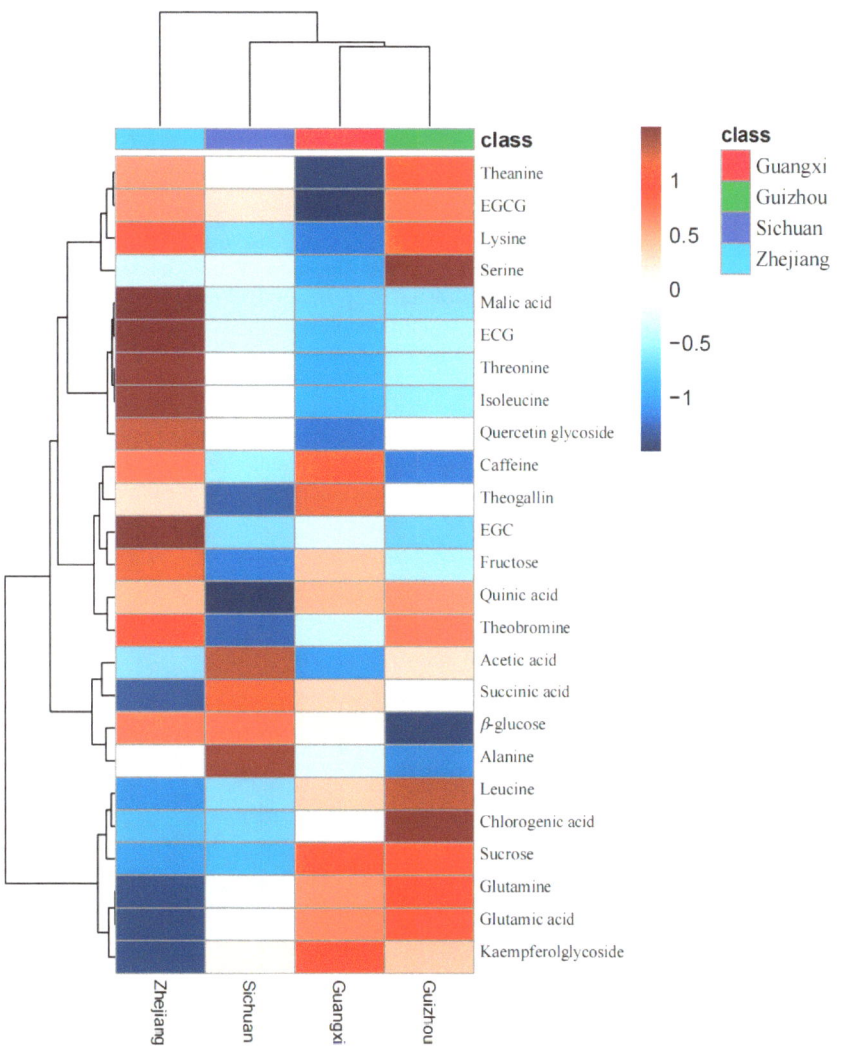

Figure 3. Geographic origin-based hierarchical clustering of LJT using ^{1}H NMR spectra.

3.4. Machine-Learning Algorithm for Longjing Tea Origins

To enhance the categorization of LJT samples originating from diverse sources, a range of classification algorithms with varying attributes (linear/non-linear) were examined to identify the most suitable method for tackling intricate pattern classification issues. LDA, a well-known linear model, aims to enhance sample discrimination by maximizing inter-class variance while minimizing intra-class variance [25]. The LDA training set achieved a classification accuracy of 96.2% (Figure 4a), while the testing set demonstrated an accuracy rate of 85.6% (Figure 4b). The classification accuracy for Zhejiang reached 85.72%, while the accuracies for Guangxi, Sichuan, and Guizhou were 60%, 66.67%, and 50%, respectively. RF is an innovative ensemble technique employed for machine-learning models, particularly those relying on nonlinear classification trees [26]. The RF algorithm builds numerous classification trees by randomly picking variables (columns) and data instances (rows), subsequently combining the outcomes of these trees for the purpose of classification or regression. The optimized RF model was utilized to distinguish LJT from four distinct sources (Figure 4c,d). In comparison to LDA, RF exhibited superior classification accuracy, achieving a discrimination rate of 100% for the training set and 92.3% for the testing set (Figure 4). Among the samples, those from Guizhou exhibited the highest classification error rate, while Zhejiang and Sichuan samples had the lowest. Specifically, one sample from Guangxi and one from Guizhou were misclassified as Zhejiang. Both of these samples originate from tea plant varieties transplanted from Zhejiang, indicating that the variety of raw material significantly impacts the final tea quality. This finding is consistent with previous research, where Cui et al. reported that the raw material used in tea processing is a major factor affecting origin-related quality differences [14]. The absence of misclassification between Sichuan and Zhejiang LJTs, which have similar dimensions, suggests that climatic conditions are not the primary determinant of tea's chemical composition. Comparing the prediction results of nonlinear algorithms with those of linear algorithms, it was found that nonlinear algorithms outperform linear algorithms in terms of predictive accuracy [14]. This finding is consistent with previous research, which indicates that metabolite levels in teas from different origins cannot be easily classified using simple linear methods due to the complex interplay of factors such as tea plant varieties, climate, management practices, and processing methods [27]. To enhance the differentiation of quality characteristics among origins, advanced machine-learning algorithms are essential.

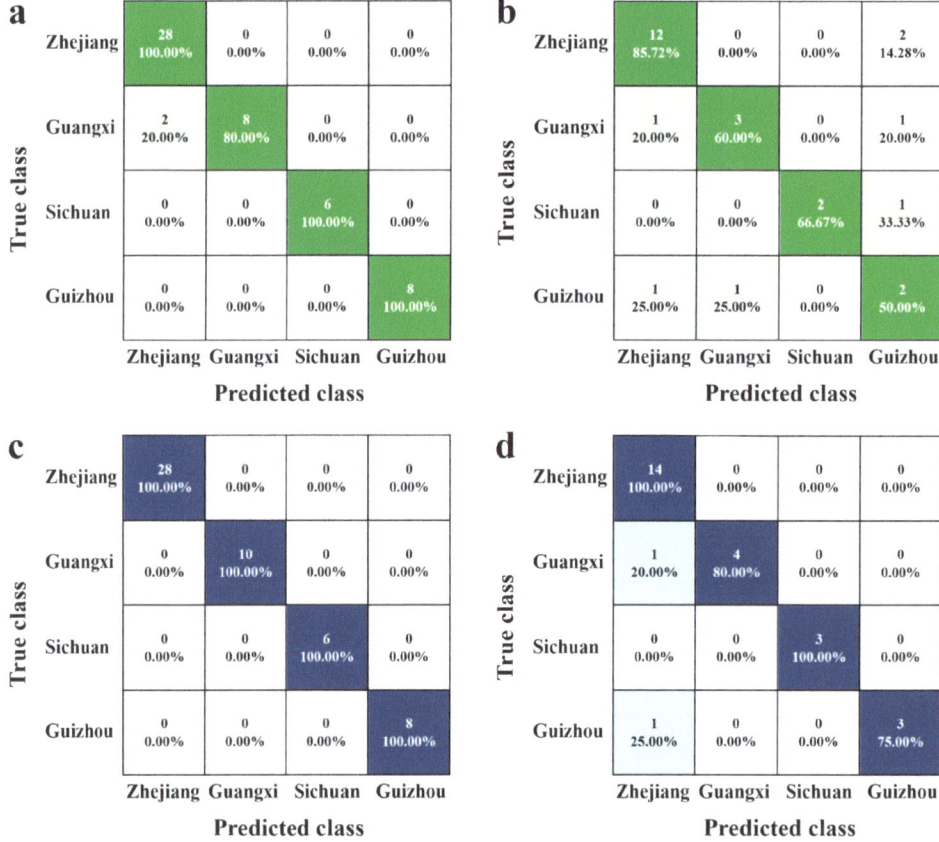

Figure 4. The confusion matrices for different models were obtained using all the data from 78 LJT samples from four production areas. (**a**) Training set of LDA. (**b**) Testing set of LDA. (**c**) Training set of RF. (**d**) Testing set of RF. The darker the green and blue colours in the matrix squares, the higher the accuracy rate.

3.5. Metabolite Biomarkers Differentiating Longjing Tea Origins

Through RF analysis (Figure 5), 15 potential chemical markers distinguishing LJT samples originating from various locales have been meticulously identified. Directly measuring the impact of each feature on the accuracy of the model is what mean decrease accuracy aims to achieve [28]. This is accomplished by rearranging the sequence of feature values and assessing the influence of changes in order on model accuracy. A higher average reduction in accuracy suggests a stronger influence of the variable on RF predictions. In terms of ranking, the metabolite that holds the utmost significance in distinguishing between the four production areas is Kaempferol glycoside. Previous research has indicated that variations in cultivation environments could potentially exert a substantial influence on the structural alterations observed in specific flavonoid metabolites within LJT of identical varieties [29]. It has been proposed that geographical origin has less impact on flavonoid metabolites compared to cultivation variety. Consistent with this, our study found that the content of Kaempferol glycoside is primarily dependent on the genetic characteristics of the tea plant, with less impact from the cultivation variety on quercetin glycoside. Quercetin glycoside and kaempferol glycoside contribute to the mild astringency of the tea brew and enhance the bitterness of caffeine, making them important components of the tea flavor [30]. Our study discovered that LJT from Zhejiang has lower levels of kaempferol glycoside compared to other regions, while quercetin glycoside content is higher than in other regions (Figure 5a). This may be due to the predominant use of specific varietal materials, although the high taste threshold of flavonoid glycosides makes it difficult for assessors or consumers to detect taste differences in the tea infusion. Previous research has utilized glutamine, a prominent umami amino acid found in tea, as a significant indicator for differentiating between various types of green tea [31]. Recent studies have shown that extended processing time and heating temperature reduce glutamine content [32]. Our study found that glutamine levels are lower in Zhejiang samples compared to other regions, possibly due to different processing conditions and temperatures, indicating that processing methods are a significant factor affecting the quality of LJT from different origins.

Furthermore, the RF model's discrimination results are affected by an additional set of five amino acids (Theanine, Alanine, Lysine, Leucine, and Isoleucine), ranked in descending order of significance. In green tea, isoleucine, leucine, and lysine contribute to bitterness, alanine is considered a sweet amino acid, and theanine is regarded as the primary umami amino acid [33]. The variation in the origin of LJT may result in differences in its taste due to variances in amino acid composition. Previous research has suggested that certain amino acids (proline, valine, and glutamic Acid) exhibit stability throughout the processing stages, whereas others (isoleucine, leucine, lysine, alanine, and theanine) are more prone to reduction during processing [34]. This suggests that differences in amino acids in LJT may be primarily influenced by processing, with these six amino acids helping to differentiate closely related geographic regions. ECG is one of the primary contributors to the bitterness and astringency of tea infusion [35]. The higher content of ECG in LJT from Zhejiang compared to other regions is primarily due to the combined effects of cultivar selection, agronomic practices, and processing methods. Glucose and fructose contribute sweetness to tea infusion. Prior research has suggested a correlation between the temperature at which tea leaves grow and the buildup of carbohydrates in them [36]. Our research found that the glucose and fructose content in tea from Zhejiang and Sichuan is higher compared to that from Guizhou and Guangxi. This disparity may be attributed to the fact that LJT from Guizhou and Guangxi is harvested from tea plants grown in southern China, where the environment features higher light intensity and temperatures, leading to lower carbohydrate accumulation in the tea plants [37]. Conversely, in the core production area of LJT, higher quality standards are typically enforced. As a result, only the new shoots from early spring, just after winter, are collected for processing into LJT. In contrast, in other regions, new tea shoots are collected and processed throughout both spring and summer, during which carbohydrate accumulation in tea leaves is lower, resulting in a reduced sweetness in the tea infusion.

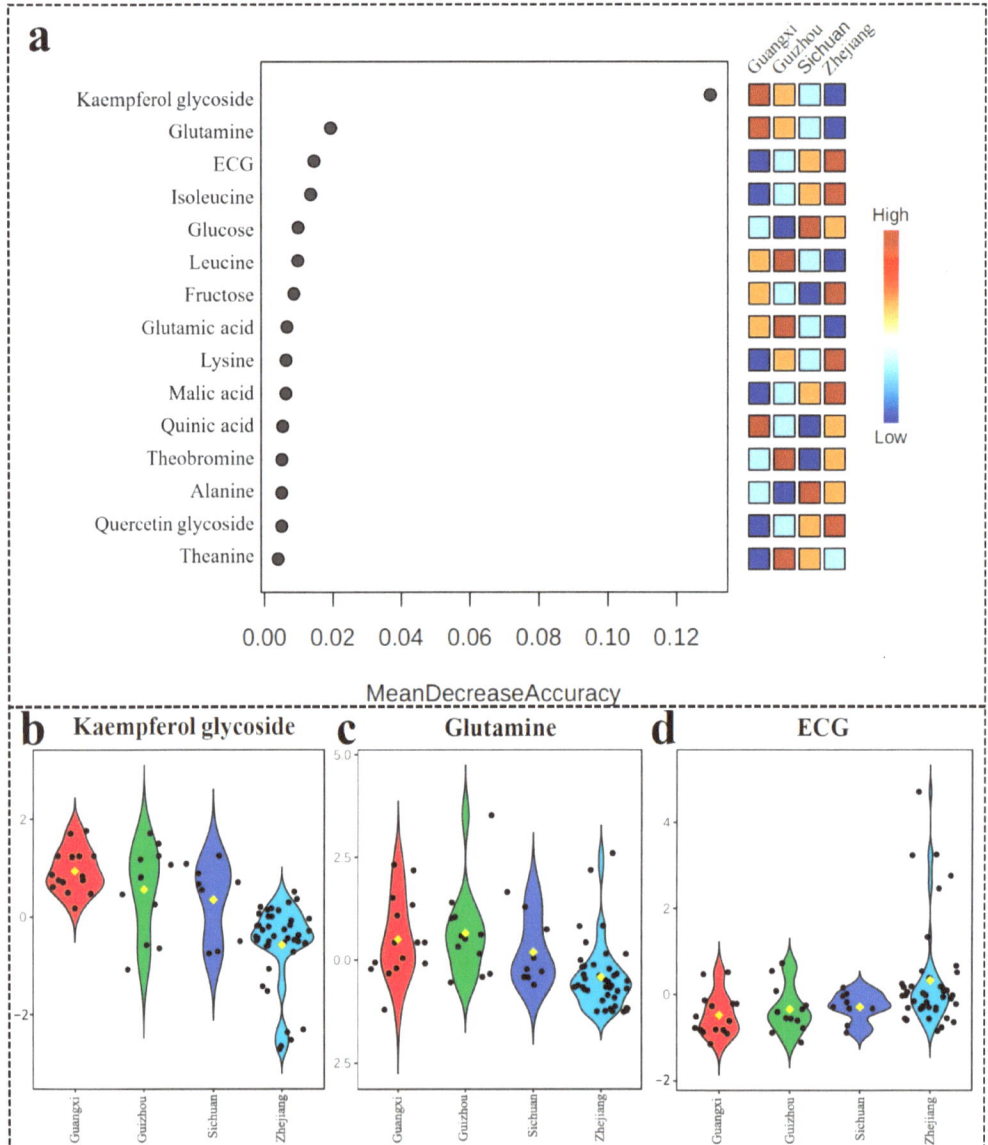

Figure 5. (**a**) Significant features identified by the random forest algorithm; (**b**) Kaempferol glycoside, (**c**) Glutamine, and (**d**) ECG box. The black dots in the fiddle diagram represent the relative content values for each sample, and the yellow dots represent the within-group average values.

In recent studies, ^{1}H NMR has been recognized as an effective method for assessing the origin of black tea [14]. Our study reveals that ^{1}H NMR also exhibits considerable potential in assessing the provenance of green tea. Previous investigations have identified glucose, sucrose, EGCG, EGC, EC, caffeine, theanine, alanine, and threonine as crucial indicators for distinguishing the source of green tea [38]. Our study confirms the significance of glucose, caffeine, and theanine in tea origin identification and reveals that, for LJT, key distinguishing compounds include kaempferol glycoside, which is significantly affected by cultivar; glutamine, which is influenced by processing; and ECG, which is impacted by multiple factors. RF modeling indicates that the key variables for differentiating the origin of LJT are predominantly influenced by cultivar and processing methods. The importance of these variables highlights that the varietal variations play a pivotal role in differentiating the source of LJT.

In brief, we have devised a quick and uncomplicated technique for determining the source and assessing the quality of Longjing tea. In contrast to the 40 min digestion period needed for identifying green tea origin through ICP-MS [8] and the 42 min detection time required for black tea origin identification using HS-GC/MS [9], our sample preparation requires only 15 min, followed by a detection time of only 2 min. This significant reduction in processing time facilitates the establishment of large datasets. In addition, the high reproducibility of NMR results compared to analytical methods such as LC-MS [39] and GC-MS [40] enhances the stability of model performance in academic research. Considering the influence of production and storage years on tea metabolites, more LJT samples from different years still need to be collected for analysis in practical applications to help optimize the machine-learning model to ensure the accuracy of the identification results.

4. Conclusions

This study employed a combination of ^{1}H NMR chemical fingerprints and machine-learning algorithms to analyze 78 Longjing tea samples from four major production regions. In these samples, a total of 30 metabolites were identified, including tea polyphenols, organic acids, carbohydrates, and alkaloids. Accurate identification of the origin of Longjing tea was achieved using ^{1}H NMR chemical fingerprint information combined with a non-linear algorithm (random forest), achieving an identification rate of 92.3%. The study thoroughly discussed the impact of raw material cultivar and processing conditions on the discrimination results. By analyzing the average decrease in random forest classification accuracy, 15 important variables were identified. Kaempferol glycoside, significantly affected by cultivar; glutamine, influenced by processing; and ECG, impacted by both cultivar and processing, were identified as major discriminatory factors. The findings suggest that the utilization of machine-learning algorithms in conjunction with ^{1}H NMR can serve as an efficient approach to assess the excellence and source of high-grade green teas, thereby contributing to quality management within the tea industry. This methodology offers a swift, consistent, and replicable means for certifying the origin of various agricultural products or food items.

Supplementary Materials: The following supporting information can be downloaded at: https://www.mdpi.com/article/10.3390/foods13172702/s1, Table S1: Detailed sources of Longjing tea samples.

Author Contributions: Conceptualization, methodology, formal analysis, investigation, resources, writing—original draft preparation, visualization, supervision, project administration, funding acquisition, Z.H.; methodology, formal analysis, data curation, writing—original draft preparation, software, Y.J.; methodology, investigation, data curation, software, Z.G.; investigation, data curation, software, R.Z.; resources, writing—review and editing, Z.S.; writing—review and editing, data curation, resources, S.L. All authors have read and agreed to the published version of the manuscript.

Funding: This research was funded by the National Natural Science Foundation of China, grant number 32302608, the Scientific Research and Development Foundation of Zhejiang A & F University, grant number 2022FR025.

Institutional Review Board Statement: Not applicable.

Informed Consent Statement: Not applicable.

Data Availability Statement: The original contributions presented in the study are included in the article/Supplementary Material, further inquiries can be directed to the corresponding author.

Conflicts of Interest: The authors declare no conflicts of interest.

References

1. Zhang, H.Y.; Zhang, J.X.; Liu, S.T.; Li, T.H.; Wei, Y.M.; Gu, Z.; Su, Z.C.; Ning, J.M.; Wang, Y.J.; Hou, Z.W. Characterization of the key volatile compounds in longjing tea (*Camellia sinensis*) with different aroma types at different steeping temperatures by GC-MS and GC-IMS. *LWT-Food Sci. Technol.* **2024**, *200*, 116183. [CrossRef]
2. GB/T 18650-2008; Product of Geographical Indication - Longjing Tea. National Standards of the People's Republic of China: Beijing, China, 2008. (In Chinese)
3. Ni, K.; Wang, J.; Zhang, Q.F.; Yi, X.Y.; Ma, L.F.; Shi, Y.Z.; Ruan, J.Y. Multi-element composition and isotopic signatures for the geographical origin discrimination of green tea in China: A case study of Xihu Longjing. *J. Food Compos. Anal.* **2018**, *67*, 104–109. [CrossRef]
4. Lu, X.H.; Wang, J.; Lu, G.D.; Lin, B.; Chang, M.Z.; He, W. Quality level identification of West Lake Longjing green tea using electronic nose. *Sens. Actuators B Chem.* **2019**, *301*, 127056. [CrossRef]
5. Wang, L.Y.; Wei, K.; Cheng, H.; He, W.; Li, X.H.; Gong, W.Y. Geographical tracing of Xihu Longjing tea using high performance liquid chromatography. *Food Chem.* **2014**, *146*, 98–103. [CrossRef]
6. He, W.; Hu, X.S.; Zhao, L.; Liao, X.J.; Zhang, Y.; Zhang, M.W.; Wu, J.H. Evaluation of Chinese tea by the electronic tongue: Correlation with sensory properties and classification according to geographical origin and grade level. *Food Res. Int.* **2009**, *42*, 1462–1467. [CrossRef]
7. Fang, S.M.; Huang, W.J.; Wei, Y.M.; Tao, M.; Hu, X.; Li, T.H.; Kalkhajeh, Y.K.; Deng, W.W.; Ning, J.M. Geographical origin traceability of Keemun black tea based on its non-volatile composition combined with chemometrics. *J. Sci. Food Agric.* **2019**, *99*, 6937–6943. [CrossRef]
8. Ma, G.C.; Zhang, Y.B.; Zhang, J.Y.; Wang, G.Q.; Chen, L.Y.; Zhang, M.L.; Liu, T.; Liu, X.; Lu, C.Y. Determining the geographical origin of Chinese green tea by linear discriminant analysis of trace metals and rare earth elements: Taking Dongting Biluochun as an example. *Food Control* **2016**, *59*, 714–720. [CrossRef]
9. Yun, J.; Cui, C.J.; Zhang, S.H.; Zhu, J.J.; Peng, C.Y.; Cai, H.M.; Yang, X.G.; Hou, R.Y. Use of headspace GC/MS combined with chemometric analysis to identify the geographic origins of black tea. *Food Chem.* **2021**, *360*, 130033. [CrossRef]
10. Gu, H.W.; Yin, X.L.; Peng, T.Q.; Pan, Y.; Cui, H.N.; Li, Z.Q.; Sun, W.Q.; Ding, B.M.; Hu, X.C.; Zhang, Z.H.; et al. Geographical origin identification and chemical markers screening of Chinese green tea using two-dimensional fingerprints technique coupled with multivariate chemometric methods. *Food Control* **2022**, *135*, 108795. [CrossRef]
11. Shuai, M.Y.; Peng, C.Y.; Niu, H.L.; Shao, D.L.; Hou, R.Y.; Cai, H.M. Recent techniques for the authentication of the geographical origin of tea leaves from *camellia sinensis*: A review. *Food Chem.* **2022**, *374*, 131713. [CrossRef]
12. Hatzakis, E. Nuclear magnetic resonance (NMR) spectroscopy in food science: A comprehensive review. *Compr. Rev. Food Sci. Food Saf.* **2019**, *18*, 189–220. [CrossRef]
13. Cui, C.J.; Xia, M.Y.; Wei, Z.Q.; Chen, J.L.; Peng, C.Y.; Cai, H.M.; Jin, L.; Hou, R.Y. ^{1}H NMR-based metabolomic approach combined with machine learning algorithm to distinguish the geographic origin of huajiao (*Zanthoxylum bungeanum* Maxim.). *Food Control* **2023**, *145*, 109476. [CrossRef]
14. Cui, C.J.; Xu, Y.F.; Jin, G.; Zong, J.F.; Peng, C.Y.; Cai, H.M.; Hou, R.Y. Machine learning applications for identify the geographical origin, variety and processing of black tea using ^{1}H NMR chemical fingerprinting. *Food Control* **2023**, *148*, 109686. [CrossRef]
15. Worley, B.; Powers, R. PCA as a practical indicator of OPLS-DA model reliability. *Curr. Metab.* **2016**, *4*, 97–103. [CrossRef]
16. Wu, X.H.; He, F.; Wu, B.; Zeng, S.P.; He, C.Y. Accurate classification of Chunmee tea grade using NIR spectroscopy and fuzzy maximum uncertainty linear discriminant analysis. *Foods* **2023**, *12*, 541. [CrossRef]
17. Zhang, L.Z.; Dai, H.M.; Zhang, J.L.; Zheng, Z.Q.; Song, B.; Chen, J.Y.; Lin, G.; Chen, L.H.; Sun, W.J.; Huang, Y. A study on origin traceability of white tea (White Peony) based on near-infrared spectroscopy and machine learning algorithms. *Foods* **2023**, *12*, 499. [CrossRef] [PubMed]
18. Jin, G.; Zhu, Y.Y.; Cui, C.J.; Yang, C.; Hu, S.D.; Cai, H.M.; Ning, J.M.; Wei, C.L.; Li, A.X.; Hou, R.Y. Tracing the origin of Taiping Houkui green tea using ^{1}H NMR and HS-SPME-GC-MS chemical fingerprints, data fusion and chemometrics. *Food Chem.* **2023**, *425*, 136538. [CrossRef]
19. Tarachiwin, L.; Ute, K.; Kobayashi, A.; Fukusaki, E. ^{1}H NMR based metabolic profiling in the evaluation of Japanese green tea quality. *J. Agric. Food Chem.* **2007**, *55*, 9330–9336. [CrossRef]
20. Lee, J.E.; Lee, B.J.; Chung, J.O.; Hwang, J.A.; Lee, S.J.; Lee, C.H.; Hong, Y.S. Geographical and climatic dependencies of green tea (*Camellia sinensis*) metabolites: A ^{1}H NMR-based metabolomics study. *J. Agric. Food Chem.* **2010**, *58*, 10582–10589. [CrossRef]
21. Boffo, E.F.; Tavares, L.A.; Ferreira, M.M.; Ferreira, A.G. Classification of Brazilian vinegars according to their ^{1}H NMR spectra by pattern recognition analysis. *LWT-Food Sci. Technol.* **2009**, *42*, 1455–1460. [CrossRef]
22. Le Gall, G.; Colquhoun, I.J.; Defernez, M. Metabolite profiling using ^{1}H NMR spectroscopy for quality assessment of green tea, *Camellia sinensis* (L.). *J. Agric. Food Chem.* **2004**, *52*, 692–700. [CrossRef] [PubMed]
23. Shevchuk, A.; Jayasinghe, L.; Kuhnert, N. Differentiation of black tea infusions according to origin, processing and botanical varieties using multivariate statistical analysis of LC-MS data. *Food Res. Int.* **2018**, *109*, 387–402. [CrossRef] [PubMed]
24. Zeng, L.; Fu, Y.Q.; Gao, Y.; Wang, F.; Liang, S.; Yin, J.F.; Fauconnier, M.L.; Ke, L.; Xu, Y.Q. Dynamic changes of key metabolites in Longjing green tea during processing revealed by widely targeted metabolomic profiling and sensory experiments. *Food Chem.* **2024**, *450*, 139373. [CrossRef]

25. Estoup, A.; Lombaert, E.; MARIN, J.M.; Guillemaud, T.; Pudlo, P.; Robert, C.P.; Cornuet, J.M. Estimation of demo-genetic model probabilities with Approximate Bayesian Computation using linear discriminant analysis on summary statistics. *Mol. Ecol. Resour.* **2012**, *12*, 846–855. [CrossRef] [PubMed]
26. Lin, Y.D.; Ma, J.; Wang, Q.J.; Sun, D.W. Applications of machine learning techniques for enhancing nondestructive food quality and safety detection. *Crit. Rev. Food Sci. Nutr.* **2023**, *63*, 1649–1669. [CrossRef] [PubMed]
27. Fraser, K.; Lane, G.A.; Otter, D.E.; Hemar, Y.; Quek, S.Y.; Harrison, S.J.; Rasmussen, S. Analysis of metabolic markers of tea origin by UHPLC and high resolution mass spectrometry. *Food Res. Int.* **2013**, *53*, 827–835. [CrossRef]
28. Xu, M.; Wang, J.; Zhu, L.Y. The qualitative and quantitative assessment of tea quality based on E-nose, E-tongue and E-eye combined with chemometrics. *Food Chem.* **2019**, *289*, 482–489. [CrossRef]
29. Yu, X.-L.; Li, J.; Yang, Y.Q.; Zhu, J.Y.; Yuan, H.B.; Jiang, Y.W. Comprehensive investigation on flavonoids metabolites of Longjing tea in different cultivars, geographical origins, and storage time. *Heliyon* **2023**, *9*, e17305. [CrossRef]
30. Ye, J.H.; Ye, Y.; Yin, J.F.; Jin, J.; Liang, Y.R.; Liu, R.Y.; Tang, P.; Xu, Y.Q. Bitterness and astringency of tea leaves and products: Formation mechanism and reducing strategies. *Trends Food Sci. Technol.* **2022**, *123*, 130–143. [CrossRef]
31. Yu, Z.M.; Yang, Z.Y. Understanding different regulatory mechanisms of proteinaceous and non-proteinaceous amino acid formation in tea (*Camellia sinensis*) provides new insights into the safe and effective alteration of tea flavor and function. *Crit. Rev. Food Sci. Nutr.* **2020**, *60*, 844–858. [CrossRef]
32. Jiang, H.; Yu, F.; Qin, L.; Zhang, N.; Cao, Q.; Schwab, W.; Li, D.X.; Song, C.K. Dynamic change in amino acids, catechins, alkaloids, and gallic acid in six types of tea processed from the same batch of fresh tea (*Camellia sinensis* L.) leaves. *J. Food Compos. Anal.* **2019**, *77*, 28–38. [CrossRef]
33. Farag, M.A.; Elmetwally, F.; Elghanam, R.; Kamal, N.; Hellal, K.; Hamezah, H.S.; Zhao, C.; Mediani, A. Metabolomics in tea products; a compile of applications for enhancing agricultural traits and quality control analysis of *Camellia sinensis*. *Food Chem.* **2023**, *404*, 134628. [CrossRef] [PubMed]
34. Chen, Q.C.; Shi, J.; Mu, B.; Chen, Z.; Dai, W.D.; Lin, Z. Metabolomics combined with proteomics provides a novel interpretation of the changes in nonvolatile compounds during white tea processing. *Food Chem.* **2020**, *332*, 127412. [CrossRef]
35. Yang, C.; Cui, C.J.; Zhu, Y.Y.; Xia, X.Y.; Jin, G.; Liu, C.J.; Li, Y.Y.; Xue, X.H.; Hou, R.Y. Effect of brewing conditions on the chemical and sensory profiles of milk tea. *Food Chem. X* **2022**, *16*, 100453. [CrossRef] [PubMed]
36. Yue, C.; Cao, H.L.; Wang, L.; Zhou, Y.H.; Huang, Y.T.; Hao, X.Y.; Wang, Y.C.; Wang, B.; Yang, Y.J.; Wang, X.C. Effects of cold acclimation on sugar metabolism and sugar-related gene expression in tea plant during the winter season. *Plant Mol. Biol.* **2015**, *88*, 591–608. [CrossRef] [PubMed]
37. Zhang, Q.W.; Li, T.Y.; Wang, Q.S.; LeCompte, J.; Harkess, R.L.; Bi, G.H. Screening tea cultivars for novel climates: Plant growth and leaf quality of *Camellia sinensis* cultivars grown in Mississippi, United States. *Front. Plant Sci.* **2020**, *11*, 280. [CrossRef]
38. Lee, J.E.; Lee, B.J.; Chung, J.O.; Kim, H.N.; Kim, E.H.; Jung, S.; Lee, H.; Lee, S.J.; Hong, Y.S. Metabolomic unveiling of a diverse range of green tea (*Camellia sinensis*) metabolites dependent on geography. *Food Chem.* **2015**, *174*, 452–459. [CrossRef]
39. Lai, G.P.; Cui, Y.Q.; Granato, D.; Wen, M.C.; Han, Z.S.; Zhang, L. Free, soluble conjugated and insoluble bonded phenolic acids in Keemun black tea: From UPLC-QQQ-MS/MS method development to chemical shifts monitoring during processing. *Food Res. Int.* **2022**, *155*, 111041. [CrossRef]
40. Hou, Z.W.; Wang, Y.J.; Xu, S.S.; Wei, Y.M.; Bao, G.H.; Dai, Q.Y.; Deng, W.W.; Ning, J.M. Effects of dynamic and static withering technology on volatile and nonvolatile components of Keemun black tea using GC-MS and HPLC combined with chemometrics. *LWT* **2020**, *130*, 109547. [CrossRef]

Disclaimer/Publisher's Note: The statements, opinions and data contained in all publications are solely those of the individual author(s) and contributor(s) and not of MDPI and/or the editor(s). MDPI and/or the editor(s) disclaim responsibility for any injury to people or property resulting from any ideas, methods, instructions or products referred to in the content.

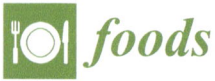

Article

Tea's Characteristic Components Eliminate Acrylamide in the Maillard Model System

Zhihao Ye [1,2,3,†], Haojie Xu [1,2,3,†], Yingying Xie [1,2,3], Ziqi Peng [1,2,3], Hongfang Li [1,2,3], Ruyan Hou [1,2,3], Huimei Cai [1,2,3], Wei Song [3], Chuanyi Peng [1,2,3,*] and Daxiang Li [1]

1. State Key Laboratory of Tea Plant Biology and Utilization, Anhui Agricultural University, Hefei 230036, China; yzh971014@163.com (Z.Y.); 18439465028@163.com (H.X.); xieyy1029@163.com (Y.X.); 15156513821@163.com (Z.P.); lihongfang@ahau.edu.cn (H.L.); hry@ahau.edu.cn (R.H.); chm@ahau.edu.cn (H.C.); song86@126.com (W.S.); dxli@ahau.edu.cn (D.L.)
2. Key Laboratory of Food Nutrition and Safety, Anhui Agricultural University, Hefei 230036, China
3. Anhui Provincial Key Laboratory of Food Safety Monitoring and Quality Control, Hefei 230036, China
* Correspondence: pcy0917@ahau.edu.cn or pcy72988@126.com; Tel./Fax: +86-0551-65786421
† These authors contributed equally to this work.

Abstract: This study investigated the effects of various characteristic components of tea—theaflavins, catechins, thearubigins, theasinensins, theanine, catechin (C), catechin gallate (CG), epicatechin (EC), epicatechin gallate (ECG), epigallocatechin (EGC), epigallocatechin gallate (EGCG), gallocatechin (GC), and gallocatechin gallate (GCG)—on acrylamide formation. The results revealed that most of tea's characteristic components could significantly eliminate acrylamide, ranked from highest to lowest as follows: GC (55.73%) > EC (46.31%) > theaflavins (44.91%) > CG (40.73%) > thearubigins (37.36%) > ECG (37.03%) > EGCG (27.37%) > theabrownine (22.54%) > GCG (16.21%) > catechins (10.14%) > C (7.48%). Synergistic elimination effects were observed with thearubigins + EC + GC + CG, thearubigins + EC + CG, thearubigins + EC + GC, theaflavins + GC + CG, and thearubigins + theaflavins, with the reduction rates being 73.99%, 72.67%, 67.62%, 71.03%, and 65.74%, respectively. Tea's components reduced the numbers of persistent free radicals to prevent acrylamide formation in the model system. The results provide a theoretical basis for the development of low-acrylamide foods and the application of tea resources in the food industry.

Keywords: acrylamide; tea's characteristic components; Maillard model; elimination effect; possible mechanism

Citation: Ye, Z.; Xu, H.; Xie, Y.; Peng, Z.; Li, H.; Hou, R.; Cai, H.; Song, W.; Peng, C.; Li, D. Tea's Characteristic Components Eliminate Acrylamide in the Maillard Model System. *Foods* **2024**, *13*, 2836. https://doi.org/10.3390/foods13172836

Academic Editor: Diego A. Moreno

Received: 29 June 2024
Revised: 7 August 2024
Accepted: 26 August 2024
Published: 6 September 2024

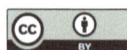

Copyright: © 2024 by the authors. Licensee MDPI, Basel, Switzerland. This article is an open access article distributed under the terms and conditions of the Creative Commons Attribution (CC BY) license (https://creativecommons.org/licenses/by/4.0/).

1. Introduction

In the thermal processing of foods, acrylamide is a harmful substance that forms during the Maillard reaction between reducing sugars and asparagine [1]. Acrylamide is not naturally present in raw foods, but usually forms during cooking at a high temperature (over 120 °C), especially when starchy and carbohydrate-rich foods are cooked [2]. In 1994, acrylamide was classified as a level 2A carcinogen by the International Agency for Research on Cancer [3], which caused global concern regarding the substance. In 2015, the European Food Safety Authority provided health-based guidance regarding the maximum permissible levels of acrylamide in foods [4], and in 2017, the European Union issued regulations specifying benchmark levels of acrylamide [5]. For example, coffee and french fries have high acrylamide levels, at 389 and 1499 μg/kg, and their recommended benchmark levels are 750 and 400 μg/kg, respectively.

An extensive research effort has been expended in attempts to minimize the amount of acrylamide that forms during food processing. The first step is assessing raw materials. Different varieties of crops, especially potatoes and cereals, contain differing levels of reducing sugars and asparagine [6], which are the precursor substances for the synthesis of acrylamide. Thus, the cultivation and selection of raw materials with low levels of sugar and asparagine play a crucial role in reducing the degree of acrylamide formation [3,7]. Second, several processing conditions—including temperature, time, and pH—strongly influence the likelihood of acrylamide formation during cooking [8,9]. Modifying these parameters can lead to major reductions in acrylamide levels. For instance, lowering the cooking temperature [10,11], extending the cooking time [11], and adjusting the pH toward acidity [12,13] have all been reported to reduce acrylamide levels in food products. Enzyme technology has also shown potential for acrylamide elimination [14,15]. Furthermore, the application of food additives, a simple strategy that can be easily implemented, can inhibit acrylamide formation without requiring a change in the raw materials or processing technologies that are used. Zamora et al. [11] found that dipalmitoylphosphatidylethanolamine reduced the amount of acrylamide produced in the glucose–asparagine (Glc-Asn) model system and that the inhibitory effect was significantly correlated with the concentration of amino phospholipid [11]. In another study, mercaptan could react with acrylamide to form stable adducts, whereas under aerobic conditions, no additional products were identified, but acrylamide formation was noticeably less severe [16].

Many plants' or extracts' pronounced antioxidant properties are known to naturally inhibit the formation of acrylamide. Liu et al. found that soaking french fries in a 1.34% sodium alginate solution reduced acrylamide production by 76.59% and had no effect on their sensory properties; this soaking resulted in the formation of a protective layer on the surface of the fries [17]. In a model system, naringin was found to inhibit acrylamide formation at a rate of 20–50%; high-performance liquid chromatography (HPLC)–tandem mass spectrometry (MS/MS) and nuclear magnetic resonance analyses revealed that this occurred because naringin reacted with the precursors of acrylamide [18]. Trujillomayol et al. [19] added 0.5% avocado peel extract to beef and vegetarian burgers to reduce the levels of acrylamide and heterocyclic amines in the cooked burgers [19]. In addition, a significant reduction in acrylamide was achieved by soaking chicken legs and wings in green tea extract before they were fried [20]; this reduction was attributed to an interaction between the precursor substances of acrylamide and the components of the green tea extract, including catechin and gallic acid. Compared with synthetic antioxidants such as butylated hydroxyanisole and butylated hydroxytoluene, plant polyphenols are more acceptable for consumers.

Plant polyphenols, which are phytochemicals, have attracted a great deal of attention because they are natural antioxidants. Tea is a polyphenol-rich food, and tea polyphenols have multiple pharmacological and physiological functionalities due to their well-known antioxidant attributes. China's overall tea production in 2023 was 3.55 million tons [21]; the production of summer and autumn teas accounts for more than 50% of Chinese tea production, but the rate of utilization of these types of tea is low because they are bitter and astringent in taste and have poor aromatic qualities. However, the leaves of these teas, which contain numerous polyphenols, have considerable potential for use in the elimination of acrylamide. In the current study, the abilities of the aforementioned teas' characteristic components—theanine, tea polyphenols and the products of their different degrees of oxidation (theaflavins, thearubigins, and theasinensins), and catechins—to eliminate acrylamide were systematically evaluated, and the possible mechanism underlying their ability to reduce acrylamide was also explored by monitoring the scavenging of free radicals.

2. Materials and Methods

2.1. Reagents and Materials

Acrylamide (C_3H_5NO, $\geq$99.90%) and $^{13}C_3$–acrylamide were purchased from Dr. Ehrenstorfer (Augsburg, Germany) and Beijing Manhage Biotechnology (Beijing, China), respectively. The asparagine, glucose, Na_2HPO_4, and K_2HPO_4 used in this study were analytical grade and obtained from Merk (Darmstadt, Germany). N-Propylethylenediamine (PSA) was purchased from Shanghai Anpel Laboratory Technologies (Shanghai, China), and deionized water (18.2 MΩ cm) was prepared using a Milli-Q Gradient system (Billerica,

MA, USA). HPLC grade characteristic components of tea—catechin (C), catechin gallate (CG), epicatechin (EC), epicatechin gallate (ECG), epigallocatechin (EGC), epigallocatechin gallate (EGCG), gallocatechin (GC), gallocatechin gallate (GCG), tea polyphenols, theaflavins, thearubigins, theabrownine, and theanine—were purchased from Shanghai Yuanye Biotechnology (Shanghai, China). Instant green tea was purchased from Zhejiang Minghuang Natural Products Development.

2.2. Glc-Asn Thermal Model Reaction

The Maillard model reaction was conducted using a previously described method with some minor modifications [22]. In brief, an equimolar solution of glucose and asparagine was accurately prepared in phosphate buffer (0.1 M, pH 6.86), and 4 mL of the solution was transferred to a 25 mL thick-walled pressurized glass tube in an oil bath (DF-1015, Shanghai Lichen Instrument Technology, Shanghai, China) at 180 °C and kept for 30 min. The sample was then allowed to cool to room temperature, and 0.1 mL of $^{13}C_3$–acrylamide standard solution (10 mg/L) was added. Subsequently, the total volume was adjusted to 100 mL by adding deionized water, and 2 mL was collected and mixed with 0.2 g of PSA. The mixture was vortexed for 2 min and then centrifuged at 8000 rpm for 5 min at 25 °C. After centrifugation, the supernatant was collected and filtered through a 0.22 μm cellulose syringe filter before undergoing liquid chromatography (LC)–mass spectrometry analysis.

2.3. Elimination Evaluation of Effects of Tea's Characteristic Components on Acrylamide in Maillard Model System

In the Maillard model system, the effects of the following substances on acrylamide levels were evaluated: instant green tea (0.01, 0.1, 1, 10, and 100 g/mol Asn), tea polyphenols (0.1, 0.25, 0.5, 1, and 2 g/mol Asn), theanine (0.1, 0.25, 0.5, 1, and 2 g/mol Asn), C (0.025, 0.05, 0.1, 0.25, and 0.5 g/mol Asn), EC (0.025, 0.05, 0.1, 0.25, and 0.5 g/mol Asn), EGC (0.025, 0.05, 0.1, 0.25, and 0.5 g/mol Asn), GC (0.05, 0.1, 0.25, 0.5, and 1 g/mol Asn), CG (0.025, 0.05, 0.1, 0.25, and 0.5 g/mol Asn), ECG (0.025, 0.05, 0.1, 0.25, and 0.5 g/mol Asn), EGCG (0.025, 0.05, 0.1, 0.25, and 0.5 g/mol Asn), GCG (0.05, 0.1, 0.25, 0.5, and 1 g/mol Asn), theaflavins (0.05, 0.1, 0.25, 0.5, and 1 g/mol Asn), thearubigins (0.05, 0.1, 0.25, 0.5, and 1 g/mol Asn), and theabrownine (0.05, 0.1, 0.25, 0.5, and 1 g/mol Asn). The optimal composition with equal weights of well-behaved characteristic components of tea was then determined using a comprehensive experimental design.

2.4. LC–Triple Quadrupole (QQQ) MS/MS Analysis of Acrylamide in the Maillard Model System

An LC-QQQ-MS/MS device equipped with an electrospray ionization source (AB SCIEX, Boston, MA, USA) coupled with a SCIEX high-performance liquid spectrometer system was used to determine the levels of acrylamide that formed in the Maillard model system [23]. The analyte was separated on a Waters Acquity UPLC BEH Shield RP18 column (1.7 μm, 1.0 mm × 50 mm, Waters, MA, USA) at 40 °C under a flow rate of 0.2 mL/min. The injection volume was 2 μL, and during isocratic elution, the mobile phase consisted of methanol/0.1% formic acid in deionized water (10:90, v/v). Acrylamide was identified and quantified using the multiple reaction monitoring mode; the transitions m/z 72→55 and m/z 72→27 indicated acrylamide, whereas m/z 75→58 and m/z 75→29 indicated $^{13}C_3$–acrylamide.

2.5. Free Radicals in the Maillard Model System

Electron paramagnetic resonance (EPR) was performed to investigate the variation in the free radicals in the Glc-Asn model system before and after the addition of the characteristic components of tea and thereby explore the possible mechanism of acrylamide reduction. The EPR process was as follows: A reacted sample was collected and prepared as a 1 mg/mL solution, and equal volumes of this solution and a radical scavenger solution were mixed. Subsequently, a capillary was employed to draw an appropriate amount of the mixed solution into a quartz tube, and the total spin number was recorded on a Bruker

EMX plus 6/1 spectrometer (Billerica, Massachusetts, USA) equipped with an Oxford Instrument. The instrument parameters were as follows: center magnetic field, 3480 G; scan time and width, 60 s and 50 G, respectively; microwave power, 6 mW; and modulation amplitude, 3.0 G.

2.6. Statistical Analysis

All experiments were performed at least in triplicate, and the data were statistically analyzed using IBM SPSS software (version 26.0, SPSS, Chicago, IL, USA). The results are presented as means ± standard deviations (SDs). Analysis of variance and the least significant difference test or Dunnett's test, selected on the basis of the results of Bartlett's test for equal variances, were used to determine the differences between means. Significance was considered at $p < 0.05$.

3. Results and Discussion

3.1. The Effects of Instant Green Tea on Acrylamide Levels in the Glc-Asn Model System

The effects of instant green tea on the profile of acrylamide in the Glc-Asn model system are illustrated in Figure 1. The level of acrylamide under the control condition (i.e., 0 g/mol Asn) was 140.58 ± 13.92 µmol/mol Asn. When the amounts of instant green tea were 0.1, 1, and 10 g/mol Asn, the levels of acrylamide in the model system were significantly lower; the rates of inhibition were 13.22–25.48%. However, the low dose (<0.1 g/mol Asn) and high dose (>10 g/mol Asn) of instant green tea did not have significantly inhibitive effects. Morales et al., Li et al., and Budryn et al. have reported that the addition of an aqueous extract of green tea or tea polyphenols could significantly reduce the levels of acrylamide in fried potatoes, bread, and fried yeast donuts, with maximum reductions of 62%, 43%, and 15%, respectively [24–26]. However, another study discovered that the addition of a high amount of green tea extract to fried yeast donuts enhanced the formation of acrylamide [26].

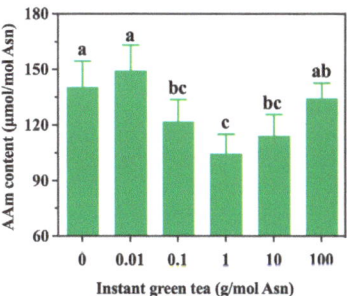

Figure 1. The effects of instant green tea on acrylamide reduction in the Glc-Asn model system. The different letters indicate significant differences at $p < 0.05$ at different instant green tea concentrations.

Tea can be classified into six basic types on the basis of its degree of fermentation with polyphenol oxidase and the microorganisms of tea polyphenols: green tea, white tea, yellow tea, oolong tea, black tea, and brick tea [27]. Green tea has the highest concentration of total catechins and the strongest antioxidant activity when it is prepared from the dried leaves of a single *Camellia sinensis* cultivar [28]. Green tea contains abundant secondary metabolites, including tea polyphenols and theanine; however, the specific characteristic component of green tea that contributes to acrylamide reduction remains unclear, as do the possible synergistic or antagonistic effects.

3.2. The Effects of Tea's Characteristic Components on Acrylamide Levels in the Glc-Asn Model System

To better understand the effects of tea's specific components on acrylamide levels, different characteristic components of tea—tea polyphenols, theanine, and catechins—were investigated in the Glc-Asn model system. As illustrated in Figure 2A,B, neither tea polyphenols nor theanine (when applied at levels of 0.1, 0.25, 0.5, 1, and 2 g/mol Asn) significantly affected acrylamide formation ($p < 0.05$). According to the performance results for instant green tea, tea polyphenols, and theanine, these substances had clear effects antagonistic to acrylamide reduction. Tea polyphenols, also called tea tannings or tea tannins, mainly comprise catechins, flavonoids, anthocyanins, and phenolic acids, with the content of catechin compounds being the highest; catechin compounds account for 60–80% of the total amount of tea polyphenols. Dozens of studies have reported that plant polyphenols with different structures have differing impacts on the formation of acrylamide [1]. Apple extract has been reported to inhibit acrylamide formation, and dragon fruit and hesperetin have been reported to enhance acrylamide formation [29,30]. Reactive carbonyl groups of plant polyphenols were reported by one study to be the major sites of acrylamide formation [1]. In the present study, eight catechin monomers were individually investigated to evaluate their roles in acrylamide elimination.

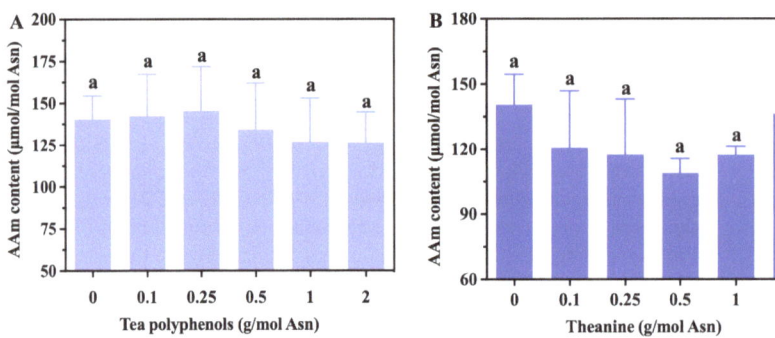

Figure 2. The effects of tea polyphenols (**A**) and theanine (**B**) on acrylamide reduction in the Glc-Asn model system. The different letters indicate significant differences at $p < 0.05$ at different concentrations.

The effects of nonester catechin monomers (C, EC, EGC, and GC) on acrylamide levels in the Glc-Asn model system are presented in Figure 3A–D. C (applied at levels of 0.025–0.5 g/mol Asn) and EGC (0.025–0.5 g/mol Asn) did not have an inhibitory effect ($p > 0.05$). By contrast, the addition of EC (0.25–0.5 g/mol Asn) and GC (0.1–1 g/mol Asn) resulted in significantly lower acrylamide content; the highest level of inhibition for EC was found to be 46.31%, achieved at 0.25 g/mol Asn, and that for GC was discovered to be 55.73%, achieved at 0.5 g/mol Asn. Figure 3E–H present the inhibition performances for ester catechin monomers (GCG, ECG, CG, and EGCG). The effect of GCG was not sufficient to achieve a significant reduction in acrylamide levels ($p > 0.05$, Figure 3E). The additions of ECG, CG, and EGCG resulted in less acrylamide when they were applied at the levels of 0.25, 0.05–0.5, and 0.05–0.25 g/mol Asn, respectively; the maximum inhibitions were 37.03%, 40.73%, and 27.37%, respectively. The effects of these catechin monomers were discovered to not be dose-dependent, implying that the inhibition of acrylamide formation may be dependent on the structure and concentration of the specific polyphenol. EC and EGCG were reported to terminate the formation of Maillard products in the model system and in UHT milk during storage [30]. Hedegaard et al. [31] discovered that 1.0 mM EC or EGCG decreased the acrylamide content in a model food system, whereas the lower concentration of 0.1 mM did not. Remarkably, numerous studies have obtained evidence indicating that the correlation between acrylamide formation and the concentration of plant polyphenols is nonlinear [1,32]. For example, a phenolic extract from virgin olive oil was found to efficiently inhibit acrylamide formation in the Glc-Asn model system, whereas the opposite effect occurred when a higher concentration of the phenolic extract was employed [33] and when apple proanthocyanidins were applied to fried potato [34].

The link between antioxidant capacity and elimination effects thus remains unclear. Plant polyphenols' prevention of the formation of acrylamide may be attributable to the reaction of these polyphenols with acrylamide, acrylamide precursors, or intermediates during thermal processing.

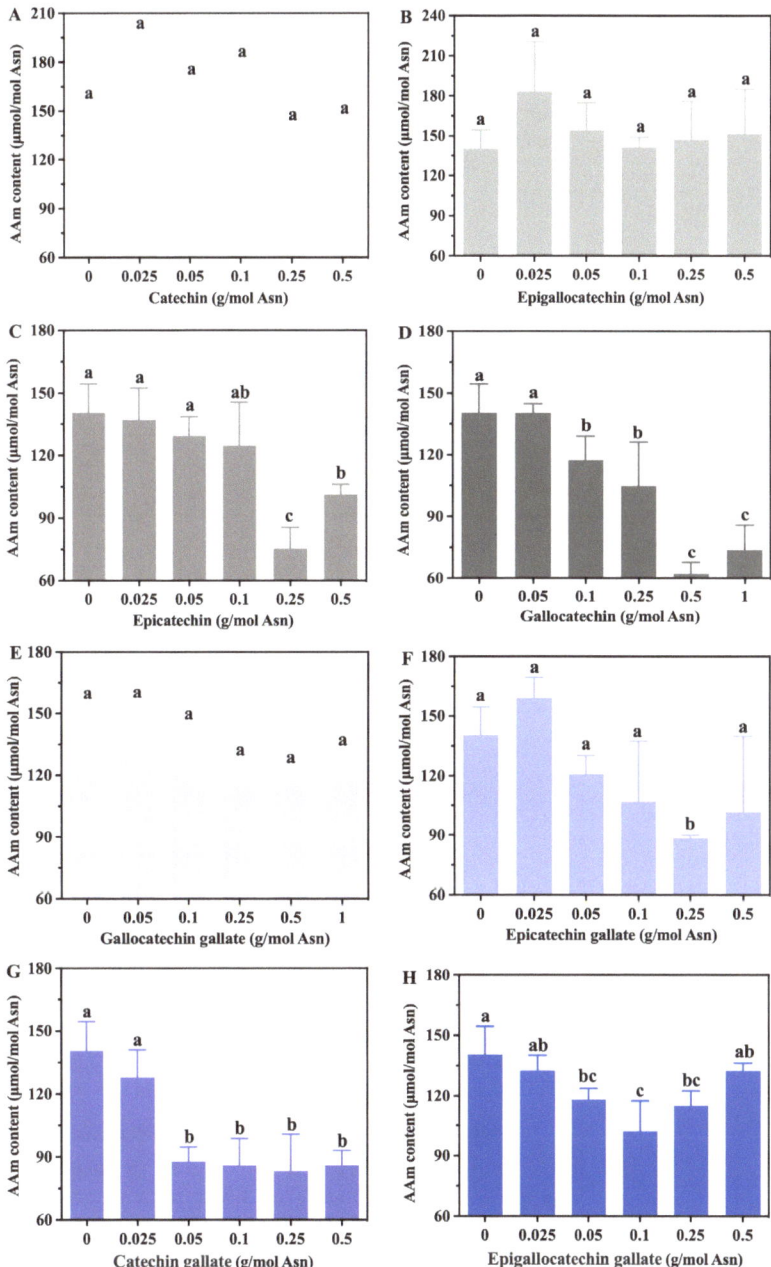

Figure 3. The effects of C (**A**), EGC (**B**), EC (**C**), GC (**D**), GCG (**E**), ECG (**F**), CG (**G**), and EGCG (**H**) on acrylamide reduction in the Glc-Asn model system. The different letters indicate significant differences at $p < 0.05$ at different concentrations.

3.3. The Effects of Tea Polyphenol Oxides on Acrylamide Levels in the Glc-Asn Model System

Tea polyphenols have multiple phenolic hydroxyl groups and are easily oxidized into theaflavins and thearubigins by polyphenol oxidase; they can also be converted into theabrownine with the assistance of microorganism fermentation. In the current study, the ability of tea polyphenol oxides to inhibit acrylamide in the model system was assessed (Figure 4). The results revealed that oxidation products of tea polyphenols (theaflavins and thearubigins) had strong inhibitory effects on acrylamide, with maximum inhibitions of 44.91% and 37.36%, respectively, when applied at 0.5 g/mol Asn. Thus, minor oxidation can improve tea polyphenols' ability to reduce the amount of acrylamide (Figure 2A). However, theabrownine did not have an inhibitory effect ($p > 0.05$, Figure 4C).

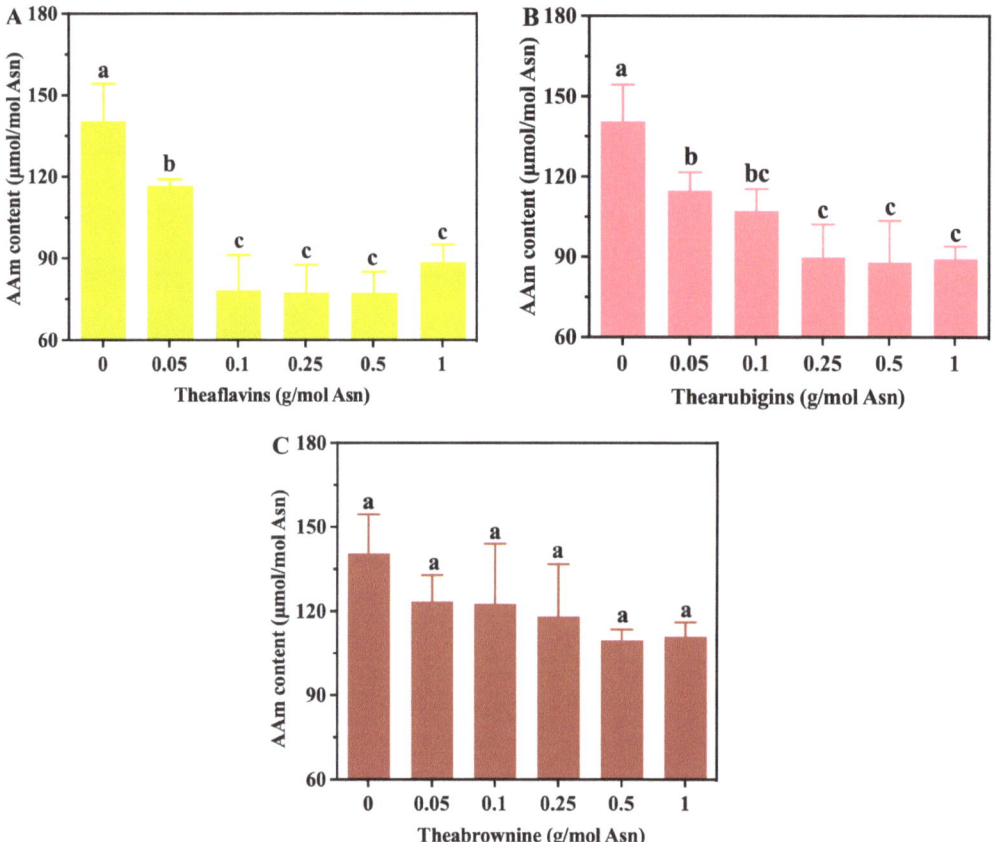

Figure 4. Effects of theaflavins (**A**), thearubigins (**B**), and theabrownine (**C**) on acrylamide reduction. The different letters indicate significant differences at $p < 0.05$ at different concentrations.

3.4. Synergistic or Antagonistic Effects of Tea's Characteristic Components on Acrylamide Formation

To investigate the possible synergistic or antagonistic effects of tea's characteristic components on acrylamide levels, five characteristic components of tea with inhibition rates higher than 35% (theaflavins, thearubigins, EC, GC, and CG) were selected and grouped in 26 combinations. Combinations with component levels of 1 g/mol Asn in equal masses were added to the Glc-Asn model system separately, and the acrylamide content in the systems with these combinations was determined; the results are presented in Table 1. Both synergistic and antagonistic effects were discovered for certain combinations. Combinations 3 (theaflavins + thearubigins + EC + CG), 4 (theaflavins + thearubigins + GC + CG), 5 (theaflavins + EC + GC + CG), 6 (thearubigins + EC + GC + CG), 7 (EC + GC + CG), 9 (thearubigins + EC + CG), 10 (thearubigins + EC + GC), 11 (theaflavins + GC + CG), and 26 (theaflavins + thearubigins) were discovered to have a synergistic effect, that is, to result in much lower acrylamide levels than the individual components did. The acrylamide reduction rates of combinations 1 (theaflavins + thearubigins + EC + GC + CG), 12 (theaflavins + EC + CG), 16 (theaflavins + thearubigins + EC), and 22 (thearubigins + EC) were only 19.52%, 10.65%, 28.19%, and 21.54%, respectively. These combinations were thus concluded to have clear antagonistic effects. However, the mechanisms underlying the synergistic and antagonistic effects of these components remain unclear.

Table 1. Effects of 26 complexes on acrylamide formation in Glc-Asn model system.

Combination	Ingredient					AAm Content (μmol/mol Asn)	Reduction Rate (%)
	Theaflavins	Thearubigins	EC	GC	CG		
Control	-	-	-	-	-	140.58 ± 13.92 [a]	ND
1	+	+	+	+	+	113.14 ± 10.80 [bc]	19.52
2	+	+	+	+	-	74.39 ± 14.61 [ghij]	47.08
3	+	+	+	-	+	55.97 ± 19.74 [jkl]	60.19
4	+	+	-	+	+	51.14 ± 5.22 [kl]	63.62
5	+	-	+	+	+	61.66 ± 3.35 [ijk]	56.14
6	-	+	+	+	+	36.56 ± 1.79 [l]	73.99
7	-	-	+	+	+	50.28 ± 3.93 [kl]	64.24
8	-	+	-	+	+	77.78 ± 13.13 [fghi]	44.67
9	-	+	+	-	+	38.42 ± 3.71 [l]	72.67
10	-	+	+	+	-	45.53 ± 3.64 [kl]	67.62
11	+	-	-	+	+	40.73 ± 2.34 [l]	71.03
12	+	-	+	-	+	125.61 ± 17.96 [ab]	10.65
13	+	-	+	+	-	82.79 ± 2.70 [efgh]	41.11
14	+	+	-	-	+	96.47 ± 5.59 [cdef]	31.38
15	+	+	-	+	-	96.75 ± 4.03 [cdef]	31.18
16	+	+	+	-	-	100.96 ± 14.17 [cde]	28.19
17	-	-	-	+	+	73.94 ± 0.96 [hij]	47.40
18	-	-	+	-	+	91.08 ± 3.86 [defg]	35.21
19	-	-	+	+	-	72.32 ± 1.99 [ghij]	48.56
20	-	+	-	-	+	72.65 ± 13.71 [ghij]	48.32
21	-	+	-	+	-	70.87 ± 11.83 [hij]	49.59
22	-	+	+	-	-	110.30 ± 24.53 [bcd]	21.54
23	+	-	-	-	+	92.51 ± 9.22 [defg]	34.19
24	+	-	-	+	-	91.70 ± 11.91 [defgh]	34.77
25	+	-	+	-	-	86.39 ± 17.54 [efgh]	38.55
26	+	+	-	-	-	48.165 ± 5.3 [kl]	65.74

Note: The data presented are the means and standard deviations of three samples (n = 3). Lowercase letters indicate significant differences ($p < 0.05$); "+" indicates added, "-" indicates not added, and "ND" indicates observations with no detection.

The elimination rates obtained in this study were compared with those previously reported. Compared with the rates for other plant polyphenols, the elimination rates of the tea characteristic components considered in the present study were favorable for their use for the elimination of acrylamide (Table 2). This provides an effective option for the high-value utilization of tea resources, especially summer and autumn tea resources.

Table 2. A comparison of the proposed tea characteristic components and the reported plant polyphenols for AAm elimination.

Plant Polyphenols	Matrix	Amount	Elimination Rate (%)	Reference
Tea characteristic components		0.25–0.5 g/mol Asn	37.36–55.73	This study
Combinations		1 g/mol Asn	65.74 / 67.62 / 71.03 / 72.67 / 73.99	
Naringin		11.6 mg/mol Asn	20	[18]
		22.3 mg/mol Asn	40	
		58.1 mg/mol Asn	60	
Apigenin	Glc-Asn model system	18.9 g/mol Asn	67.17	[35]
Cyanidenon		20.02 g/mol Asn	84.17	
Quercetin		2.11 g/mol Asn	80.11	
Glycyrrhizin		0.18 g/mol Asn	88.77	
Liquiritin		0.29 g/mol Asn	81.65	
Genistein		1.89 g/mol Asn	86.51	
Silymarin		3.37 mg/mol Asn	83.99	
Garlic powder (freeze-dry)		41.67 g/mol Asn	41	[36]
Garlic powder (oven-dry)			37.3	
Garlicin		9.1 mg/mol Asn	71.3	
Antioxidant of bamboo leaves	Potato chips	0.1% (w/w)	74.1	[37]
	French fries	0.01% (w/w)	76.1	
	Chinese fried dough stick	0.1% (w/w)	82.9	
	Fried chicken wings	0.5% (w/w)	59	

3.5. The Effects of Tea's Characteristic Components on Free Radical Generation in the Glc-Asn Model System

EPR is the most straightforward and practical method for detecting free radicals. In EPR, different spectral peaks occur when different scavengers are added to samples, and the nature of the free radicals that are present can be determined by their spectral characteristics. Figure S1 presents the EPR spectra of the persistent radicals in the Glc-Asn model system before and after the addition of tea's characteristic components. The amplitude of the spectra obtained after this addition is smaller than that of the spectra obtained before the addition. The total number of spins before addition was 1.37×10^{14}; after EC, CG, GC, and thearubigins were added, the total numbers of spins were 5.60×10^{13}, 3.93×10^{13}, 4.46×10^{13}, and 5.21×10^{13}, respectively. This finding suggests that the mechanism through which acrylamide formation is prevented by tea's characteristic components may involve the prevention of the formation of persistent free radicals. The protection mechanism of plant polyphenols is likely strongly related to the scavenging of free radicals from the Maillard reaction [26,38]. Plant polyphenols are a large group of naturally occurring polyphenolic hydroxyl groups, the hydrogen atoms of which can scavenge free radicals and terminate the propagation of free radical chain reactions [1].

4. Conclusions

The comprehensive influence of tea and its characteristic components on the formation of acrylamide in the Glc-Asn model system was investigated. Within the selected ranges of addition levels, all characteristic components of tea, with the exception of EGC, were discovered to negatively affect the formation of acrylamide in the model system. The components, ranked from highest to lowest rate, had the following acrylamide reduction rates: GC (55.73%) > EC (46.31%) > theaflavins (44.91%) > CG (40.73%) > thearubigins (37.36%) > ECG (37.03%) > EGCG (27.37%) > green tea (25.48%) > theanine (22.54%) > GCG (16.21%) > catechins (10.14%) > C (7.48%). Combinations 7 (EC + GC + CG), 9 (thearubigins + EC + CG), 10 (thearubigins + EC + GC), 11 (theaflavins + GC + CG), and 26 (theaflavins + thearubigins) were found to have favorable negative effects on acrylamide. These combinations achieved acrylamide reduction rates higher than 65% and rates that were 11.89–36.63% higher than those achieved for the individual components. Tea's characteristic components reduce the amount of acrylamide that forms by preventing the formation of persistent free radicals. This study provides a practical strategy and useful guidelines for controlling the amounts of acrylamide in thermally processed foods using tea and its characteristic components as food ingredients.

Supplementary Materials: The following supporting information can be downloaded at: https://www.mdpi.com/article/10.3390/foods13172836/s1, Figure S1: Effects of EC, CG, GC, and thearubigins on free radicals in model system.

Author Contributions: Z.Y.: methodology, formal analysis, investigation, writing—original draft. H.X.: formal analysis, writing—review and editing. Y.X.: investigation. Z.P.: data curation. H.L.: writing—review and editing. W.S.: writing—review and editing. R.H.: formal analysis, writing—review and editing. H.C.: formal analysis, writing—review and editing. C.P.: conceptualization, formal analysis, data curation, writing—review and editing, project administration, D.L.: writing—review and editing. All authors have read and agreed to the published version of the manuscript.

Funding: The present work was financially supported by the China Agriculture Research System of MOF and MARA (CARS-19) and Anhui Province Excellent Research and Innovation Team (2022AH010055).

Data Availability Statement: The original contributions presented in the study are included in the article/Supplementary Material, further inquiries can be directed to the corresponding author.

Conflicts of Interest: The authors declare that they have no known competing financial interests or personal relationships that could have appeared to influence the work reported in this paper.

References

1. Liu, Y.; Wang, P.; Chen, F.; Yuan, Y.; Zhu, Y.; Yan, H.; Hu, X. Role of plant polyphenols in acrylamide formation and elimination. *Food Chem.* **2015**, *186*, 46–53. [CrossRef]
2. Maan, A.A.; Anjum, M.A.; Khan, M.K.I.; Nazir, A.; Saeed, F.; Afzaal, M.; Aadil, R.M. Acrylamide formation and different mitigation strategies during food processing—A review. *Food Rev. Int.* **2022**, *38*, 70–87. [CrossRef]
3. Bertuzzi, T.; Martinelli, E.; Mulazzi, A.; Rastelli, S. Acrylamide determination during an industrial roasting process of coffee and the influence of asparagine and low molecular weight sugars. *Food Chem.* **2020**, *303*, 125372. [CrossRef] [PubMed]
4. EFSA CONTAM Panel (EFSA Panel on Contaminants in the Food Chain). Scientific Opinion on acrylamide in food. *EFSA J.* **2015**, *13*, 4104.
5. Commission, E. Establishing Mitigation Measures and Benchmark Levels for the Reduction of the Presence of Acrylamide in Food. 2017. Eur-Lex. Available online: https://eur-lex.europa.eu/eli/reg/2017/2158 (accessed on 20 November 2017).
6. Capuano, E.; Ferrigno, A.; Acampa, I.; Serpen, A.; Açar, Ö.; Gökmen, V.; Fogliano, V. Effect of flour type on Maillard reaction and acrylamide formation during toasting of bread crisp model systems and mitigation strategies. *Food Res. Int.* **2009**, *42*, 1295–1302. [CrossRef]
7. Pedreschi, F.; Kaack, K.; Granby, K. Reduction of acrylamide formation in potato slices during frying. *LWT—Food Sci. Technol.* **2004**, *37*, 679–685. [CrossRef]
8. Lim, P.K.; Jinap, S.; Sanny, M.; Tan, C.P.; Khatib, A. The influence of deep frying using various vegetable oils on acrylamide formation in sweet potato (*ipomoea batatas* L. lam) chips. *J. Food Sci.* **2014**, *79*, T115–T121. [CrossRef]
9. Tepe, T.K.; Kadakal, C. Temperature and slice size dependences of acrylamide in potato fries. *J. Food Process. Preserv.* **2019**, *43*, e14270. [CrossRef]
10. Chan, D.S. Computer Simulation with a Temperature-Step Frying Approach to Mitigate Acrylamide Formation in French Fries. *Foods* **2020**, *9*, 200. [CrossRef] [PubMed]
11. Zamora, R.; Delgado, R.M.; Hidalgo, F.J. Amino phospholipids and lecithins as mitigating agents for acrylamide in asparagine/glucose and asparagine/2,4-decadienal model systems. *Food Chem.* **2011**, *126*, 104–108. [CrossRef]
12. Ma, Y.J.; Huang, H.R.; Zhang, Y.; Li, F.; Gan, B.; Yu, Q.; Xie, J.H.; Chen, Y. Soluble dietary fiber from tea residues with inhibitory effects against acrylamide and 5-hydroxymethylfurfural formation in biscuits: The role of bound polyphenols. *Food Res. Int.* **2022**, *159*, 111595. [CrossRef] [PubMed]
13. Mestdagh, F.; Maertens, J.; Cucu, T.; Delporte, K.; Van Peteghem, C.; De Meulenaer, B. Impact of additives to lower the formation of acrylamide in a potato model system through pH reduction and other mechanisms. *Food Chem.* **2008**, *107*, 26–31. [CrossRef]
14. Aiswarya, R.; Baskar, G. Enzymatic mitigation of acrylamide in fried potato chips using asparaginase from Aspergillus terreus. *Int. J. Food Sci. Technol.* **2018**, *53*, 491–498. [CrossRef]

15. Liu, C.; Luo, L.J.; Lin, Q.L. Antitumor activity and ability to prevent acrylamide formation in fried foods of asparaginase from soybean root nodules. *J. Food Biochem.* **2019**, *43*, e12756. [CrossRef]
16. Hidalgo, F.J.; Delgado, R.M.; Zamora, R. Role of mercaptans on acrylamide elimination. *Food Chem.* **2010**, *122*, 596–601. [CrossRef]
17. Liu, H.; Li, X.N.; Yuan, Y. Mitigation effect of sodium alginate on acrylamide formation in fried potato chips system based on response surface methodology. *J. Food Sci.* **2020**, *85*, 2615–2621. [CrossRef] [PubMed]
18. Cheng, K.W.; Zeng, X.H.; Tang, Y.S.; Wu, J.J.; Liu, Z.W.; Sze, K.H.; Chu, I.K.; Chen, F.; Wang, M.F. Inhibitory mechanism of naringenin against carcinogenic acrylamide formation and nonenzymatic browning in maillard model reactions. *Chem. Res. Toxicol.* **2009**, *22*, 1483–1489. [CrossRef]
19. Trujillo-Mayol, I.; Sobral, M.M.C.; Viegas, O.; Cunha, S.C.; Alarcón-Enos, J.; Pinho, O.; Ferreira, I. Incorporation of avocado peel extract to reduce cooking-induced hazards in beef and soy burgers: A clean label ingredient. *Food Res. Int.* **2021**, *147*, 110434. [CrossRef]
20. Demirok, E.; Kolsarici, N. Effect of green tea extract and microwave pre-cooking on the formation of acrylamide in fried chicken drumsticks and chicken wings. *Food Res. Int.* **2014**, *63*, 290–298. [CrossRef]
21. NBSC (National Bureau of Statistics of China). Statistical Communiqué of the People's Republic of China on The 2023 National Economic and Social Development. 2024. Available online: https://www.stats.gov.cn/english/PressRelease/202402/t20240228_1947918.html (accessed on 28 February 2023).
22. Knol, J.J.; van Loon, W.A.M.; Linssen, J.P.H.; Ruck, A.L.; van Boekel, M.A.J.S.; Voragen, A.G.J. Toward a kinetic model for acrylamide formation in a glucose-asparagine reaction system. *J. Agric. Food Chem.* **2005**, *53*, 6133–6139. [CrossRef]
23. GB 5009.204; Determination of Acrylamide in Food. SAPRC (Standardization Administration of the People's Republic of China): Beijing, China, 2014.
24. Morales, G.; Jimenez, M.; Garcia, O.; Mendoza, M.R.; Beristain, C.I. Effect of natural extracts on the formation of acrylamide in fried potatoes. *LWT—Food Sci. Technol.* **2014**, *58*, 587–593. [CrossRef]
25. Li, D.; Chen, Y.; Zhang, Y.; Lu, B.; Jin, C.; Wu, X.; Zhang, Y. Study on mitigation of acrylamide formation in cookies by 5 antioxidants. *J. Food Sci.* **2012**, *77*, C1144–C1149. [CrossRef]
26. Budryn, G.; Żyżelewicz, D.; Nebesny, E.; Oracz, J.; Krysiak, W. Influence of addition of green tea and green coffee extracts on the properties of fine yeast pastry fried products. *Food Res. Int.* **2013**, *50*, 149–160. [CrossRef]
27. Peng, C.Y.; Ren, Y.F.; Ye, Z.H.; Zhu, H.Y.; Liu, X.Q.; Chen, X.T.; Hou, R.Y.; Granato, D.; Cai, H.M. A comparative UHPLC-Q/TOF-MS-based metabolomics approach coupled with machine learning algorithms to differentiate Keemun black teas from narrow-geographic origins. *Food Res. Int.* **2022**, *158*, 111512. [CrossRef]
28. Xie, G.; Yan, J.; Lu, A.; Kun, J.; Wang, B.; Song, C.; Tong, H.; Meng, Q. Characterizing relationship between chemicals and in vitro bioactivities of teas made by six typical processing methods using a single *Camellia sinensis* cultivar, Meizhan. *Bioengineered* **2021**, *12*, 1251–1263. [CrossRef] [PubMed]
29. Cheng, J.; Chen, X.; Zhao, S.; Zhang, Y. Antioxidant-capacity-based models for the prediction of acrylamide reduction by flavonoids. *Food Chem.* **2015**, *168*, 90–99. [CrossRef] [PubMed]
30. Oral, R.A.; Dogan, M.; Sarioglu, K. Effects of certain polyphenols and extracts on furans and acrylamide formation in model system, and total furans during storage. *Food Chem.* **2014**, *142*, 423–429. [CrossRef] [PubMed]
31. Hedegaard, R.V.; Granby, K.; Frandsen, H.; Thygesen, J.; Skibsted, L.H. Acrylamide in bread-Effect of prooxidants and antioxidants. *Eur. Food Res. Technol.* **2007**, *227*, 519–525. [CrossRef]
32. Zhang, Y.; Ying, T.; Zhang, Y. Reduction of acrylamide and its kinetics by addition of antioxidant of bamboo leaves (AOB) and extract of green tea (EGT) in asparagine–Glucose Microwave Heating System. *J. Food Sci.* **2008**, *73*, C60–C66. [CrossRef]
33. Kotsiou, K.; Tasioula-Margari, M.; Kukurová, K.; Ciesarová, Z. Impact of oregano and virgin olive oil phenolic compounds on acrylamide content in a model system and fresh potatoes. *Food Chem.* **2010**, *123*, 1149–1155. [CrossRef]
34. Cheng, K.W.; Shi, J.J.; Ou, S.Y.; Wang, M.; Jiang, Y. Effects of fruit extracts on the formation of acrylamide in model reactions and fried potato crisps. *J. Agric. Food Chem.* **2010**, *58*, 309–312. [CrossRef] [PubMed]
35. Yu, Z. Studies on Reduction Mechanism and Structure-Activity Relationship of Acrylamide in Foods by Bio-Flavonoids. Ph.D. Thesis, Zhejiang University, Hangzhou, China, 2008.
36. Salazar, R.; Arámbula-Villa, G.; Hidalgo, F.J.; Zamora, R. Mitigating effect of piquin pepper (*Capsicum annuum* L. var. Aviculare) oleoresin on acrylamide formation in potato and tortilla chips. *LWT—Food Sci. Technol.* **2012**, *48*, 261–267. [CrossRef]
37. Huang-you, L. Inhibition of Acrylamide and 5-Hydroxymethylfurfural Formation by Natural Plant Flavonoids in the Maillard Systems. Ph.D. Thesis, Jilin University, Changchun, China, 2018.
38. Li, X.D.; Teng, W.D.; Liu, G.M.; Guo, F.Y.; Xing, H.Z.; Zhu, Y.H.; Li, J.W. Allicin promoted reducing effect of garlic powder through acrylamide formation stage. *Foods* **2022**, *11*, 2394. [CrossRef] [PubMed]

Disclaimer/Publisher's Note: The statements, opinions and data contained in all publications are solely those of the individual author(s) and contributor(s) and not of MDPI and/or the editor(s). MDPI and/or the editor(s) disclaim responsibility for any injury to people or property resulting from any ideas, methods, instructions or products referred to in the content.

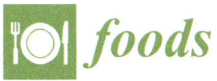

Article

Impact of Mild Field Drought on the Aroma Profile and Metabolic Pathways of Fresh Tea (*Camellia sinensis*) Leaves Using HS-GC-IMS and HS-SPME-GC-MS

Xiaohui Liu [1,2,3], Fabao Dong [3], Yucai Li [3], Fu Lu [3], Botao Wang [3], Taicen Zhou [3], Degang Zhao [1,2,*], Mingzheng Huang [3,*] and Feifei Wang [4]

[1] Plant Conservation & Breeding Technology Center, Guizhou Key Laboratory of Agricultural Biotechnology, Guizhou Institute of Pratuculture, Guizhou Academy of Agricultural Sciences, Guiyang 550006, China; liuxiaohui0908@hotmail.com

[2] Key Laboratory of Plant Resources Conservation and Germplasm Innovation in Mountainous Region (Ministry of Education), College of Tea Sciences, Guizhou University, Guiyang 550025, China

[3] College of Food and Pharmaceutical Engineering, Guizhou Institute of Technology, Guiyang 550025, China; fabao1234@163.com (F.D.); liyucai2860@hotmail.com (Y.L.); 17586454497@163.com (F.L.); 17585632907@163.com (B.W.); a1747632830@163.com (T.Z.)

[4] Key Laboratory of Plant Functional Genomics of the Ministry of Education, Jiangsu Key Laboratory of Crop Genomics and Molecular Breeding, Jiangsu Co-Innovation Center for Modern Production Technology of Grain Crops, Institutes of Agricultural Science, Yangzhou University, Yangzhou 225009, China; feifei.wang@yzu.edu.cn

* Correspondence: dgzhao@gzu.edu.cn (D.Z.); huangmingzheng@git.edu.cn (M.H.)

Citation: Liu, X.; Dong, F.; Li, Y.; Lu, F.; Wang, B.; Zhou, T.; Zhao, D.; Huang, M.; Wang, F. Impact of Mild Field Drought on the Aroma Profile and Metabolic Pathways of Fresh Tea (*Camellia sinensis*) Leaves Using HS-GC-IMS and HS-SPME-GC-MS. *Foods* **2024**, *13*, 3412. https://doi.org/10.3390/foods13213412

Academic Editor: Ricard Boqué

Received: 6 October 2024
Revised: 21 October 2024
Accepted: 23 October 2024
Published: 26 October 2024

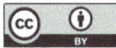

Copyright: © 2024 by the authors. Licensee MDPI, Basel, Switzerland. This article is an open access article distributed under the terms and conditions of the Creative Commons Attribution (CC BY) license (https://creativecommons.org/licenses/by/4.0/).

Abstract: Aroma plays a pivotal role in defining tea quality and distinctiveness, and tea producers have often observed that specific drought conditions are closely associated with the formation and accumulation of characteristic aroma compounds in tea leaves. However, there is still limited understanding of the differential strategies employed by various tea cultivars in response to drought stress for the accumulation of key volatile aroma compounds in fresh tea leaves, as well as the associated metabolic pathways involved in aroma formation. In this study, two widely cultivated tea cultivars in China, Fuding Dabai (FD) and Wuniuzao (WNZ), were examined to assess the impact of mild field drought stress on the composition and accumulation of key volatile aroma compounds in fresh leaves using headspace gas chromatography–ion mobility spectrometry (HS-GC-IMS) and headspace solid phase micro-extraction gas chromatography–mass spectrometry (HS-SPME-GC-MS) technologies. Results revealed that drought stress led to a substantial increase in the diversity of volatile compounds (VOCs) in FD, while WNZ exhibited a notable rise in low-threshold VOC concentrations, amplifying sweet, floral, fruity, and earthy aroma profiles in post-drought fresh leaves. Through partial least squares discriminant analysis (PLS-DA) of HS-GC-IMS and HS-SPME-GC-MS data, integrating variable importance projection (VIP) scores and odor activity values (OAVs) above 1, 9, and 13, key odor-active compounds were identified as potential markers distinguishing the drought responses in the two cultivars. These compounds serve as crucial indicators of the aromatic profile shifts induced by drought, providing insights into the differential metabolic strategies of the cultivars. Additionally, KEGG enrichment analysis revealed 12 metabolic pathways, such as terpenoid biosynthesis, fatty acid synthesis, cutin, suberine, and wax biosynthesis, and phenylalanine metabolism, which may play crucial roles in the formation and accumulation of VOCs in tea leaves under drought stress. These findings provide a comprehensive framework for understanding the cultivar-specific mechanisms of aroma formation and accumulation in tea leaves under mild drought conditions.

Keywords: *Camellia sinensis* cultivar; drought stress; fresh tea leaves; gas chromatography–ion mobility spectrometry (GC-IMS); headspace solid-phase micro-extraction gas chromatography–mass spectrometry (HS-SPME-GC-MS); aroma profile; odor activity values (OAVs); odor-active aroma compounds

1. Introduction

Tea is a globally popular beverage known for its distinctive flavor and health-promoting properties [1–3]. Tea products are primarily derived from the buds and young or mature leaves of the tea plant (*Camellia sinensis*) [4]. Consequently, the bioactive compounds responsible for tea's flavor and health qualities are predominantly found in these buds and leaves. Several factors, including tea plant cultivar [5–7], environmental growing conditions [8–12], and post-harvest processing methods [13–16], significantly influence the production and accumulation of these active metabolites, thereby affecting the overall quality of the tea. The quality of fresh tea leaves is a fundamental factor in determining the final quality of the processed tea product. It is generally accepted that only high-quality fresh leaves can produce premium tea. The accumulation of bioactive compounds in fresh tea leaves is closely related to both the tea plant cultivar and its growing environment. Among environmental factors, drought is a common stressor that significantly affects tea plant growth and the accumulation of metabolites in young shoots [17–19]. Some studies have shown that moderate drought can enhance tea flavor by balancing specific metabolite levels in fresh leaves [19], while slight drought stress has been found to promote polyphenol synthesis, leading to improved tea flavor quality [20]. In addition, drought stress is also known to influence the formation of tea's unique aromatic compounds. For example, the characteristic aromas of Keemun black tea from China, high-aroma Ceylon tea from Sri Lanka, and Darjeeling tea from India have been associated with short-term drought conditions [21]. In China's Yunnan province, local tea plantation smallholders also observe that spring drought positively influences the aroma of tea [22]. In a previous study on *Lingtou Dancong* tea plants under drought stress, it was found that different levels of drought can induce the synthesis of varying types of aromatic compounds, with the number of aroma compounds in fresh tea leaves increasing as drought stress intensifies [23]. Additionally, research indicates that slight drought stress can lead to the enrichment of metabolic pathways involved in linoleic acid and butyric acid metabolism, further suggesting drought's role in modulating tea aroma [20].

Despite the existing research on the positive effects of moderate or slight drought on tea flavor and aroma, the mechanisms by which drought stress specifically influences the formation of key aroma compounds in tea remain insufficiently explored. Volatile compounds (VOCs) in tea, although comprising only 0.01% of the dry weight, are crucial for its aroma [24]. To date, over 700 VOCs have been identified in tea, predominantly alcohols, aldehydes, ketones, and terpenes [4]. However, only a limited number of these compounds, with odor activity values (OAVs) exceeding 1, are considered to make significant contributions to the overall aroma, thus being classified as key odor-active aroma compounds [25,26]. Most previous research has focused on identifying key odor-active aroma compounds in processed tea [13,27–29], with limited attention given to fresh tea leaves prior to processing, particularly concerning the effects of abiotic stresses like drought on the formation of key odor-active aroma compounds in fresh tea leaves. This study aims to address this gap by evaluating the effects of field drought stress on the key odor-active aroma compounds in fresh leaves from two widely cultivated tea cultivars in China, Fuding Dabai (FD) and Wuniuzao (WNZ). The primary objective is to assess the impact of drought on the volatile profile and aroma characteristics of fresh tea leaves and to elucidate the differential metabolic pathways involved in aroma formation under drought conditions between the two cultivars.

Gas chromatography–mass spectrometry (GC-MS) is a widely used technique for the identification and quantification of VOCs in tea [4,14,30]. With advances in technology, pre-concentration techniques for VOCs and methods for their separation and identification, centered around GC-MS, have been improved. In particular, headspace solid-phase micro-extraction (HS-SPME) technology offers significant advantages for collecting and concentrating VOCs from tea leaves. This method allows for the efficient extraction of trace aroma compounds in a highly sensitive and rapid manner, enabling ultra-trace (nanogram-level) quantification when combined with GC-MS [13,30–32]. Additionally, gas chromatography–ion mobility spectrometry (GC-IMS), a novel technique for the separation, identification, and quantification of VOCs, has also gained prominence in tea research. Compared to HS-SPME-GC-MS, GC-IMS offers the advantage of direct extraction and analysis of volatiles from tea samples without the need for extensive pretreatment, making it particularly effective in separating isomers and complementing HS-SPME-GC-MS in volatile aroma profiling [24,33].

In this study, both HS-GC-IMS and HS-SPME-GC-MS were employed to comprehensively analyze the effects of drought stress on the volatile profiles of fresh tea leaves from FD and WNZ cultivars. Key odor-active aroma compounds were identified based on their OAVs, and differences in key aroma markers between the two tea cultivars under drought conditions were assessed using variable importance in projection (VIP) scores in a partial least squares discriminant analysis (PLS-DA) model. Furthermore, KEGG pathway enrichment analysis was performed to investigate the differential metabolic strategies adopted by the two cultivars in response to drought stress. The findings from this study offer valuable insights into how drought stress affects the composition and presentation of key odor-active aroma compounds in fresh tea leaves, particularly via terpenoid biosynthesis, phenylalanine metabolism, fatty acid synthesis, and cutin, suberine, and wax biosynthesis. These results contribute to our understanding of the mechanisms responsible for aroma formation, particularly in cultivar-specific responses to drought stress, while also providing a foundation for optimizing water management in tea cultivation and refining processing techniques to enhance tea quality.

2. Materials and Methods

2.1. Experimental Design and Collection of Tea Samples

The experimental tea garden is situated at Hongfengshanyun Tea Farm, Qingzhen, Guizhou Province, China (106°22′ E, 26°31′ N). Eight-year-old 'Fuding Dabai' (FD) and 'Wuniuzao' (WNZ) tea plants were used as the experimental materials. Tea plants grown under field conditions were subjected to a 20-day natural drought treatment without irrigation, representing the drought-stressed groups (FD-D and WNZ-D, with soil water content at 55% ± 2.5%). In contrast, the control groups (FD-CK and WNZ-CK) were maintained under normal irrigation conditions, with soil water content at 75% ± 2.5%. Tea samples were randomly collected on 26 July 2022, with three biological replicates for each sample. The collected samples, consisting of one bud and two leaves, were promptly frozen in liquid nitrogen and stored at −80 °C in an ultra-low temperature freezer for subsequent aroma analysis.

2.2. Chemical Reagents

Aroma internal standard ethyl decanoate (98%) was purchased from TCI (Shanghai, China). Aroma standards of linalool (98%), geraniol (98%), citronellol (95%), phenethyl alcohol (99.10%), 1-octanol (99.5%), citral (95%), decanal (98%), undecanal (97%), hexadecanal (97%), benzaldehyde (99.50%), methyl heptenone (99.50%), ionone (95%), and methyl hexanoate (99.5%) were purchased from Macklin (Shanghai, China). Aroma standards of 2,4-di-tert-butylphenol (98%), (+)-limonene (99%), nerol (98%), and coumarin (98%) were purchased from Yuanye (Shanghai, China). Tea infusion blank matrix standards of epicatechin (EC, 95%), (−)-epigallocatechin gallate (EGCG, 95%), (+)-catechin (C, 95%), and L-theanine (98%) were provided by Macklin (Shanghai, China). Tea infusion blank matrix standards of epigallocatechin (EGC, 98%) and epicatechin gallate (ECG, 98%) were provided by Bidepharm (Shanghai, China). The tea infusion blank matrix standard for caffeine (99.7%) was provided by TMstandard (Beijing, China). Analytical reagents sodium chloride and ethanol absolute were obtained from Jinshan (Chengdu, China). Distilled water was bought from Wahaha Group (Hangzhou, China) and a mixture of n-alkanes (C7–C30) was purchased from Sigma-Aldrich (St. Louis, MO, USA). n-Alkanes (C4–C9), including 2-butanone (99.5%), 2-pentanone (99.5%), 2-hexanone (99.5%), 2-heptanone (98%), 2-octanone (99%), and 2-nonanone (99%), were sourced from Sinopharm (Shanghai, China).

2.3. HS-GC-IMS Analysis

The VOCs and polymers of low molecular weight in the sample were detected using the FlavourSpec® (Melbourne, Australia) flavor analyzer, which employs GC-IMS technology. The FlavourSpec® flavor analyzer was equipped with a gas-phase ion mobility spectrometry unit and an automatic headspace sampling unit. The sample preparation procedure was as follows: 1 g of the sample was weighed and placed in a 20 mL headspace vial, followed by the addition of 20 µL of the internal standard ethyl decanoate (100 ppm) and mixing. The sample was then incubated at 60 °C for 15 min before injecting 500 µL of the headspace. The incubation speed was set to 500 rpm, and the headspace injection needle temperature was maintained at 85 °C. Each sample was analyzed in triplicate to ensure reproducibility.

The gas chromatography conditions were as follows: an MXT-5 column (15 m × 0.53 mm × 1.0 µm, Restek, Bellefonte, PA, USA) was used. The column temperature was maintained at 60 °C, with nitrogen (purity 99.999%) as the carrier gas. The total chromatographic run time was 20 min, with the carrier gas flow rate gradient set to an initial flow rate of 2 mL/min maintained for 2 min, and then linearly increased to 100 mL/min over the remaining 18 min. For ion mobility spectrometry, the drift tube temperature was set at 45 °C, and nitrogen (purity ≥99.999%) was used as the drift gas, with a flow rate of 150 mL/min.

The qualitative analysis of volatile substances was conducted using the VOCal software integrated with the National Institute of Standards and Technology (NIST), Flavors and Fragrances of Natural and Synthetic Compounds (FFNSC) library, and the IMS database from G.A.S. (Dortmund, Germany). Retention index (RI) values of the target VOCs were calculated using n-alkanes (C4–C9) as external standards. The identification of VOCs was achieved by matching RI and drift time (Dt) against the NIST and IMS database. The internal standard method was used for quantitative analysis.

2.4. HS-SPME-GC-MS Analysis

HS-SPME-GC-MS provides significant advantages in the qualitative and quantitative analysis of VOCs in complex samples, such as superior enrichment, heightened sensitivity, and enhanced selectivity. This technique is particularly effective for the dissociative qualitative analysis of high-molecular-weight VOCs. Consequently, the Shimadzu GCMS-TQ8040 NX triple quadrupole GC-MS system (Shimadzu, Kyoto, Japan), combined with HS-SPME, was utilized for the analysis of VOCs in tea leaf samples. The gas chromatographic separation was conducted using an InertCap 5MS capillary column (30 m × 0.25 mm, 0.25 µm, Shimadzu, Kyoto, Japan), with the AOC-6000 Plus Multifunctional Autosampler (Shimadzu, Kyoto, Japan) facilitating fully automated sample injection. The extraction and analysis of VOCs were performed following the published experimental protocol, with certain modifications [34,35].

2.4.1. Sample Preparation

An appropriate amount of tea leaf sample was placed in a mortar and ground with liquid nitrogen. Precisely 0.5 g of the ground sample was then transferred into a 20 mL headspace vial, followed by the addition of 1.5 g of NaCl and 5 mL of boiled ultrapure water. Additionally, 4 µL of ethyl decanoate (1 mg/L, diluted in anhydrous ethanol) was incorporated as an internal standard. The vial was promptly sealed with a screw cap fitted with a PTFE–silicon spacer and positioned in the AOC-6000 Plus (Shimadzu, Kyoto, Japan) sample tray in preparation for detection.

2.4.2. HS-SPME Extraction of VOCs

The HS-SPME procedure was configured as follows: the sample was equilibrated at 70 °C for 5 min, after which the SPME fiber (50/30 µm DVB/CAR/PDMS, CTC Analytics, Zwingen, Switzerland) was exposed to the headspace for extraction at 70 °C for 30 min, with the agitator set to 600 rpm. The fiber was then inserted into the GC injection port in splitless mode for desorption for 5 min, followed by a post-conditioning time of 5 min.

2.4.3. GC-MS Analysis of VOCs

The separation of VOCs was performed using an InertCap 5MS capillary column (30 m × 0.25 mm, 0.25 μm) with helium (purity >99.999%) as the carrier gas. The GC program was set as follows: an initial temperature of 40 °C was maintained for 3 min, followed by a ramp of 2 °C/min to 190 °C, held for 1 min, and then a second ramp of 10 °C/min to 230°C, held for 2 min. The flow rate of the carrier gas was set to 1 mL/min, and the column oven cooling rate was adjusted to medium. The MS conditions were as follows: an electron impact (EI) ion source was operated at an electron energy of 70 eV. The ion source and interface temperatures were both set to 280 °C. A solvent delay time of 2 min was applied, and the mass scanning range was established from m/z 33 to 600. Each sample was subjected to triplicate injections for analysis.

2.4.4. Identification and Quantification of VOCs

All VOCs were initially identified using the NIST 17 and FFNSC1.3 library match, selecting aroma compounds with a similarity score exceeding 80%. These VOCs were further confirmed through their RI and authentic standards. n-Alkane (C7-C30) standards were utilized to determine the RI of VOCs. Each aroma standard compound, at a specified concentration, was mixed with the 'volatile-free' blank matrix and subjected to qualitative and quantitative analysis via HS-SPME-GC-MS to obtain calibration curves. For compounds lacking available standards, estimation was conducted using standards with analogous functional groups and comparable carbon atom counts [34,35]. The standard curve method was employed for the absolute quantitative analysis of certain VOCs, while the internal standard method was utilized for the semi-quantitative analysis of other VOCs. The details of the 'volatile-free' blank matrix model stock solution and the calibration standard curves are shown in Tables S1 and S2.

2.4.5. Odor Activity Value (OAV) Analysis of VOCs

OAV is a critical indicator for determining key aroma-active compounds in a sample. The OAV is calculated as the ratio of the concentration of each volatile compound to its odor threshold (OT) in water, with the thresholds primarily referenced from early relevant studies [4,36–38]. When multiple data points are available for the threshold, the selection criteria prioritize using data from aqueous systems and the most recent data. Generally, when the OAV exceeds 1, the compound significantly influences the tea's overall flavor. With an OAV between 0.1 and 1, the compound acts as a modifying aroma, subtly enhancing the flavor profile [39]. The higher the OAV, the greater the compound's contribution to the overall flavor, and vice versa.

2.5. Data Analysis

All experiments were performed in triplicate and the corresponding results are presented as the mean ± standard deviation (SD). Statistical analysis of VOC differences among the groups was conducted using one-way analysis of variance (ANOVA) with SPSS software 26 (IBM, Armonk, NY, USA), and p-values < 0.05 were considered statistically significant. Multivariate statistical analysis of the experimental data was performed using MetaboAnalyst 6.0 (https://www.metaboanalyst.ca/, accessed on 7 September 2024) and SIMCA 14.1 (Umetrics, Umea, Sweden), focusing on Principal Component Analysis (PCA) and partial least squares discriminant analysis (PLS-DA) to analyze the similarities and differences in VOCs across different samples. The variable importance in projection (VIP) method, derived from PLS-DA models, was utilized to identify the key aroma compounds responsible for distinguishing between different tea cultivars and the effects of drought treatments. The alterations in VOCs following drought treatment were illustrated using a volcano plot. Significant changes were defined by a p-value < 0.05 (t-test) and a fold change

(FC) of ≥2 or ≤0.5. The volcano plot was generated with MetaboAnalyst 6.0. Graphical representations of the data were created using OriginPro 2021 (OriginLab, Northampton, MA, USA), MetaboAnalyst 6.0, Reporter and Gallery Plot plug (G.A.S., Dortmund, Germany), and the Biodeep cloud platform from Panomix (Suzhou, China).

3. Results and Discussion

3.1. Qualitative and Quantitative Analysis of the VOCs by HS-GC-IMS

Aroma volatiles of fresh tea leaves were identified and analyzed through HS-GC-IMS, employing retention indexes (RIs), retention times, and drift times referenced from the NIST library. A total of 50 peaks were detected across four groups, with 44 peaks successfully identified as specific chemical compounds, while 6 peaks remained unidentified and were classified as unknown substances, requiring further validation. The detailed analysis results are provided in Table S3. The detected VOCs were categorized into several groups, including aldehydes, ketones, esters, terpenes, furans, alcohols, aromatics, and pyrazines (Figure 1A). Among these, aldehydes, ketones, and terpenes were the three most dominant volatile groups, collectively constituting over 60% of the total volatiles (Figure 1B), with 12, 7, and 6 aroma compounds, respectively (Table S3).

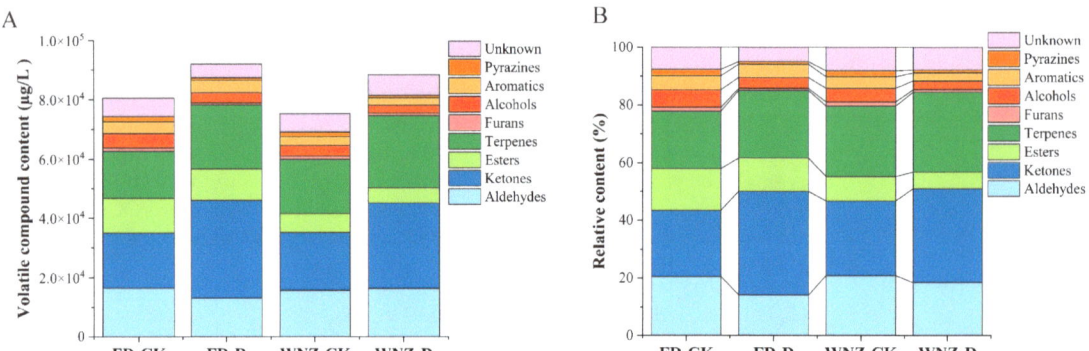

Figure 1. Comparison of VOCs in 4 groups detected by HS-GC-IMS. (**A**) Stacked column graph of VOC content; (**B**) 100% stacked column graph of VOC relative content.

The VOC content exhibited variation between different tea cultivars. Overall, the FD cultivar demonstrated higher VOC levels compared to the WNZ cultivar. Drought stress led to an increase in VOC levels in both cultivars. Notably, in the FD cultivar, ketones, terpenes, and aromatics showed a substantial increase under drought conditions, while aldehydes, esters, furans, alcohols, and pyrazines decreased. In comparison, in the WNZ cultivar, aldehydes, ketones, and terpenes exhibited a marked increase under drought stress, while the levels of esters, furans, alcohols, aromatics, and pyrazines decreased. The results indicate that the differential accumulation of aroma compounds under drought stress is related to the varying drought adaptability of different tea cultivars [40].

In summary, across both cultivars, drought stress induced a notable increase in ketones and terpenes, contributing to enhanced citrus, floral, sweet, earthy, and herbal aroma characteristics in fresh tea leaves. These results suggest that ketones and terpenes play a key role not only in the drought resilience of tea plants but also in the modulation of tea flavor under environmental stress. Interestingly, tea plantation smallholders serving as informants from tea production communities in Yunnan Province, China, also observed that the aroma of spring tea becomes more intense during drought periods, which they believed positively influences the market price of the tea [22]. This observation aligns with the findings of our study, where the content of volatile compounds increased in both FD and WNZ tea cultivars following drought stress (shown in Figure 1A).

Drought stress influences the differential accumulation of VOCs in the fresh leaves of tea plants. Compared to the control group, drought-stressed plants exhibited higher levels of ketone VOCs, including methyl-5-hepten-2-one, 3-octanone, mesityl oxide, 2-pentanone, 2-butanone, and acetone. Additionally, methylated VOCs ((E)-4-methyl-2-(pent-1-enyl)-1,3-dioxolane, methyl acetate, 5-methylfurfural, 2-furanmethanol, 5-methyl-, and 3-methyl-3-buten-1-ol), linalool oxides (trans-linalool oxide, cis-linalool oxide), (E)-2-hexenyl acetate-D, oct-1-en-3-ol, p-xylene, and benzaldehyde were also elevated (Figure 2A–C). These VOCs contribute predominantly to sweet, caramel-like, floral, earthy, and fruity aroma characteristics (shown in Table S3).

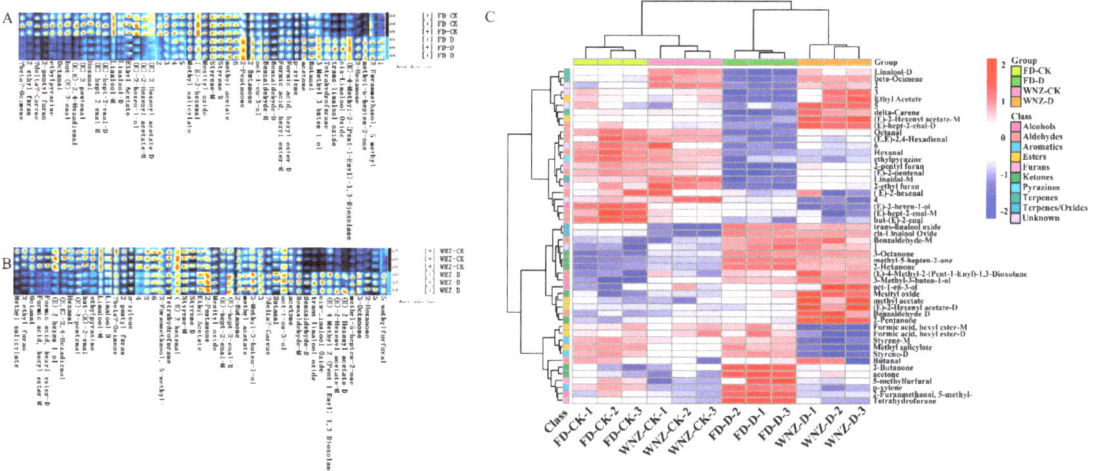

Figure 2. Comparisons of the identified VOCs in 4 groups by HS-GC-IMS. (**A**) The VOC fingerprint comparisons of FD-CK and FD-D; (**B**) the VOC fingerprint comparisons of WNZ-CK and WNZ-D; (**C**) heatmap clustering of VOCs in FD-CK, FD-D, WNZ-CK, and WNZ-D.

It is important to note that certain VOCs exhibited distinct accumulation patterns across different tea cultivars. For example, VOCs such as (E)-hept-2-enal-D, butanal, (E)-2-hexenyl acetate-M, ethyl acetate, and delta-carene were present in significantly higher concentrations in the WNZ cultivar under drought stress (Figure 2B), whereas their levels decreased in the FD cultivar under the same conditions (Figure 2A). Conversely, formic acid, hexyl ester-M, formic acid, hexyl ester-D, and styrene-D concentrations were elevated in cultivar FD following drought stress but decreased in WNZ (Figure 2A,B). These variations in VOC accumulation between cultivars are likely linked to differences in their metabolic adaptations to drought stress.

Moreover, an intriguing finding from this study was the increase in methylated volatile compounds under drought stress, which contributed to the enhanced sweet and fruity characteristics of fresh tea leaves. However, due to the absence of molecular and epigenetic data, the specific mechanisms by which drought conditions regulate the biosynthesis of methylated VOCs in tea remain unclear. Previous studies have suggested that environmental stresses, such as cold and drought, as well as postharvest processing, can induce changes in 5-methylcytosine (5mC) DNA methylation [17,41,42]. These epigenetic modifications are known to affect the expression of key genes involved in flavor biosynthesis, subsequently influencing the accumulation of compounds such as theanine, catechins, terpenoid [41], and indoles [42]. Investigating DNA methylation as a potential regulator of increased methylated VOCs in response to drought stress in tea could serve as a promising avenue for future research.

It is noteworthy that the alteration in linalool oxide levels observed under drought stress may be indicative of its role as a signaling molecule in the tea plant's stress response.

Previous research has demonstrated that linalool can be converted to linalool oxides via 6,7-epoxylinalool, and that infestations by green leafhoppers activate the metabolic flux from linalool to linalool oxides and their glycosides [43]. These findings may shed light on the regulatory mechanisms underlying linalool oxide accumulation in response to stress in tea plants.

In conclusion, the present study identifies several VOCs as potential metabolic markers for breeding drought-resistant tea cultivars with enhanced aroma profiles. These insights may also provide a basis for improving tea quality through targeted manipulation of metabolic pathways involved in aroma compound biosynthesis.

3.2. Identification of VOCs by HS-SPME-GC-MS

The volatile organic compounds (VOCs) from four tea sample groups were identified using HS-SPME-GC-MS, revealing a total of 144 distinct VOCs. The number of volatiles detected varied across the groups, with 85, 82, 83, and 100 volatiles identified in WNZ-CK, WNZ-D, FD-CK, and FD-D, respectively. These identified volatiles were categorized into 10 classes, namely esters, alcohols, ketones, aldehydes, terpenoids, acids, alkanes, alkenes, aromatics, and heterocyclics (as detailed in Table S4 and Figure 3B). To provide a clearer visualization of the variations in and characteristics of VOCs between groups, the total content, number, and proportion of VOCs in each category were summarized and presented through chord graphs, bar plots, and Venn diagrams (Figure 3). In terms of total VOC content, WNZ samples exhibited higher levels compared to FD samples (Figure 3A). The primary VOC classes in WNZ-CK and WNZ-D were terpenoids, alcohols, and ketones, accounting for 95% and 89% of the total concentration, respectively (Figure 3C). In contrast, FD-CK and FD-D were dominated by alcohols, terpenoids, and aldehydes, with these three categories comprising 97% of the total concentration (Figure 3D).

Following drought stress, a decrease in VOC concentration was observed in both the FD and WNZ cultivars (Figure 3A). Regarding VOC diversity, FD exhibited a greater increase in component richness after drought stress, whereas the variation in WNZ was less pronounced (Figure 3B). In both cultivars, terpenoids, alcohols, ketones, aldehydes, and esters were the predominant VOC classes, collectively contributing 85%, 85%, 87%, and 90% in FD-CK, FD-D, WNZ-CK, and WNZ-D, respectively. In the FD cultivar, drought stress led to an increase in the number of alcohols, aldehydes, and ketones, while the numbers of terpenoids and esters decreased. In comparison, the WNZ cultivar experienced a rise in aldehydes and ketones, but a reduction in alcohols, terpenoids, and esters under drought conditions (Figure 3D).

Furthermore, 44 volatiles were found to be common across all four groups, while 5, 26, 12, and 8 volatiles were exclusively detected in FD-CK, FD-D, WNZ-CK, and WNZ-D, respectively (Figure 3E). It is noteworthy that while the total VOC content in WNZ-CK exceeded that in FD-CK, the difference in VOC variety between these groups was marginal. Under drought stress, although both cultivars showed a reduction in total VOC content, FD-D exhibited a smaller decrease, along with a notable increase in component richness. By contrast, WNZ-D displayed only a slight reduction in VOC variety but experienced a more significant decline in total VOC content.

These findings are not entirely congruent with those obtained through HS-GC-IMS, likely due to differences in the target compounds and detection principles of the two methodologies. Therefore, employing a complementary, multi-technique approach is essential for achieving a more comprehensive and nuanced characterization of sample attributes [31,44].

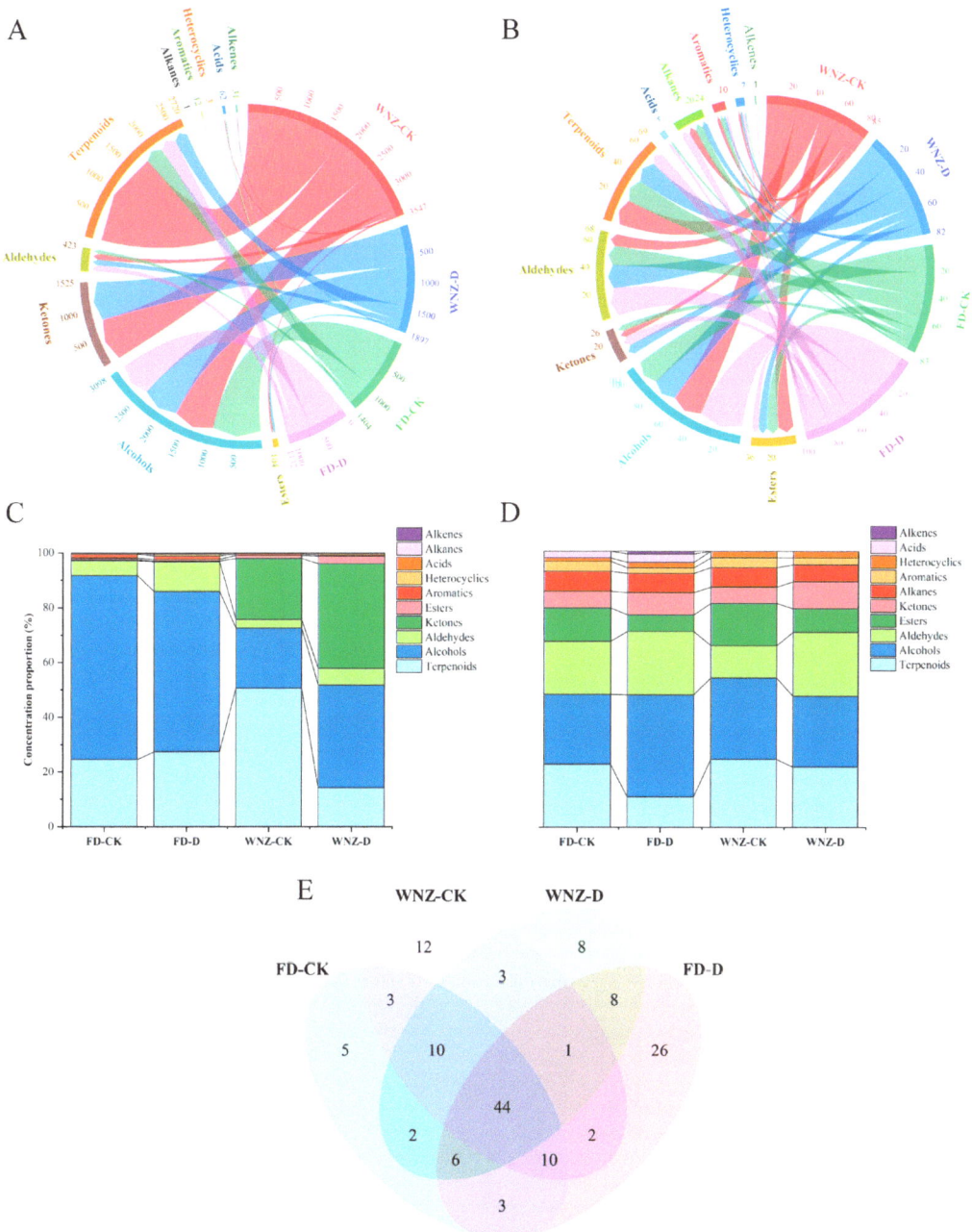

Figure 3. Volatile profiles across the four groups detected by HS-SPME-GC-MS. (**A**) Chord plot of aggregate VOC concentrations by category; (**B**) chord plot of total VOC numbers in each category; (**C**) 100% stacked graph of concentration proportions for different VOC categories; (**D**) 100% stacked graph of number proportions for different VOC categories; and (**E**) Venn diagram depicting VOC differences across the four groups.

3.3. OAV Analysis of HS-SPME-GC–MS Data

The contribution of VOCs to the overall aroma profile of tea is influenced not only by their concentrations but also by their respective odor thresholds. The ratio between an odorant's concentration and its detection threshold, commonly referred to as the odor activity value (OAV), serves as a critical determinant of its impact on the sample's aroma [4,26,28]. Comprehensive details regarding the concentration, odor threshold, odor descriptions, and OAVs of VOCs across the four sample groups are presented in Table S4. VOCs with OAVs ≥ 1, as well as those with OAVs between 0.1 and 1, are selectively highlighted and discussed in Table 1.

Table 1. The main aroma-active compounds with an odor activity value (OAV) ≥ 0.1 in 4 groups.

NO.	Volatile Compounds	Odor Characteristics	OT (μg/L)	OAVs FD-CK	FD-D	WNZ-CK	WNZ-D
1	Hex-(3Z)-enyl acetate	Green, fruity	13	0.19	-	1.58	0.25
2	Methyl salicylate	Minty, green	40	0.12	0.17	0.27	1.18
3	1-Hexanol	Herbal, fruity	5.6	0.62	0.63	0.64	0.64
4	1-Heptanol	Green, leafy, violet	5.4	0.68	0.79	0.7	0.7
5	1-Octen-3-ol	Earthy, mushroom	1.5	2.36	2.53	2.35	2.76
6	(Z)-Hex-3-en-1-ol	Green, grassy	3.9	1.66	-	-	-
7	1-Octanol	Waxy, green, orange	125.8	0.03	0.06	0.1	-
8	Linalool	Floral, citrus, rose	0.22	3155.46	1577.42	2307.87	2190.92
9	1-Nonanol	Floral, rose, orange	45.5	-	-	0.16	-
10	Geraniol	Floral, rose	1.1	119.45	115.99	130.9	99.64
11	6-methyl-5-Hepten-2-one	Citrus, lemon	0.16	-	1.68	-	3.06
12	1-Octen-3-one	Earthy, herbal, mushroom	0.003	-	-	-	113.76
13	(Z)-Jasmone	Floral, woody, herbal	0.26	9.31	0.16	-	1.81
14	(E)-alpha-Ionone	Violet	0.1	-	5.09	2.76	29.44
15	beta-Damascone	Fruity, floral, berry	0.002	9.32	19.18	60.44	157.58
16	(E)-beta-Ionone	Foral, fruity, woody	0.007	217.88	8.6	746.08	658.21
17	Hexanal	Green, grassy	5	0.61	1.34	0.81	1.24
18	2-Hexenal	Green, almond, fruity	30	0.16	0.66	0.14	0.67
19	Heptanal	Green, fatty, herbal	2.8	0.71	0.7	-	0.68
20	(E)-2-Heptenal	Green, vegetable, fatty	13	-	0.14	-	0.16
21	(E,E)-2,4-Heptadienal	Fatty, green	0.032	-	58.5	-	59.41
22	Octanal	Aldehydic, citrus	0.587	4.02	4.45	-	4.13
23	Oct-(2E)-enal	Fatty, green, herbal	0.2	-	-	-	9.83
24	Benzeneacetaldehyde	Green, floral, hyacinth	5.2	-	0.19	-	0.2
25	Nonanal	Aldehydic, orange, rose	1.1	2.79	3.18	2.78	-
26	(E)-2-Nonenal	Fatty, cucumber, citrus	0.19	10.01	-	-	10.78
27	Decanal	Aldehydic	3	0.74	0.96	0.71	0.91
28	(E)-2-Decenal	Fatty, earthy, green	0.3	7.9	7.82	7.48	10.78
29	Nona-(2E,4E)-dienal	Fatty, melon, green	0.1	-	-	-	19.16
30	Neral	Citrus, lemon	53	0.04	0.04	0.62	-
31	Citral	Citrus, lemon, sweet	40	1.06	1.43	1.42	1.43

Table 1. Cont.

NO.	Volatile Compounds	Odor Characteristics	OT (µg/L)	OAVs FD-CK	OAVs FD-D	OAVs WNZ-CK	OAVs WNZ-D
32	Undecanal	Aldehydic, floral, citrus	12.5	0.16	-	-	-
33	Dodecanal	Aldehydic, floral, citrus	0.13	-	16.5	-	-
34	Tridecanal	Aldehydic, citrus, grapefruit	10	-	0.19	-	-
35	beta-Myrcene	Spicy, peppery, woody	1.2	3.85	2.83	3.85	3.1
36	D-Limonene	Citrus, orange	34	0.1	0.09	0.1	-
37	(E)-beta-Ocimene	Herbal, citrus, woody	34	0.13	0.09	0.11	0.16
38	alpha-Farnesene	Woody, citrus, herbal	87	-	-	-	0.24
39	delta-Cadinene	Woody, spicy, burnt	1.5	2.36	-	3.38	2.4
40	Cedrol	Woody, cedarwood	0.5	6.54	6.03	5.75	-
41	Linalool oxide I	Woody, flowery, earthy	100	0.98	1.4	1.3	6.41
42	Linalool oxide II	Woody, flowery	190	0.76	0.95	0.36	5.72
43	Coumarin	Tonka	25	0.14	-	0.15	0.17
44	Naphthalene	Pungent, dry resinous	6	0.59	0.6	0.58	0.59
45	Indole	Flowery	40	-	-	0.13	0.13

Notes: odor characteristics and odor threshold (OT) were referenced from sources denoted as in Table S4.

In total, 45 VOCs exhibited OAVs ≥0.1, with 27 of these compounds showing OAVs greater than 1 across the four groups. Specifically, 15, 16, 14, and 22 VOCs with OAVs ≥1 were identified in FD-CK, FD-D, WNZ-CK, and WNZ-D, respectively. These findings suggest that drought stress prompted an increase in the number of VOCs with OAVs ≥1 in both cultivars, with WNZ-D experiencing a marked 57.14% rise compared to WNZ-CK.

Notably, seven VOCs shared across all four groups exhibited OAVs ≥1, including 1-octen-3-ol (earthy, mushroom), linalool (floral), geraniol (floral), β-damascone (fruity), (E)-β-ionone (floral), citral (citrus), and β-myrcene (spicy). These volatiles contribute significantly to the floral and fruity aromatic characteristics of tea leaves. Linalool, which had the highest OAV, is ubiquitous in a wide range of teas, including green tea, black tea, oolong tea, white tea, and yellow tea. Its production is predominantly linked to the light fermentation and drying phases of tea processing, where it imparts a fresh floral fragrance. In addition, geraniol, β-damascone, (E)-β-ionone, and β-myrcene are typically more abundant in black and oolong teas, particularly during fermentation, oxidation, and rolling processes. In contrast, 1-octen-3-ol and citral are more frequently detected in green and white teas, especially during the light fermentation and drying stages.

Upon drought stress, 10 key VOCs in the FD cultivar with OAVs exceeding 1 showed a notable increase, including 1-octen-3-ol, 6-methyl-5-hepten-2-one, (E)-α-ionone, β-damascone, (E,E)-2,4-heptadienal, octanal, nonanal, citral, dodecanal, and linalool oxide I. These compounds predominantly contribute to enhanced fruity, citrus, and orange aroma profiles. Conversely, nine volatiles demonstrated a decline in OAVs, such as (Z)-hex-3-en-1-ol, linalool, geraniol, (Z)-jasmone, (E)-β-ionone, (E)-2-nonenal, β-myrcene, δ-cadinene, and cedrol, primarily associated with green, grassy, floral, and spicy aromatic characteristics. In contrast, the WNZ cultivar under drought stress exhibited an increase in 15 volatiles with OAVs exceeding 1, including methyl salicylate, 1-octen-3-ol, 6-methyl-5-hepten-2-one, 1-octen-3-one, (E)-α-ionone, β-damascone, hexanal, (E,E)-2,4-heptadienal, octanal, (E)-2-nonenal, (E)-2-decenal, nona-(2E,4E)-dienal, linalool oxide I, and linalool oxide II, which contribute to heightened minty, earthy, citrus, violet, fruity, fatty, spicy, floral and woody aroma notes. On the other hand, eight VOCs displayed reduced OAVs, including hex-(3Z)-enyl acetate, linalool, geraniol, (Z)-jasmone, (E)-β-ionone, nonanal, β-myrcene, and δ-cadinene, characterized by green, floral, orange, spicy, and woody aromas. In summary, these findings suggest that drought stress predominantly intensified citrus and fruity aromas, while diminishing green and grassy notes. A consistent trend across both cultivars was the elevation of OAVs for aldehyde and ketone VOCs, whereas certain alcohol and terpene VOCs exhibited decreased OAVs. Particularly noteworthy is the observed reduction in linalool's OAV, accompanied by a corresponding increase in linalool oxide's OAV, indicating a potential conversion of linalool to its oxides in response to environmental stressors, thus contributing to floral and woody aroma characteristics. This phenomenon aligns with the results derived from HS-GC-IMS analyses.

Synthesis of the data presented in Figure 3 and Table S4 underscores the distinct adaptive responses of the two tea cultivars to drought stress. The FD cultivar's response was characterized by an expansion in the number of VOCs, while the WNZ cultivar exhibited a strategy of enhancing the concentrations of low-threshold, aroma-active compounds, thereby augmenting their OAVs and leading to a more pronounced aromatic profile. This differential response between cultivars presents an intriguing avenue for future exploration.

3.4. Comparative Analysis of HS-GC-IMS and HS-SPME-GC-MS in Identifying VOCs

3.4.1. Comparative Analysis of VOC Quantities and Categories

As illustrated in Figure 4A, a total of 178 VOCs were identified in this study using two distinct analytical methodologies. Specifically, HS-GC-IMS detected 44 VOCs, while HS-SPME-GC–MS identified 144 VOCs. Among these, 10 volatiles were found to be common across both methods, namely linalool, linalool oxide II, linalool oxide I, 6-methyl-5-hepten-2-one, benzaldehyde, methyl salicylate, octanal, (E)-2-heptenal, 1-octen-3-ol, and hexanal. These shared compounds are integral to the aroma profiles of fresh tea leaves and various tea products [4,24].

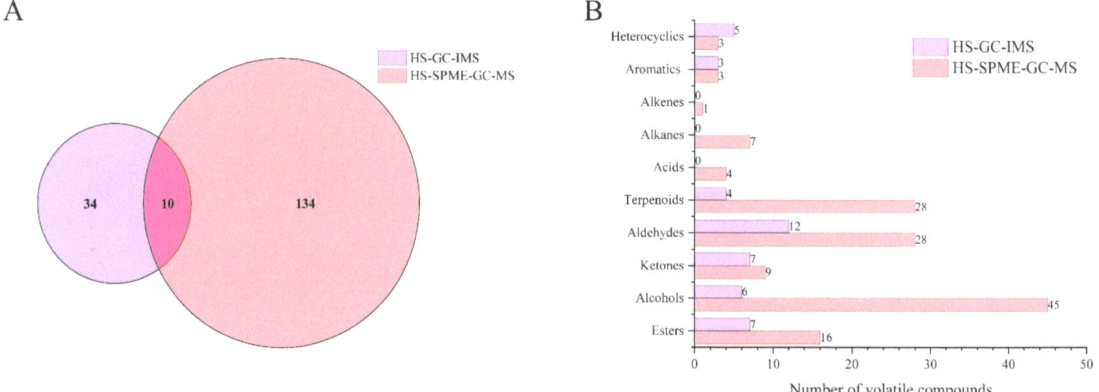

Figure 4. Comparative analysis of VOC quantities and categories: (**A**) Venn diagram of VOC numbers; (**B**) column graph of VOC categories.

VOC classification further revealed that HS-GC-IMS grouped the detected volatiles into seven categories, with aldehydes representing the most abundant class. By contrast, the VOCs identified via HS-SPME-GC–MS were categorized into ten groups, with alcohols being the dominant class. Notably, HS-GC-IMS did not to detect acids, alkanes, or alkenes, and the number of VOCs in most other categories, except for heterocyclic and aromatic compounds, was significantly lower compared to those identified by HS-SPME-GC–MS (Figure 4B). This disparity aligns with previous findings in the literature, wherein the two techniques were applied for the analysis of tea aroma compounds. HS-GC-IMS predominantly detects highly volatile and low-boiling-point compounds, whereas HS-SPME-GC–MS is more proficient in enriching and identifying higher-boiling-point volatiles. Moreover, the limited selectivity of IMS, attributed to ion–molecule and ion–ion competition reactions within the ionization chamber [45,46], may further contribute to the lower number of detected volatiles in comparison to HS-SPME-GC–MS.

3.4.2. PCA of All VOCs

In order to comprehensively evaluate the discriminative capacity of the two analytical methods applied to the four sample groups, as well as to elucidate the VOCs most strongly correlated with each group, unsupervised PCA analyses were conducted on both datasets, as depicted in Figure 5A,B. Figure 5A illustrates the PCA score plot (Figure 5A(a)) and the corresponding bi-plot (Figure 5A(b)) based on VOC concentration data obtained via HS-GC-IMS. The first two principal components account for 81.8% of the total variance, effectively segregating the four sample groups into distinct quadrants. Control groups are primarily located along the positive axis of PC1, whereas drought-stressed groups occupy the negative axis of PC1. Similarly, WNZ cultivars are positioned on the positive side of PC2, and FD cultivars on the negative side. The above results indicate that both tea cultivars experienced drought stress-induced significant variations in volatile profiles.

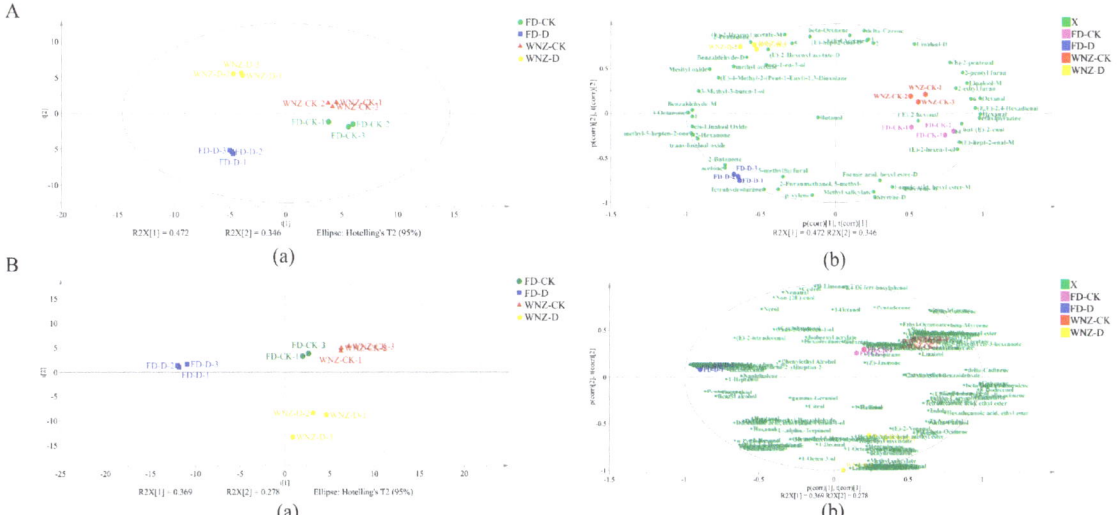

Figure 5. PCA plot and bioplot HS-GC-IMS and HS-SPME-GC-MS. (**A**) PCA (**a**) and biplot (**b**) of VOC intensity detected by HS-GC-IMS; (**B**) PCA (**a**) and biplot (**b**) of VOC concentration detected by HS-SPME-GC–MS.

Furthermore, Figure 5A(b) identifies several key VOCs strongly associated with WNZ-CK, including 2-pentyl furan (fruity and green), linalool-M (citrus and floral), 2-ethyl furan (Beany, ethereal, and cocoa), (E)-2-pentenal (green and fruity), (E,E)-2,4-Hexadienal (sweet and green), and octanal (waxy and citrus). Collectively, these compounds contribute to the characteristic green, fruity, and citrus aroma of WNZ-CK. In contrast, WNZ-D, situated in the second quadrant, is closely associated with 2-pentanone (sweet, and fruity), (E)-2-hexenyl acetate-D (sweet privet), benzaldehyde-D (bitter, almond, cherry, and burnt sugar), (E)-2-hexenyl acetate-M (sweet privet), oct-1-en-3-ol (mushroom, earthy, and green), and methyl acetate (sweet and fruity), contributing sweet, fruity, and earthy notes to the aroma profile of WNZ-D.

In parallel, FD-D exhibits a strong correlation with VOCs such as 2-butanone (fruity, and camphoraceous), acetone (apple and pear), tetrahydrofuran, 5-methylfurfural (sweet and caramellic), and 2-furanmethanol, 5-methyl- (sweet and caramellic), which collectively imbue FD-D with distinctive fruity, sweet, and caramel-like aromas. On the other hand, FD-CK is highly correlated with (E)-2-hexenal (leafy, green), ethylpyrazine (nutty and coffee), (E)-2-enal, (E)-hept-2-enal-M (green, vegetable), and (E)-2-hexen-1-ol (fresh green and leafy), lending a predominantly leafy, green, and nutty aromatic profile to FD-CK.

Figure 5B illustrates the PCA of VOCs in the four sample groups, as determined by HS-SPME-GC-MS. PC1 and PC2 explain 36.9% and 27.8% of the total variance, respectively. The sample groups are distributed across three quadrants, demonstrating clear discrimination between the control and drought-stressed groups. FD-CK and WNZ-CK are both situated in the first quadrant, while FD-D occupies the second quadrant, and WNZ-D the fourth quadrant (Figure 5B(a)). Notably, PC1 effectively separates the control and treatment groups of the FD cultivar, while PC2 discriminates between the control and treatment groups of the WNZ cultivar. Although FD-CK and WNZ-CK both reside within the first quadrant, their confidence ellipses differ, with FD-CK falling within the 50% confidence interval and WNZ-CK within the 75% confidence interval.

Compared to the HS-GC-IMS results, the HS-SPME-GC-MS analysis reveals a broader range of VOCs (Figure 5B(b)). The results from Figure S1 and Figure 5(Bb) illustrate that VOCs highly correlated with the control groups (WNZ-CK and FD-CK) are predominantly linked to floral, herbal, green, and fruity aroma characteristics. Notable compounds include (Z)-jasmone (floral), theaspirane (tea herbal), delta-elemene (herbal), hexyl isobutyrate (green), linalool oxide IV (tea-like, woody, and floral), undecanal (floral), (Z)-2-hepten-1-ol (fatty), (Z)-hex-3-en-1-ol (green), and nonanoic acid (waxy). In contrast, linalool (floral), (E)-beta-farnesene (herbal), neral (citrus), 1-nonanol (floral), cyclohexanol (green and rummy), alpha-calacorene (woody), (E)-3-hexen-1-ol (green), hex-(3Z)-enyl butyrate (green), acetic acid hexyl ester (fruity), T-cadinol (balsamic), and (Z)-3-hexenyl hexanoate (green) show a strong association with FD-CK.

On the other hand, VOCs significantly correlated with FD-D include caryophyllene oxide (woody), pinocarveol (herbal and woody), perilla alcohol (green, cumin, and spicy), dodecanal (soapy, waxy, and citrus), 1-tetradecanol (waxy), Z-5-decen-1-ol (waxy, fatty, and rose), 10-undecen-1-ol (citrus), dodecanoic acid (fatty and coconut), exo-Isocitral (lemongrass), tetradecanal (waxy, citrus, and fatty), (Z)-9-octadecen-1-ol (fatty), dehydrolinalool (floral), 1-undecanol (fresh, waxy, and rose), 6-hepten-1-ol (herbal), 2-undecenal (fruity), and tridecanal (citrus and grapefruit peel). Conversely, VOCs closely linked to WNZ-D predominantly include linalool oxide I (woody and floral), linalool oxide II (woody and floral), linalool oxide III (woody, floral, and citrus), alpha-farnesene (woody, and citrus), oct-(2E)-enal (fatty), nona-(2E,4E)-dienal (fatty, melon, and waxy), (3Z)-beta-ocimene (floral), (E)-2-decenal (waxy, fatty, and earthy), methyl salicylate (minty), alpha-guaiene (sweet and woody), gamma-muurolene (woody), beta-damascone (fruity and floral), dehydrolinalool (floral), hexadecanoic acid methyl ester (waxy), and 1-octen-3-one (earthy and mushroom). A holistic analysis of these findings indicates that the drought-treated groups (FD-D and WNZ-D) are more closely associated with woody, floral, rose, waxy, fatty, fruity, citrus, and earthy VOCs. Notably, the drought-treated groups exhibit a wider diversity of VOCs, leading to more complex and enriched aroma profiles. One particularly interesting observation is that VOCs correlated with the oxidation and dehydrogenation products of linalool are more prevalent in WNZ-D, primarily in the form of four distinct compounds: linalool oxide I, linalool oxide II, linalool oxide III, and dehydrolinalool. These compounds significantly enhance the floral and woody aroma characteristics in WNZ-D.

3.4.3. Identification of Aroma Markers Based on HS-GC-IMS and HS-SPME-GC–MS Data

In the PCA model, sample data visualization is enhanced by projecting the observations into a reduced dimensional space that captures the variance in the first few principal components, thereby highlighting classification trends across the samples. In contrast, the supervised PLS-DA model seeks to maximize the discrimination between different groups by focusing on the most influential differential metabolites across samples [47]. Specifically, VOCs with VIP > 1 were selected as the key discriminatory features in the PLS-DA model [48], as these VOCs substantially contribute to the overall aroma profile.

Figure 6 illustrates the effectiveness of PLS-DA modeling in distinguishing the VOC content differences detected via HS-GC-IMS and HS-SPME-GC-MS, alongside the critical aroma volatiles that contribute prominently to sample discrimination. The PLS-DA score plots derived from HS-GC-IMS (Figure 6(Aa)) and HS-SPME-GC-MS (Figure 6(Ba)) datasets explain 68.5% and 58.9% of the total variance, respectively. Both score plots exhibit clear separation of the sample groups, demonstrating the capability of PLS-DA to effectively distinguish between the different sample groups. To validate the accuracy and robustness of the PLS-DA models, cross-validation (CV) was performed, and the statistical parameters—accuracy, R^2, and Q^2—all exceeded 0.95 (Figure 6A(c),B(c)), confirming the reliability of the PLS-DA models employed.

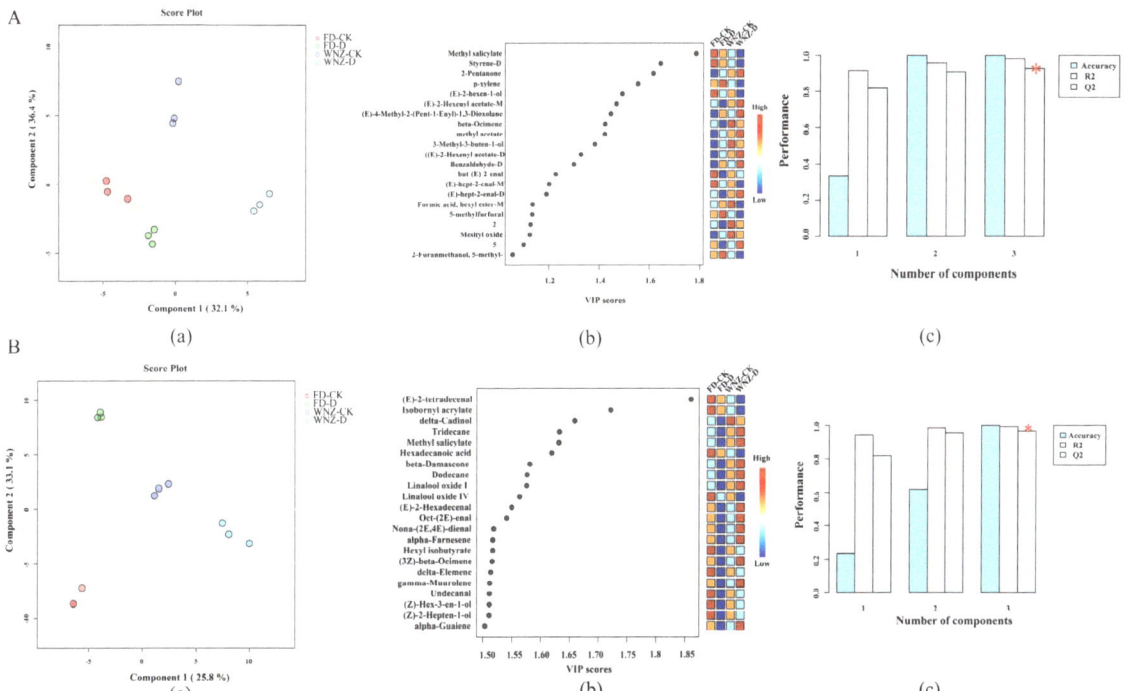

Figure 6. PLS-DA analysis on data obtained from HS-GC-IMS and HS-SPME-GC-MS. (**A**) PLS-DA score plot (**a**), VIP score plot (**b**), and model prediction accuracy for HS-GC-IMS data (**c**); (**B**) PLS-DA score plot (**a**), VIP score plot (**b**), and model prediction accuracy (**c**) for HS-SPME-GC-MS data. Filled circles in panel (a) represent the 95% confidence region and the red star in panel (c) represents the best classifier.

Furthermore, in the VIP score plot (Figure 6A(b)), 21 VOCs with VIP > 1 were identified as potential characteristic compounds in the PLS-DA model based on HS-GC-IMS data. Given that aroma presentation is ultimately related to the OAV of VOCs, nine volatiles—including methyl salicylate, Styrene-D, 2-pentanone, (E)-2-hexen-1-ol, β-ocimene, 3-Methyl-3-buten-1-ol, but-(E)-2-enal, (E)-hept-2-enal-M and (E)-hept-2-enal-D—had OAVs all >1, indicating their potential as key aroma markers that drive the discrimination in the HS-GC-IMS PLS-DA model. In comparison, for the PLS-DA model based on HS-SPME-GC-MS data, a total of 52 VOCs had VIP > 1, with 22 VOCs exhibiting VIP > 1.5 (Table S5). Thus, a VIP score plot was generated for these 22 VOCs (Figure 6(Bb)), which could serve as potential characteristic VOCs for the PLS-DA model based on HS-SPME-GC-MS data. Combining the criteria of VIP > 1 and OAV > 1, 13 VOCs—methyl salicylate, β-damascone, linalool oxide I, oct-(2E)-enal, nona-(2E,4E)-dienal, (Z)-hex-3-en-1-ol, (E,E)-2,4-heptadienal, linalool oxide II, cedrol, nonanal, (Z)-jasmone, hexanal, and 1-octen-3-one—were highlighted as critical aroma markers for the HS-SPME-GC-MS-based PLS-DA model.

3.4.4. VOC Change of Different Tea Cultivars Following Drought Stress

To gain deeper insights into the effects of field drought on the VOCs profiles of fresh tea leaves from different cultivars, a within-group comparative analysis was conducted between control and drought-treated samples of the FD and WNZ cultivars, respectively. Specifically, differential VOCs were screened using T-test analysis (p-value < 0.05) and fold change (FC $\geq$ 2 or $\leq$ 0.5) as the selection criteria. As illustrated in Figure 7, the volcano plots clearly depict the upregulation and downregulation of VOCs between drought-stressed and control samples.

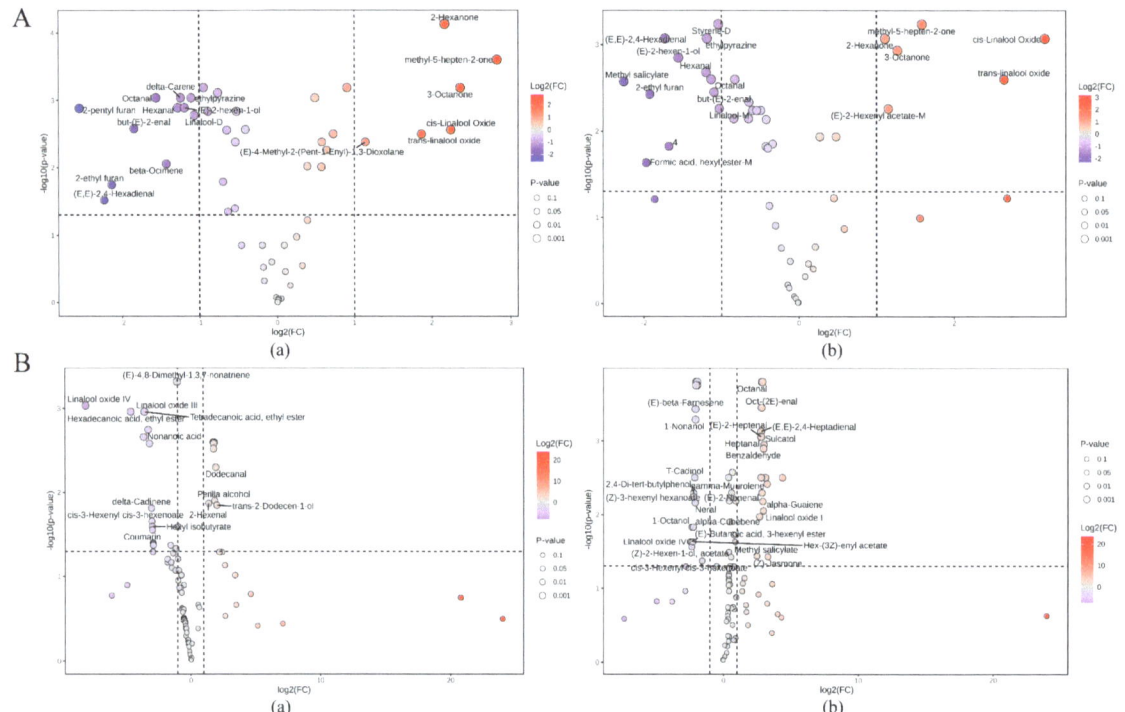

Figure 7. Volcanic map of differential VOCs detected by HS-GC-IMS (**A**) and HS-SPME-GC-MS (**B**). (**a**) FD-D vs. FD-CK; (**b**) WNZ-D vs. WNZ-CK.

A total of 17 and 18 differential VOCs were identified between the FD-D vs. FD-CK group and the WNZ-D vs. WNZ-CK group using HS-GC-IMS data (Figure 7A). In the FD-D vs. FD-CK comparison, six VOCs were significantly increased, including 2-hexanone, methyl-5-hepten-2-one, 3-octanone, cis-linalool oxide, trans-linalool oxide, and (E)-4-methyl-2-(pent-1-enyl)-1,3-dioxolane. Meanwhile, 11 VOCs were significantly decreased, namely octanal, delta-carene, ethylpyrazine, hexanal, (E)-2-hexen-1-ol, 2-pentyl furan, linalool-D, but-(E)-2-enal, β-ocimene, 2-ethyl furan, and (E,E)-2,4-hexadienal. In contrast, the WNZ cultivar exhibited significant alterations in VOCs under drought stress, with six VOCs showing marked upregulation. These included methyl-5-hepten-2-one, cis-linalool oxide, 2-hexanone, 3-octanone, trans-linalool oxide, and (E)-2-hexenyl acetate-M. Meanwhile, 12 VOCs were significantly decreased, such as styrene-D, (E,E)-2,4-hexadienal, ethylpyrazine, (E)-2-hexen-1-ol, hexanal, octanal, methyl salicylate, but-(E)-2-enal, 2-ethyl furan, linalool-M, an unidentified volatile compound, and formic acid hexyl ester-M. From the above analysis, it is evident that the increased volatiles in both tea cultivars under drought stress exhibited a high degree of similarity, while the decreased VOCs showed some variations. Overall, the significantly increased volatiles predominantly displayed sweet, floral, earthy, fruity, and citrus aroma characteristics, whereas the decreased VOCs were mainly associated with fresh green, grassy, and leafy aromas.

Figure 7B provides the volcano plots for VOCs in the FD-D vs. FD-CK and WNZ-D vs. WNZ-CK groups as measured by HS-SPME-GC-MS, with increased and decreased VOCs highlighted in red and blue, respectively. A total of 55 VOCs were significantly elevated, and 47 VOCs were reduced in the drought-treated groups compared to the control groups for the FD and WNZ cultivars. Detailed information regarding these VOCs is available in Tables S6 and S7.

For the FD-D vs. FD-CK comparison, 30 VOCs were significantly elevated, including dodecanamide, dihydro-β-ionol, benzaldehyde, benzeneacetaldehyde, 2-hexenal, alkenes, medium- and long-chain fatty alcohols, and unsaturated fatty alcohols. In contrast, 25 VOCs were significantly reduced, primarily consisting of linalool oxide IV, linalool oxide III, coumarin, sesquiterpenes, and several green-odor-type alcohols and esters. In the WNZ-D vs. WNZ-CK comparison, 23 VOCs were significantly elevated and 24 VOCs were significantly reduced. The elevated VOCs mainly exhibited sweet, floral, and fruity odors, including volatile terpenoids (VTs), volatile phenylpropanoids/benzenoids (VPBs), and medium- to long-chain volatile fatty acid derivatives (VFADs, including fatty acid aldehydes, fatty acid alcohols, and fatty acid esters). Examples include benzeneacetaldehyde, 2,4,6-trimethyl-benzaldehyde, linalool oxide I, linalool oxide II, linalool oxide III, (3Z)-β-ocimene, α-farnesene, γ-muurolene, α-guaiene, methyl salicylate, (Z)-jasmone, and sulcatol. On the other hand, significantly downregulated VOCs mainly displayed citrus, woody, and herbal aromas, such as (E)-β-farnesene, D-limonene, linalool oxide IV, α-calacorene, δ-guaiene, cedrol, α-cubebene, δ-3-carene, as well as citrus/green-odor-type VFADs (fatty acid alcohols and fatty acid esters), such as non-(2E)-enol, cyclohexanol, cycloheptanol, (E)-3-hexen-1-ol, 1-octanol, (Z)-3-hexenyl hexanoate, (E)-butanoic acid 3-hexenyl ester, hex-(3Z)-enyl acetate, cis-3-hexenyl cis-3-hexenoate, and nonanal.

In comparison to HS-GC-IMS, HS-SPME-GC-MS detected a greater diversity of VOCs, with more pronounced up- and downregulation. The elevated VOCs detected by both methods mainly featured sweet, floral, and fruity characteristics, whereas the reduced VOCs were predominantly associated with green and herbal aromas. Notably, our findings on major differences in linalool oxides, jasmone, α-farnesene [23], methyl salicylate [18], 2-hexenal [49], alkenes, medium- and long-chain fatty alcohols, and unsaturated fatty alcohols [50–52] are consistent with previous reports. It is also noteworthy that methyl salicylate has been reported to induce stomatal closure in guard cells [53], which may aid in plant self-protection during drought stress.

Furthermore, compared to the control groups, the drought-stressed groups displayed a significant reduction in sesquiterpenes but an increase in monoterpenes, monoterpene oxides, and medium- to long-chain VFADs, particularly fatty alcohols. Similarly, drought has been reported to induce significant increases in alkanes and fatty alcohols in wheat leaves during both the seedling and flowering stages [54]. Numerous studies suggest that fatty alcohols may enhance drought resistance by modulating gene expression related to drought response, potentially through interactions with transcription factors. For instance, the OsFAR1 gene in rice has been implicated in primary fatty alcohol biosynthesis and plays a critical role in drought stress response [52]. Additionally, fatty alcohols act as organic solutes that help reduce cellular osmotic potential, thereby maintaining turgor pressure and supporting normal physiological processes under drought conditions. Long-chain VFADs, including fatty alcohols, have been shown to reduce water loss by forming cuticular waxes, thereby enhancing plant drought tolerance [50,51]. In conclusion, the accumulation of medium- and long-chain fatty alcohols, unsaturated fatty alcohols, and alkanes represents a key physiological adaptation to drought stress in plants, playing an essential role in osmotic regulation and the modulation of drought-responsive gene expression.

3.5. Analysis of Differential Metabolite KEGG Enrichment Pathways in Different Tea Cultivars Subjected to Drought Stress

To further elucidate the pivotal metabolic pathways associated with the alterations in VOCs for different tea cultivars subjected to drought stress, we performed a comprehensive VOC metabolite pathway enrichment analysis. This analysis enabled the visualization of pathway significance and weight through the enrichment of volatiles with analogous functions. As depicted in Figure 8, KEGG metabolic pathway analysis identified a total of 12 and 14 differential metabolic pathways for the comparisons of FD-D vs. FD-CK and WNZ-D vs. WNZ-CK, respectively. Comprehensive details regarding p-values, false discovery rates (FDRs), impact factors, compound names, and pathway links are provided in Tables S8 and S9. The identified pathways encompassed monoterpenoid biosynthesis, butanoate metabolism, phenylalanine metabolism, fatty acid degradation, fatty acid biosynthesis, caffeine metabolism, cutin, suberine, and wax biosynthesis, sesquiterpenoid and triterpenoid biosynthesis, fatty acid elongation, alpha-linolenic acid metabolism, the biosynthesis of unsaturated fatty acids, and the biosynthesis of various secondary metabolites. Notably, these 12 pathways were consistently observed in both FD and WNZ. In addition, the WNZ-D vs. WNZ-CK comparison revealed two supplementary enriched pathways: phenylalanine, tyrosine, and tryptophan biosynthesis, alongside tryptophan metabolism, primarily attributed to the differential accumulation of the target compound indole.

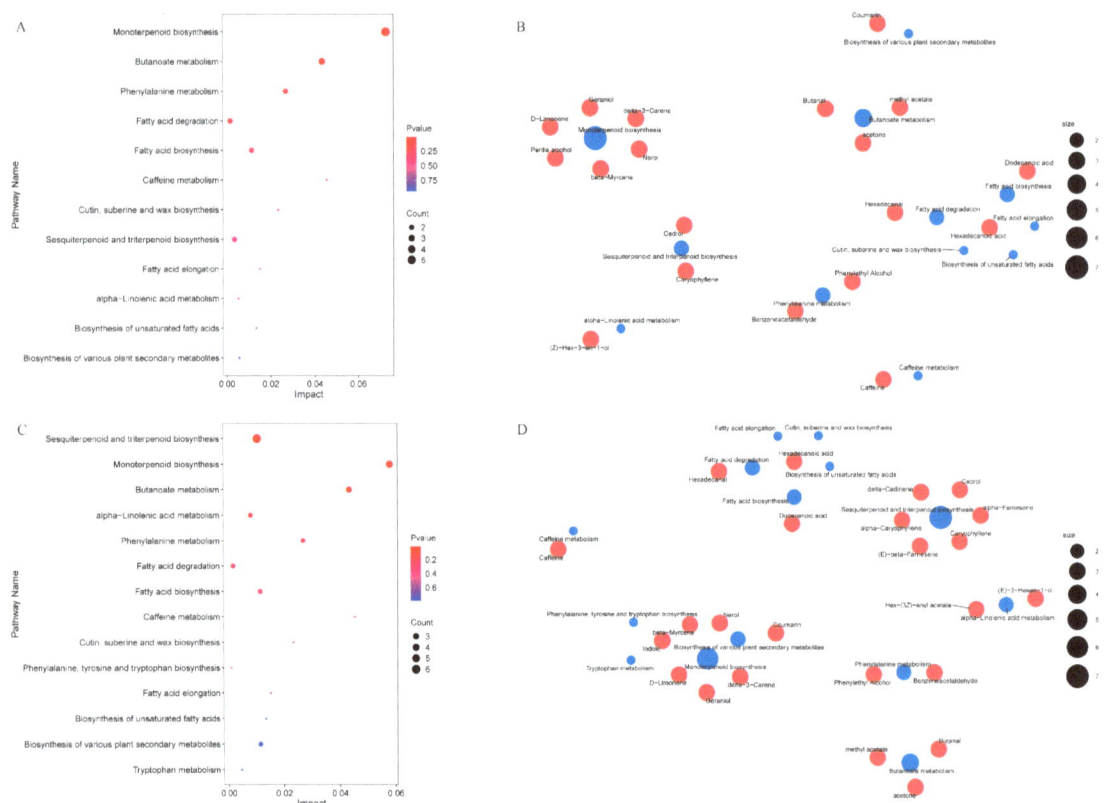

Figure 8. Pathway enrichment analysis of significantly altered VOCs of FD-D vs. FD-CK and WNZ-D vs. WNZ-CK. Differential VOC KEGG enrichment pathway bubble maps (**A**,**C**) and network maps of key target volatiles (**B**,**D**) of FD-D vs. FD-CK and WNZ-D vs. WNZ-CK, respectively.

As depicted in Figure 8A,B, the pathways enriched in FD-D vs. FD-CK involved 19 differential VOCs across eight metabolic network pathways. The most significantly enriched metabolic pathway ($p < 0.05$) was monoterpenoid biosynthesis, which included six differentially accumulated volatiles: nerol, geraniol, perilla alcohol, beta-myrcene, D-limonene, and delta-3-carene. Remarkably, nerol and perilla alcohol levels increased in the FD-D group, whereas geraniol, beta-myrcene, D-limonene, and delta-3-carene were more abundant in the FD-CK group. Moreover, in the WNZ-D vs. WNZ-CK analysis, 23 differential VOCs were linked to seven metabolic networks. The pathways of sesquiterpenoid and triterpenoid biosynthesis, as well as monoterpenoid biosynthesis, were significantly enriched ($p < 0.05$). Within the sesquiterpenoid and triterpenoid biosynthesis pathway, the differentially accumulated VOCs included delta-cadinene, caryophyllene, alpha-farnesene, (E)-beta-farnesene, alpha-caryophyllene, and cedrol. In contrast, the enriched VOCs in the monoterpenoid biosynthesis pathway included nerol, geraniol, beta-myrcene, D-limonene, and delta-3-carene. Following drought stress, the only VOC exhibiting increased expression in the WNZ-D cultivar within these two enriched terpenoid metabolic pathways was alpha-farnesene, while the remaining enriched VOCs were found in higher concentrations in the WNZ-CK group. The findings suggest that drought stress markedly influences the accumulation of sesquiterpenes, resulting in a greater prevalence of terpene oxides, including linalool oxides and caryophyllene oxides.

In conclusion, both FD and WNZ cultivars were implicated in fatty acid degradation, fatty acid biosynthesis, fatty acid elongation, the biosynthesis of unsaturated fatty acids, and cutin, suberine, and wax biosynthesis post-drought stress. This indicates that tea plants may sustain cellular osmotic pressure and physiological functionality through the synthesis of medium-chain VFADs and unsaturated fatty acids, while simultaneously mitigating water loss via cutin, suberine, and wax biosynthesis to endure drought conditions [50–52,54]. Additionally, phenylalanine metabolism is closely linked to plant growth and environmental interactions [55]. Extensive research has demonstrated that numerous phenylpropanoids play critical roles in the response to drought stress [56–58]. Phenylpropanoids are vital aromatic compounds in tea leaves, significantly influencing quality formation and stress response [59]. Our study identified notable differences in the enrichment of benzeneacetaldehyde and phenylethyl alcohol within the phenylalanine metabolism pathway, particularly in the WNZ cultivar, where drought stress markedly elevated these compounds. This observation aligns with prior findings highlighting the significant increase in phenylethyl alcohol under drought conditions [18], contributing to enhanced rose floral aroma characteristics in tea leaves.

Collectively, these results indicate that these metabolic pathways and their associated metabolites are crucial determinants influencing the VOC composition and aroma expression of tea leaves under drought stress.

4. Conclusions

By employing HS-GC-IMS and HS-SPME-GC-MS techniques alongside PLS-DA modeling, this study delineated significant alterations in the VOCs of FD and WNZ tea cultivars subjected to drought stress. The drought-stressed groups exhibited a marked increase in both the concentration and diversity of VOCs associated with sweet, fruity, caramel-like, floral, and earthy notes, while green, grassy, leafy, woody, herbal, and floral aromas were diminished. Notably, there was an elevated presence of methylated compounds, linalool oxides, and medium- to long-chain VFADs in the drought-treated samples. Conversely, sesquiterpenoid content and diversity were substantially reduced. The varietal responses to drought stress were distinct, with FD-D showing an increased diversity of VOCs, whereas WNZ exhibited a greater increase in the concentrations of low-threshold VOCs.

Among the four sample groups, key aroma-active compounds (OAV > 1) included 1-Octen-3-ol, linalool, geraniol, β-damascone, (E)-β-ionone, citral, and β-myrcene, with linalool exhibiting the highest OAV, underscoring its role as a primary aroma contributor in both tea cultivars. Based on VIP > 1 and OAV > 1 thresholds, 8 and 13 potential key aroma markers were identified for distinguishing between the different cultivars and treatments using the PLS-DA model for HS-GC-IMS and HS-SPME-GC-MS, respectively. Additionally, KEGG enrichment analysis revealed significant alterations in 12 metabolic pathways following drought stress. The sesquiterpenoid and triterpenoid biosynthesis pathways, as well as monoterpenoid biosynthesis, exhibited significant changes ($p < 0.05$). Furthermore, pathways related to fatty acid synthesis, elongation, degradation, the biosynthesis of unsaturated fatty acids, linalool oxides, cutin, suberine and wax biosynthesis, and phenylalanine metabolism were also enriched, further validating the observed increases in the abundance and diversity of linalool oxides and medium- to long-chain VFADs, along with the pronounced reduction in sesquiterpenoid compounds under drought stress.

Overall, these results provide a comprehensive insight into how drought stress affects VOC accumulation in fresh tea leaves across different cultivars, while highlighting the corresponding alterations in key metabolic pathways. This knowledge establishes a foundation for optimizing water management strategies in tea plant cultivation, aiming to enhance flavor quality. The current study relies on metabolomics and flavoromics to analyze key volatile aroma compounds and their metabolic pathways in tea leaves subjected to 20 days of continuous field drought stress. However, the absence of physiological or genetic data linking VOC changes to drought resistance presents a limitation. Future research will aim to integrate physiology, transcriptomics, and DNA methylation data to elucidate the molecular mechanisms governing VOC accumulation and aroma formation in tea under drought stress.

Supplementary Materials: The following supporting information can be downloaded at: https://www.mdpi.com/article/10.3390/foods13213412/s1, Figure S1. Close-up view of a PCA biplot displaying VOCs concentrations detected by HS-SPME-GC–MS.; Table S1: Composition of model stock solution for volatile-free tea infusion blank matrix; Table S2: Calibration standards curves of the key VOCs; Table S3: The information of volatile compounds identified by HS-GC-IMS; Table S4: Identification and quantification of the VOCs, odor description, and OAV analysis in this study by HS-SPME-GC–MS; Table S5: Importance features within PLS-DA using VIP values for HS-SPME-GC-MS data; Table S6: Significant change profiles in the accumulation of VOCs for FD-D vs. FD-CK based on HS-SPME-GC-MS data; Table S7: Significant change profiles in the accumulation of VOCs for WNZ-D vs. WNZ-CK based on HS-SPME-GC-MS data; Table S8: Detailed information on KEGG-enriched metabolic pathways for FD-CK and FD-D with reference to *Arabidopsis*; Table S9: Detailed information on KEGG-enriched metabolic pathways for WNZ-CK and WNZ-D with reference to *Arabidopsis*. References [60–68] are cited in the supplementary materials

Author Contributions: Conceptualization, X.L., F.D., F.W. and D.Z.; methodology, X.L., F.D., M.H., F.W. and D.Z.; software, X.L. and Y.L.; validation, X.L., F.D., Y.L. and M.H.; formal analysis, X.L., Y.L. and F.D.; investigation, X.L., F.D., Y.L., B.W. and T.Z.; resources and data curation, X.L., Y.L., F.L., B.W. and T.Z.; writing—original draft preparation, X.L.; writing—review and editing, X.L. and F.D.; visualization, X.L., Y.L. and F.D.; supervision, D.Z., M.H. and F.W.; project administration, X.L., F.D. and D.Z.; funding acquisition, X.L. All authors have read and agreed to the published version of the manuscript.

Funding: This research was funded by the China Postdoctoral Science Foundation, grant number 2021M693807, the Science and Technology Plan Project of Guizhou province, grant number QKHJC-ZK[2022] YB180, the Open Fund Project of the Key Laboratory of Plant Resources Conservation and Germplasm Innovation in Mountainous Region, Ministry of Education (Gui-zhou University), grant number QJH-KY-Z [2020]255, the Young Scientists Fund of the National Natural Science Foundation of China, grant number 32001463, Guizhou Fruit Wine Brewing Engineering Research Center, grant number [2022]050 and Guizhou Provincial Science and Technology Department, grant number KXJZ[2024]021. The APC was funded by the China Postdoctoral Science Foundation (2021M693807) and the Science and Technology Plan Project of Guizhou province, grant number QKHJC-ZK[2022] YB180.

Institutional Review Board Statement: Not applicable.

Informed Consent Statement: Not applicable.

Data Availability Statement: The original contributions presented in this study are included in the article/Supplementary Materials; further inquiries can be directed to the corresponding authors.

Acknowledgments: We express our gratitude to Weimin Zhang, the legal representative of Hongfengshanyun Tea Farm Co., Ltd., Qingzhen, Guizhou province, China, for providing us with the experimental site and tea plant experimental materials.

Conflicts of Interest: The authors declare no conflicts of interest.

References

1. Chen, L.; Zhang, S.; Feng, Y.; Jiang, Y.; Yuan, H.; Shan, X.; Zhang, Q.; Niu, L.; Wang, S.; Zhou, Q.; et al. Seasonal variation in non-volatile flavor substances of fresh tea leaves (*Camellia sinensis*) by integrated lipidomics and metabolomics using UHPLC-Q-Exactive mass spectrometry. *Food Chem.* **2025**, *462*, 140986. [CrossRef]
2. Liu, X.; Zhao, Y.; Zhao, D. Next-Generation Tea Beverages: Innovations in Formulation and Processing. *J. Tea Sci. Res.* **2024**, *14*, 112–122. [CrossRef]
3. Xiang, L.; Zhu, C.; Qian, J.; Zhou, X.; Wang, M.; Song, Z.; Chen, C.; Yu, W.; Chen, L.; Zeng, L. Positive contributions of the stem to the formation of white tea quality-related metabolites during withering. *Food Chem.* **2024**, *449*, 139173. [CrossRef] [PubMed]
4. Zhai, X.; Zhang, L.; Granvogl, M.; Ho, C.T.; Wan, X. Flavor of tea (Camellia sinensis): A review on odorants and analytical techniques. *Compr. Rev. Food Sci. Food Saf.* **2022**, *21*, 3867–3909. [CrossRef]
5. Fang, R.; Redfern, S.P.; Kirkup, D.; Porter, E.A.; Kite, G.C.; Terry, L.A.; Berry, M.J.; Simmonds, M.S.J. Variation of theanine, phenolic, and methylxanthine compounds in 21 cultivars of *Camellia sinensis* harvested in different seasons. *Food Chem.* **2017**, *220*, 517–526. [CrossRef] [PubMed]
6. Qin, X.; Zhou, J.; He, C.; Qiu, L.; Zhang, D.; Yu, Z.; Wang, Y.; Ni, D.; Chen, Y. Non-targeted metabolomics characterization of flavor formation of Lichuan black tea processed from different cultivars in Enshi. *Food Chem. X* **2023**, *19*, 100809. [CrossRef]
7. Niu, M.; Li, R.; Li, X.; Yang, H.; Ding, J.; Zhou, X.; He, Y.; Xu, Y.; Qu, Q.; Liu, Z.; et al. Insights into the Metabolite Profiles of Two Camellia (Theaceae) Species in Yunnan Province through Metabolomic and Transcriptomic Analysis. *Biomolecules* **2024**, *14*, 1106. [CrossRef]
8. Zheng, C.; Wang, Y.; Ding, Z. Global transcriptional analysis reveals the complex relationship between tea quality, leaf senescence and the responses to cold-drought combined stress in Camellia sinensis. *Front. Plant Sci.* **2016**, *7*, 227252. [CrossRef]
9. Zhang, Q.; Cai, M.; Yu, X.; Wang, L.; Guo, C.; Ming, R.; Zhang, J. Transcriptome dynamics of Camellia sinensis in response to continuous salinity and drought stress. *Tree Genet. Genomes* **2017**, *13*, 1–17. [CrossRef]
10. Zhang, C.; Wang, M.; Chen, J.; Gao, X.; Shao, C.; Lv, Z.; Jiao, H.; Xu, H.; Shen, C. Survival strategies based on the hydraulic vulnerability segmentation hypothesis, for the tea plant [*Camellia sinensis* (L.) O. Kuntze] in long-term drought stress condition. *Plant Physiol. Biochem.* **2020**, *156*, 484–493. [CrossRef]
11. Li, Y.; Chen, Y.; Chen, J.; Shen, C. Flavonoid metabolites in tea plant (Camellia sinensis) stress response: Insights from bibliometric analysis. *Plant Physiol. Biochem.* **2023**, *202*, 107934. [CrossRef] [PubMed]
12. Ran, W.; Li, Q.; Hu, X.; Zhang, D.; Yu, Z.; Chen, Y.; Wang, M.; Ni, D. Comprehensive analysis of environmental factors on the quality of tea (*Camellia sinensis* var. *sinensis*) fresh leaves. *Sci. Hortic.* **2023**, *319*, 112177. [CrossRef]
13. Xie, J.; Wang, L.; Deng, Y.; Yuan, H.; Zhu, J.; Jiang, Y.; Yang, Y. Characterization of the key odorants in floral aroma green tea based on GC-E-Nose, GC-IMS, GC-MS and aroma recombination and investigation of the dynamic changes and aroma formation during processing. *Food Chem.* **2023**, *427*, 136641. [CrossRef] [PubMed]
14. Wen, S.; Sun, L.; Zhang, S.; Chen, Z.; Chen, R.; Li, Z.; Lai, X.; Zhang, Z.; Cao, J.; Li, Q.; et al. The formation mechanism of aroma quality of green and yellow teas based on GC-MS/MS metabolomics. *Food Res. Int.* **2023**, *172*, 113137. [CrossRef]
15. Wei, F.; Luo, L.; Zeng, L. Characterization of key sweet taste compounds in *Camellia nanchuanica* black tea. *LWT* **2023**, *182*, 114858. [CrossRef]
16. Wang, J.-Q.; Dai, Z.-S.; Gao, Y.; Wang, F.; Chen, J.-X.; Feng, Z.-H.; Yin, J.-F.; Zeng, L.; Xu, Y.-Q. Untargeted metabolomics coupled with chemometrics for flavor analysis of Dahongpao oolong tea beverages under different storage conditions. *LWT* **2023**, *185*, 115128. [CrossRef]
17. Yue, C.; Cao, H.; Zhang, S.; Shen, G.; Wu, Z.; Yuan, L.; Luo, L.; Zeng, L. Multilayer omics landscape analyses reveal the regulatory responses of tea plants to drought stress. *Int. J. Biol. Macromol.* **2023**, *253*, 126582. [CrossRef]
18. Jin, J.; Zhao, M.; Gao, T.; Jing, T.; Zhang, N.; Wang, J.; Zhang, X.; Huang, J.; Schwab, W.; Song, C. Amplification of early drought responses caused by volatile cues emitted from neighboring tea plants. *Hortic. Res.* **2021**, *8*, 243. [CrossRef]
19. Li, M.; Liu, J.; Zhou, Y.; Zhou, S.; Zhang, S.; Tong, H.; Zhao, A. Transcriptome and metabolome profiling unveiled mechanisms of tea (*Camellia sinensis*) quality improvement by moderate drought on pre-harvest shoots. *Phytochemistry* **2020**, *180*, 112515. [CrossRef]
20. Wang, Y.; Fan, K.; Wang, J.; Ding, Z.-T.; Wang, H.; Bi, C.-H.; Zhang, Y.-W.; Sun, H.-W. Proteomic analysis of *Camellia sinensis* (L.) reveals a synergistic network in the response to drought stress and recovery. *J. Plant Physiol.* **2017**, *219*, 91–99. [CrossRef]
21. Huafu, W. Characteristic aroma components of Qimen Black Tea. *J. Tea Sci.* **1993**, *13*, 61–68.

22. Ahmed, S.; Stepp, J.R.; Orians, C.; Griffin, T.; Matyas, C.; Robbat, A.; Cash, S.; Xue, D.; Long, C.; Unachukwu, U.; et al. Effects of Extreme Climate Events on Tea (*Camellia sinensis*) Functional Quality Validate Indigenous Farmer Knowledge and Sensory Preferences in Tropical China. *PLoS ONE* **2014**, *9*, e109126. [CrossRef] [PubMed]
23. Cao, P.; Liu, C.; Liu, K. Aromatic constituents in fresh leaves of Lingtou Dancong tea induced by drought stress. *Front. Agric. China* **2007**, *1*, 81–84. [CrossRef]
24. Guo, X.; Schwab, W.; Ho, C.-T.; Song, C.; Wan, X. Characterization of the aroma profiles of oolong tea made from three tea cultivars by both GC–MS and GC-IMS. *Food Chem.* **2022**, *376*, 131933. [CrossRef] [PubMed]
25. Wang, C.; Li, J.; Wu, X.; Zhang, Y.; He, Z.; Zhang, Y.; Zhang, X.; Li, Q.; Huang, J.; Liu, Z. Pu-erh tea unique aroma: Volatile components, evaluation methods and metabolic mechanism of key odor-active compounds. *Trends Food Sci. Technol.* **2022**, *124*, 25–37. [CrossRef]
26. Zeng, L.; Watanabe, N.; Yang, Z. Understanding the biosyntheses and stress response mechanisms of aroma compounds in tea (*Camellia sinensis*) to safely and effectively improve tea aroma. *Crit. Rev. Food Sci. Nutr.* **2019**, *59*, 2321–2334. [CrossRef]
27. Liang, Y.; Wang, Z.; Zhang, L.; Dai, H.; Wu, W.; Zheng, Z.; Lin, F.; Xu, J.; Huang, Y.; Sun, W. Characterization of volatile compounds and identification of key aroma compounds in different aroma types of Rougui Wuyi rock tea. *Food Chem.* **2024**, *455*, 139931. [CrossRef]
28. Wu, Y.; Li, T.; Huang, W.; Liu, Q.; Deng, G.; Zhang, J.; Wei, Y.; Wang, Y.; Ning, J. Investigation of the aroma profile and blending strategy of Lu'an Guapian teas during grain rain period by sensory evaluation combined with SBSE-GC–MS, GC–O and OAV. *Food Chem.* **2025**, *463*, 141167. [CrossRef]
29. Ouyang, J.; Jiang, R.; Chen, H.; Liu, Q.; Yi, X.; Wen, S.; Huang, F.; Zhang, X.; Li, J.; Wen, H.; et al. Characterization of key odorants in 'Baimaocha' black teas from different regions. *Food Chem. X* **2024**, *22*, 101303. [CrossRef]
30. Xiong, Z.; Feng, W.; Xia, D.; Zhang, J.; Wei, Y.; Li, T.; Huang, Y.; Wang, Y.; Ning, J. Distinguishing raw pu-erh tea production regions through a combination of HS-SPME-GC-MS and machine learning algorithms. *LWT* **2023**, *185*, 115140. [CrossRef]
31. Xu, J.; Zhang, Y.; Yan, F.; Tang, Y.; Yu, B.; Chen, B.; Lu, L.; Yuan, L.; Wu, Z.; Chen, H. Monitoring Changes in the Volatile Compounds of Tea Made from Summer Tea Leaves by GC-IMS and HS-SPME-GC–MS. *Foods* **2023**, *12*, 146. [CrossRef] [PubMed]
32. Zhang, S.; Sun, L.; Wen, S.; Chen, R.; Sun, S.; Lai, X.; Li, Q.; Zhang, Z.; Lai, Z.; Li, Z.; et al. Analysis of aroma quality changes of large-leaf black tea in different storage years based on HS-SPME and GC–MS. *Food Chem. X* **2023**, *20*, 100991. [CrossRef] [PubMed]
33. Zhang, H.; Zhang, J.; Liu, S.; Li, T.; Wei, Y.; Gu, Z.; Su, Z.; Ning, J.; Wang, Y.; Hou, Z. Characterization of the key volatile compounds in longjing tea (*Camellia sinensis*) with different aroma types at different steeping temperatures by GC-MS and GC-IMS. *LWT* **2024**, *200*, 116183. [CrossRef]
34. Qiao, D.; Zhu, J.; Mi, X.; Xie, H.; Shu, M.; Chen, M.; Li, R.; Liu, S.; Wei, C. Effects of withering time of fresh leaves on the formation of flavor quality of Taiping Houkui tea. *LWT* **2023**, *182*, 114833. [CrossRef]
35. Zhu, J.; Chen, F.; Wang, L.; Niu, Y.; Yu, D.; Shu, C.; Chen, H.; Wang, H.; Xiao, Z. Comparison of aroma-active volatiles in oolong tea infusions using GC–olfactometry, GC–FPD, and GC–MS. *J. Agric. Food Chem.* **2015**, *63*, 7499–7510. [CrossRef]
36. Wang, J.-Q.; Fu, Y.-Q.; Chen, J.-X.; Wang, F.; Feng, Z.-H.; Yin, J.-F.; Zeng, L.; Xu, Y.-Q.J.F.C. Effects of baking treatment on the sensory quality and physicochemical properties of green tea with different processing methods. *Food Chem.* **2022**, *380*, 132217. [CrossRef]
37. Wang, Y.; Deng, G.; Huang, L.; Ning, J. Sensory-directed flavor analysis reveals the improvement in aroma quality of summer green tea by osmanthus scenting. *Food Chem. X* **2024**, *23*, 101571. [CrossRef] [PubMed]
38. Van Gemert, L.J. *Odour Thresholds: Compilations of Odour Threshold Values in Air, Water and Other Media*; Oliemans Punter: Utrecht, The Netherlands, 2011.
39. Yang, J.; Liang, G.; Li, Z.; Liang, X.; Chen, Y. Analysis of aroma characteristics of fermented lingyun baihao tea based on odor activity value. *J. Food Sci.* **2023**, *44*, 336–343. [CrossRef]
40. Munivenkatappa, N.; Sarikonda, S.; Rajagopal, R.; Balakrishnan, R.; Krishnappa Nagarathana, C. Variations in quality constituents of green tea leaves in response to drought stress under south Indian condition. *Sci. Hortic.* **2018**, *233*, 359–369. [CrossRef]
41. Kong, W.; Zhu, Q.; Zhang, Q.; Zhu, Y.; Yang, J.; Chai, K.; Lei, W.; Jiang, M.; Zhang, S.; Lin, J. 5mC DNA methylation modification-mediated regulation in tissue functional differentiation and important flavor substance synthesis of tea plant (*Camellia sinensis* L.). *Hortic. Res.* **2023**, *10*, uhad126. [CrossRef]
42. Yang, J.; Zhou, X.; Wu, S.; Gu, D.; Zeng, L.; Yang, Z. Involvement of DNA methylation in regulating the accumulation of the aroma compound indole in tea (*Camellia sinensis*) leaves during postharvest processing. *Food Res. Int.* **2021**, *142*, 110183. [CrossRef] [PubMed]
43. Xiao, Y.; Tan, H.; Huang, H.; Yu, J.; Zeng, L.; Liao, Y.; Wu, P.; Yang, Z. Light synergistically promotes the tea green leafhopper infestation-induced accumulation of linalool oxides and their glucosides in tea (*Camellia sinensis*). *Food Chem.* **2022**, *394*, 133460. [CrossRef] [PubMed]
44. Feng, X.; Wang, H.; Wang, Z.; Huang, P.; Kan, J. Discrimination and characterization of the volatile organic compounds in eight kinds of huajiao with geographical indication of China using electronic nose, HS-GC-IMS and HS-SPME-GC–MS. *Food Chem.* **2022**, *375*, 131671. [CrossRef]
45. He, J.; Wu, X.; Yu, Z. Microwave pretreatment of camellia (*Camellia oleifera* Abel.) seeds: Effect on oil flavor. *Food Chem.* **2021**, *364*, 130388. [CrossRef]

46. Chen, J.; Wang, W.; Jin, J.; Li, H.; Chen, F.; Fei, Y.; Wang, Y. Characterization of the flavor profile and dynamic changes in Chinese traditional fish sauce (Yu-lu) based on electronic nose, SPME-GC-MS and HS-GC-IMS. *Food Res. Int.* **2024**, *192*, 114772. [CrossRef]
47. Worley, B.; Halouska, S.; Powers, R. Utilities for quantifying separation in PCA/PLS-DA scores plots. *Anal. Biochem.* **2013**, *433*, 102–104. [CrossRef]
48. Mahieu, B.; Qannari, E.M.; Jaillais, B. Extension and significance testing of Variable Importance in Projection (VIP) indices in Partial Least Squares regression and Principal Components Analysis. *Chemom. Intell. Lab. Syst.* **2023**, *242*, 104986. [CrossRef]
49. Hu, S.; Chen, Q.; Guo, F.; Wang, M.; Zhao, H.; Wang, Y.; Ni, D.; Wang, P. (Z)-3-Hexen-1-ol accumulation enhances hyperosmotic stress tolerance in Camellia sinensis. *Plant Mol. Biol.* **2020**, *103*, 287–302. [CrossRef] [PubMed]
50. Zhang, D.; Yang, H.; Wang, X.; Qiu, Y.; Tian, L.; Qi, X.; Qu, L.Q. Cytochrome P450 family member CYP96B5 hydroxylates alkanes to primary alcohols and is involved in rice leaf cuticular wax synthesis. *New Phytol.* **2020**, *225*, 2094–2107. [CrossRef]
51. Xue, D.; Zhang, X.; Lu, X.; Chen, G.; Chen, Z.-H. Molecular and evolutionary mechanisms of cuticular wax for plant drought tolerance. *Front. Plant Sci.* **2017**, *8*, 621. [CrossRef]
52. Guan, L.; Xia, D.; Hu, N.; Zhang, H.; Wu, H.; Jiang, Q.; Li, X.; Sun, Y.; Wang, Y.; Wang, Z. OsFAR1 is involved in primary fatty alcohol biosynthesis and promotes drought tolerance in rice. *Planta* **2023**, *258*, 24. [CrossRef] [PubMed]
53. Agurla, S.; Sunitha, V.; Raghavendra, A.S. Methyl salicylate is the most effective natural salicylic acid ester to close stomata while raising reactive oxygen species and nitric oxide in Arabidopsis guard cells. *Plant Physiol. Biochem.* **2020**, *157*, 276–283. [CrossRef] [PubMed]
54. He, J.; Li, C.; Hu, N.; Zhu, Y.; He, Z.; Sun, Y.; Wang, Z.; Wang, Y. ECERIFERUM1-6A is required for the synthesis of cuticular wax alkanes and promotes drought tolerance in wheat. *Plant Physiol.* **2022**, *190*, 1640–1657. [CrossRef] [PubMed]
55. Xu, W.; Dou, Y.; Geng, H.; Fu, J.; Dan, Z.; Liang, T.; Cheng, M.; Zhao, W.; Zeng, Y.; Hu, Z.; et al. OsGRP3 Enhances Drought Resistance by Altering Phenylpropanoid Biosynthesis Pathway in Rice (*Oryza sativa* L.). *Int. J. Mol. Sci.* **2022**, *23*, 7045. [CrossRef]
56. Fini, A.; Guidi, L.; Ferrini, F.; Brunetti, C.; Di Ferdinando, M.; Biricolti, S.; Pollastri, S.; Calamai, L.; Tattini, M. Drought stress has contrasting effects on antioxidant enzymes activity and phenylpropanoid biosynthesis in Fraxinus ornus leaves: An excess light stress affair? *J. Plant Physiol.* **2012**, *169*, 929–939. [CrossRef]
57. Shi, J.; Wang, Y.; Fan, X.; Li, R.; Yu, C.; Peng, Z.; Gao, Y.; Liu, Z.; Duan, L. A novel plant growth regulator B2 mediates drought resistance by regulating reactive oxygen species, phytohormone signaling, phenylpropanoid biosynthesis, and starch metabolism pathways in Carex breviculmis. *Plant Physiol. Biochem.* **2024**, *213*, 108860. [CrossRef]
58. Geng, D.; Shen, X.; Xie, Y.; Yang, Y.; Bian, R.; Gao, Y.; Li, P.; Sun, L.; Feng, H.; Ma, F.; et al. Regulation of phenylpropanoid biosynthesis by MdMYB88 and MdMYB124 contributes to pathogen and drought resistance in apple. *Hortic. Res.* **2020**, *7*, 102. [CrossRef] [PubMed]
59. Zhao, M.; Jin, J.; Wang, J.; Gao, T.; Luo, Y.; Jing, T.; Hu, Y.; Pan, Y.; Lu, M.; Schwab, W.; et al. Eugenol functions as a signal mediating cold and drought tolerance via UGT71A59-mediated glucosylation in tea plants. *Plant J.* **2022**, *109*, 1489–1506. [CrossRef]
60. The Good Scents Company Information System. Available online: http://www.thegoodscentscompany.com/search2.html (accessed on 7 September 2024).
61. Wu, W.; Jiang, X.; Zhu, Q.; Yuan, Y.; Chen, R.; Wang, W.; Liu, A.; Wu, C.; Ma, C.; Li, J.; et al. Metabonomics analysis of the flavor characteristics of Wuyi Rock Tea (Rougui) with "rock flavor" and microbial contributions to the flavor. *Food Chem.* **2024**, *450*, 139376. [CrossRef]
62. Lapczynski, A.; Bhatia, S.P.; Letizia, C.S.; Api, A.M. Fragrance material review on dehydrolinalool. *Food Chem. Toxicol.* **2008**, *46*, S117–S120. [CrossRef]
63. Wang, B.; Yu, M.; Tang, Y.; Wang, Y.; Xia, T.; Song, H. Characterization of odor-active compounds in Dahongpao Wuyi Rock Tea (*Camellia sinensis*) by sensory-directed flavor analysis. *J. Food Compos. Anal.* **2023**, *123*, 105612. [CrossRef]
64. Zhang, X.; Gao, P.; Xia, W.; Jiang, Q.; Liu, S.; Xu, Y. Characterization of key aroma compounds in low-salt fermented sour fish by gas chromatography-mass spectrometry, odor activity values, aroma recombination and omission experiments. *Food Chem.* **2022**, *397*, 133773. [CrossRef] [PubMed]
65. Wang, D.; Liu, Z.; Lan, X.; Wang, C.; Chen, W.; Zhan, S.; Sun, Y.; Su, W.; Lin, C.-C.; Liu, W.; et al. Unveiling the aromatic intricacies of Wuyi Rock Tea: A comparative study on sensory attributes and odor-active compounds of Rougui and Shuixian varieties. *Food Chem.* **2024**, *435*, 137470. [CrossRef] [PubMed]
66. Zhang, C.; Su, J.; Wang, J.; Zhao, Z. Identification of volatile and odor-active compounds in Maojian herbal tea (Dracocephalum rupestre Hance). *J. Food Compos. Anal.* **2024**, *135*, 106643. [CrossRef]
67. Chen, W.; Hu, D.; Miao, A.; Qiu, G.; Qiao, X.; Xia, H.; Ma, C. Understanding the aroma diversity of Dancong tea (*Camellia sinensis*) from the floral and honey odors: Relationship between volatile compounds and sensory characteristics by chemometrics. *Food Control.* **2022**, *140*, 109103. [CrossRef]
68. Xu, J.; Zhang, Y.; Hu, C.; Yu, B.; Wan, C.; Chen, B.; Lu, L.; Yuan, L.; Wu, Z.; Chen, H. The flavor substances changes in Fuliang green tea during storage monitoring by GC–MS and GC-IMS. *Food Chem. X* **2024**, *21*, 101047. [CrossRef]

Disclaimer/Publisher's Note: The statements, opinions and data contained in all publications are solely those of the individual author(s) and contributor(s) and not of MDPI and/or the editor(s). MDPI and/or the editor(s) disclaim responsibility for any injury to people or property resulting from any ideas, methods, instructions or products referred to in the content.

MDPI AG
Grosspeteranlage 5
4052 Basel
Switzerland
Tel.: +41 61 683 77 34

Foods Editorial Office
E-mail: foods@mdpi.com
www.mdpi.com/journal/foods

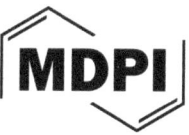

Disclaimer/Publisher's Note: The title and front matter of this reprint are at the discretion of the Collection Editors. The publisher is not responsible for their content or any associated concerns. The statements, opinions and data contained in all individual articles are solely those of the individual Editors and contributors and not of MDPI. MDPI disclaims responsibility for any injury to people or property resulting from any ideas, methods, instructions or products referred to in the content.

www.ingramcontent.com/pod-product-compliance
Lightning Source LLC
LaVergne TN
LVHW072343090526
838202LV00019B/2467